NURSING
DOCUMENTATION

Charting, Recording, and Reporting

Ellen Thomas Eggland, RN, MN

Vice President
Healthcare Personnel, Inc.
Naples, Florida

Denise Skelly Heinemann, RN, DrPH

Assistant Professor
College of Nursing
University of South Florida
Fort Myers, Florida

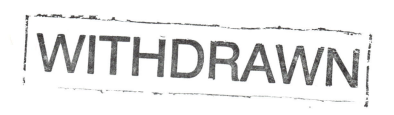

J.B. Lippincott Company
Philadelphia

Acquisitions Editor: Donna L. Hilton, RN, BSN
Coordinating Editorial Assistant: Susan M. Keneally
Project Editor: Barbara Ryalls
Indexer: David Amundson
Design Coordinator: Kathy Kelley-Luedtke
Designer: Holly Reid McLaughlin
Cover Designer: Larry Pezzato
Production Manager: Helen Ewan
Production Coordinator: Nannette Winski
Compositor: Circle Graphics
Printer/Binder: Courier Kendallville, Inc.

6 5 4 3 2

Library of Congress Cataloging-in-Publication Data

Eggland, Ellen Thomas.
    Nursing documentation : charting, recording, and reporting / Ellen
Thomas Eggland, Denise Skelly Heinemann. — 1st ed.
        p.   cm.
    Includes bibliographical references and index.
    ISBN 0-397-55010-3
    1. Nursing records.   2. Communication in nursing.   I. Heinemann,
Denise Skelly.   II. Title.
    [DNLM: 1. Documentation—nurses' instruction.   2. Nursing Care.
3. Nursing Records.   4. Nursing Process.   WY 100.5 E29n   1994]
RT50.E439   1994
610.73—dc20
DNLM/DLC
for Library of Congress   93-6172
                                                                    CIP

Any procedure or practice described in this book should be applied by the
health care practitioner under appropriate supervision in accordance with
professional standards of care used with regard to the unique circumstances
that apply in each practice situation. Care has been taken to confirm the accuracy of information presented and to describe generally accepted practices. However, the authors, editors, and publisher cannot accept any
responsibility for errors or omissions or for any consequences from application of the information in this book and make no warranty, express or implied, with respect to the contents of the book.

Every effort has been made to ensure drug selections and dosages are in accordance with current recommendations and practice. Because of ongoing
research, changes in government regulations, and the constant flow of information on drug therapy, reactions, and interactions, the reader is cautioned
to check the package insert for each drug for indications, dosages, warnings,
and precautions, particularly if the drug is new or infrequently used.

To my five brothers and sisters who gave me my earliest opportunities to "teach"; and to my two college-bound teens who give me my best practice.

Ellen Eggland, RN, MN

To my family, colleagues, and friends who gave me encouragement as I wrote: Bless you. To the students who will read this book: May you find joy and satisfaction in nursing.

Denise Heinemann, RN, DrPH

Preface

Professional nursing focuses on the "diagnosis and treatment of human responses to actual or potential health problems" (American Nurses Association, 1973), which requires many nursing activities, including the coordination of patient care provided by other health care providers. A nurse cannot accomplish this task alone. Nursing communication forms the link between and among nurses and other health care workers to facilitate coordination and continuity of care and to enhance clinical decision-making and problem-solving. Sharing information about a patient's health status, needs, treatments, outcomes, and responses assures quality care that is appropriate for each person's needs.

Communication in nursing can be in the form of written or oral documentation of nursing care. Recording involves written documentation—the charting of the pertinent and significant aspects of all facets of daily care as well as the status of the patient's condition throughout that time period. Reporting is a form of oral documentation that summarizes this care and the patient's status. Both forms of documentation facilitate continuity of care. Reporting allows rapid sharing of patient data that assures the use of current information in clinical decision making, while recording provides a permanent and complete record of patient care activity.

Skillful communication in the form of recording and reporting establishes the need for nursing care, reflects the quality of care provided, and serves as a basis for evaluation of that care. *Nursing Documentation: Charting, Recording, and Reporting* presents the essential concepts, processes, and skills to help students build a solid foundation for communicating about nursing care.

Special Chapters

Three chapters describe basic concepts of communication and their relationship to the documentation of nursing care, showing the link between communication in the nursing process and clinical decision-making.

Chapter Two, *Communication Concepts and Documentation*, provides a strong foundation for understanding the role that communication techniques play in documenting nursing care. This understanding is the key to accurate, useful recording and reporting. The chapter discusses the process of communication, factors that affect this process, and the role of communication in documentation and other nursing activities.

Chapter Nine, *Comparing Documentation Methods*, is a comparison of various contemporary documentation formats. The chapter provides the student with a basic understanding of each format and highlights the advantages, disadvantages, and applications of each method. Critical pathways, the newest method of outlining patient care, reflect an overview of managed care and are explained in detail and shown in helpful displays. Information about computerized documentation focuses on the present technology, orienting the student to the application of computerization in nursing practice, while looking to the future with forecasts for applying information technology to the health care industry.

Chapter Ten, *The Reporting Process*, is unique in that no other text dedicates an entire chapter to this critical daily nursing activity. Learning what, how, and why to report are essential professional skills for students to master. The chapter discusses types of oral reports and presents different methods of reporting such as shift reporting, audiotape reporting, walking rounds, and telephone reporting.

Key Features

Nursing Documentation: Charting, Recording, and Reporting provides a solid base of knowledge and an awareness of how this information is applied to the clinical setting. To achieve this goal, the text incorporates the following key features:

▲ Provides a strong nursing process and nursing diagnosis framework
▲ Emphasizes the role of communication as the primary purpose of recording and reporting
▲ Applies communication concepts to the documentation process
▲ Presents all forms and methods of current documentation
▲ Discusses ethical considerations in documentation
▲ Simplifies legal concepts in recording and reporting

Teaching Features

To enable students to better understand the material in this book, numerous teaching aids are used.

▲ Learning Objectives, Key Terms, and Key Points clarify and organize the content for more effective learning.
▲ In-text extracts of actual documentation show students how various types of documentation actually appear in a patient chart.
▲ Boxed displays and examples of actual chart forms emphasize essential material, clarify the text, and enhance understanding.
▲ Practice Sessions at the end of each chapter provide hands-on learning that requires students to interact with the book, reinforcing key concepts learned in the chapter.
▲ Blank chart forms in the Learning to Document sections of the Practice Sessions allow students to simulate actual documentation.
▲ Challenge for Critical Thinking sections in the Practice Sessions encourage students to analyze and apply what they have learned.
▲ Answers to the Practice Sessions provided at the back of the book provide immediate feedback and evaluation of critical thinking.
▲ Separate Reference and Bibliography lists provide students with a broad base of authoritative resources for further study.

To some nurses, recording and reporting may represent a time-consuming, unstructured communication process that takes time away from patient care. The authors of this book present this communication process as a focused, organized, and highly successful means to assure coordinated, effective nursing care. Nursing documentation involves essential skills for students to learn and to continually fine tune. *Nursing Documentation: Charting, Recording, and Reporting* is the first book of its kind to address these skills through such a diversified and interactive process.

Ellen Thomas Eggland, RN, MN
Denise Skelly Heinemann, RN, DrPH

Acknowledgments

With special thanks to the following nurses and health care organizations for their time and for sharing documentation information:

Healthcare Personnel, Naples, FL; Berit Jasion, MA, RN, CS, of Duke University Medical Center, Durham, NC; Barbara Bamberg, RN, MPA, of Robinson Memorial Hospital, Ravenna, OH; John Crossley, RN, PhD, MBA, of University Hospitals of Cleveland, Cleveland, OH; Sharon Coulter, RN, MN, MBA, of Cleveland Clinic Foundation, Cleveland, OH; Lakeside Plantation, Naples, FL; Kathleen Moehring, RN, MS, of St. Vincent Charity Hospital and Health Center, Cleveland, OH; Nancy Sword, RN, of Lee Memorial Hospital, Ft. Myers, FL; and Naples Community Hospital, Naples, FL.

Sincere appreciation is also extended to:

Mary Agnes Kendra, PhD, RN, CS, of the Cleveland State University, Cleveland, Ohio, who contributed to the practice sessions at the end of the chapters.

Donna Hilton of J.B. Lippincott Co., who provided invaluable ideas, editing, and enthusiasm to this project.

Joyce Thornton, RN, EdD, of the University of South Florida, Ft. Myers, FL, who provided cheerful support and a ready resource for information.

Contents

Appendix A:

Appendix B:

Development of Nursing Documentation

LEARNING OBJECTIVES

After studying this chapter, the learner should be able to:

▲ Describe nursing in the Nightingale era in terms of the nurse's responsibility for reporting and recording.

▲ Cite three sociopolitical or economic events that affected the development of professional nursing in the United States.

▲ Give an example of the recording and reporting responsibilities of the nurse in functional, team, and primary models of nursing care delivery.

▲ List three trends in health care delivery that will have an impact on professional communication.

KEY TERMS

Accountability	Communication	Joint documentation	Primary nursing
Case assignment	Continuity	Magnet hospital	Quality management
Case management	Documentation	Nurse practice acts	Responsibility
Charting by exception	Flow sheets	Nursing process	Team nursing
Collaboration	Functional nursing		

Eggland ET, Heinemann DS. NURSING DOCUMENTATION:
CHARTING, RECORDING, AND REPORTING.
© 1994 J.B. Lippincott Company.

The most important practical lesson that can be given to nurses is to teach them what to observe: how to observe, what symptoms indicate improvement, what the reverse, which are of importance, which are of none, which are the evidence of neglect, and of what kind of neglect. (Nightingale, 1859, p. 59)

Only when we see the whole can we adequately appreciate the significance of the nurse's contributions to patient care. (Benner, 1984, p. 41)

In the 125 years separating Nightingale and Benner, the context within which nursing is practiced has changed, education for nursing has changed, and the needs of the consumer of nursing services have changed. What has remained relatively stable is the focus of nursing—the patient or client as an individual, family, group, or community. Nursing has been and remains client centered. This chapter explores the development of reporting and recording in nursing practice within the context of the evolution of the practice of nursing, the role of communication in nursing practice and health care delivery, and current issues in nursing documentation and communication. It is our hope that the reader will appreciate the importance of recording and reporting as essential components of professional nursing and will strive to develop the requisite knowledge and skills in these aspects of professional practice.

Evolution of Nursing Communication

Nightingale Era

In the Commemorative Edition of *Notes on Nursing*, Schuyler (1992) points out that Florence Nightingale wrote the book for *all* women, not just nurses, to teach them how to care for their families. The principles of nursing she discussed, such as providing a therapeutic environment for patients, caring for them with empathy, maintaining their confidentiality, and helping them regain their independence as soon as possible, are still basic to nursing (pp. 8, 9). Each of these activities depended on the relationship between the nurse and the patient and their ability to communicate with each other.

This era was characterized by care given at home under the supervision of the patient's physician. Because the cities of Europe were well developed by the mid 19th century, access to medical care was easier than in the isolated rural communities of the United States, where transportation was a major obstacle to the delivery of

medical care. The development of the telephone, the automobile, and hard roads in this country enabled physicians of the late 19th century to see more patients at home and for patients to make office visits (Starr, 1982). It is important to recognize that there was little social stratification between the patient and the health care practitioner of 19th century America. This made it easier for patients to talk with the physician, who had little formal education beyond that of the average layman and came from middle as well as upper income families.

The American Civil War had a profound effect on hospital care of the sick and injured. As a result of the war, additional hospitals were built and the theories and practices developed by Nightingale in the Crimean War were applied in Union field hospitals. It was not until 1873, however, that the first formal educational programs to prepare nurses in the United States were opened at the urging of socially conscious upper class women who were appalled at the conditions prevalent in the hospitals of the era. Organized according to Nightingale's model, these schools created a viable occupation for women of good upbringing. By 1910, there were 1129 training schools for nurses in the United States (Ashley, 1976).

Starr (1982) credits this professionalization of nursing with bringing order and sanitary conditions to American hospitals of the day. Hospital services continued to expand in response to scientific, social, cultural, political, and economic developments in the larger society. Explication of the germ theory, the development of antisepsis and anesthesia, industrialization and urbanization, and changes in the structure of the family created a need for care of the sick in institutions devoted to that purpose.

Nurses who cared for the sick in hospitals functioned much as some primary nurses do today, that is, they were responsible for *all* aspects of the patient's care and had a direct reporting relationship to the physician in charge of a case. Nightingale (1859) referred to disease as a "reparative process" (p. 5); the role of the nurse was to manage the patient's responses to this process and to use fresh air, light, warmth, cleanliness, quiet, and proper diet to enable the patient to regain health. Nightingale recognized the need for nurses to exercise critical thinking in their practice, chiding them to select a proper source of fresh air, for instance, because all sources were not desirable. This call to manage the patient's *human responses to health problems* is reflected in the contemporary definition of nursing established by the American Nurses Association (ANA) in 1980 and articulated in the **nurse practice acts** of many states in the United States today (see display, New York State Nurse Practice Act).

▲ NEW YORK STATE NURSE PRACTICE ACT

The practice of the profession of nursing as a registered professional nurse is defined as diagnosing and treating human responses to actual or potential health problems through such services as casefinding, health teaching, health counseling, and provision of care supportive to or restorative of life and well-being, and executing medical regimens prescribed by a licensed physician, dentist, or other licensed health care provider legally authorized under this title and in accordance with the Commissioner's regulations. A nursing regimen shall be consistent with and shall not vary any existing medical regimen.

EARLY NURSING MANAGEMENT

Nightingale exhorted nurse managers of her day to make daily rounds "of every hole and corner" (p. 17) to inspect those under their jurisdiction. It is inconceivable that a great deal of communication did not occur during such rounds as the nurse sought to assure herself of the quality of the workmanship in her charge. Written documentation of nursing care was not emphasized. Addressing the verbal reports nurses typically gave to the physician in charge of a case, Nightingale warned nurses not to speak out of ignorance or to embellish from their imaginations what they actually observed.

THE BIRTH OF NURSING PROCESS

As one who recognized the importance of patterns in human responses, Nightingale recommended that nurses evaluate the patient, not at a single point in time, but over the episode of care, reporting to the physician the current status of the patient within that frame of reference. She cautioned against collecting superfluous data or "curious" facts, an issue in health care today as we move to minimize the amount of recording the nurse must do while strengthening its quality. Nightingale emphasized careful observation and assessment of the patient and the need to ask proper questions to collect valid data about the individual's status. This role of the nurse in evaluation of the patient is essential in the conduct of care today, given the changing nature of the client in the hospital setting and the expanding functions of nurses in community settings. Although patients in the Nightingale era were cared for by one nurse for the duration of their care, today's hospital patient is cared for by many individuals. Patients in the acute care setting are older, sicker, and in the hospital for shorter and shorter periods of time. Clients in the community are receiving in-home therapeutic interventions that were previously available only in hospitals, including complex antibiotic therapy, chemotherapy, and parenteral nutrition. Care has become more complex and communication more circuitous.

The explosion of knowledge since the Nightingale era has resulted in specialization in medical practice, which, in turn, has caused medical care to become compartmentalized, each specialist focusing on the body system in his or her purview. This specialization has created a void of leadership of the care enterprise; no one quite knows "who's in charge." The nurse has stepped in to coordinate the disparate elements of health care for the benefit of the consumer. Nightingale observed that the only person truly qualified to judge the condition of the patient was the person who had continued contact with him—the nurse. That is even more true today than it was then and is evidenced by the intense interest in **case management** by nurses, a nursing care delivery system of the 1990s.

Twentieth Century Nursing Before World War II

By the turn of the century, most health care was still being given in the patient's home; hospitals offered a limited armamentarium of healing. Community health nurses visited the sick in their homes, cared for mothers and their families after childbirth, taught health maintenance and disease prevention, and developed programs to meet the needs of the communities they served—a realization of Nightingale's desire to see district nurses who would visit the homes of the poor and teach them sanitation and hygiene (Nightingale, 1859).

NURSING IN THE COMMUNITY

Lillian Wald and Mary Brewster, classmates and graduates of the New York Hospital School of Nursing, opened the House on Henry Street, which became the Henry Street Visiting Nurse Service, offering a wide range of health, social, cultural, and educational services to the surrounding community. This service later became a clinical laboratory for public health nursing students enrolled in courses developed by Miss Wald and Adelaide Nutting of Teachers' College, Columbia University.

In 1902, the New York City Health Department placed nurses in the city schools to refer children to physicians, treat minor problems, teach, confer with parents, and do follow-up. Starr (1982) notes that referred children frequently were not treated because the cost of medical care was prohibitive for their families. This problem exists in this last decade of the 20th century; school nurses report increasing incidence of untreated health problems evident in school children, particularly among the millions of American families who have no health insurance.

Hospital care was still not a dominant force in health care nor did an organized system of services exist to meet the needs of the public at the turn of the century (Fitzpatrick, 1991). Local health departments as we know them today did not materialize until the 1930s. Early efforts to deliver health care and social services were the result of privately organized philanthropy and volunteerism.

World War I created an additional demand for nurses beyond the pressing needs of a growing population fueled by immigration, epidemics of infectious diseases, and the deleterious effects of industrialization. Lay volunteers and nonprofessional workers were hired to meet the need for additional personnel (Fitzpatrick, 1991). This substitution of untrained individuals for health professionals—nurses, in particular—continued to occur throughout the 20th century in response to recurring shortages of trained workers. The educational preparation of American physicians had come under scrutiny during the first decade of the 20th century, and many medical schools of lesser quality had been forced to close. Impressed with the improvements achieved in medical education as a result of the Flexnor Report in 1910, Nutting secured Rockefeller Foundation support for a study of education for public health nurses—a study that actually examined *all* nursing education. The study results, known as the Goldmark Report, were published in 1923 and called for the establishment of schools of nursing that were independent of hospitals and that offered a liberal education. Two years later, the first collegiate program in nursing opened at Yale University.

THE EFFECTS OF THE GREAT DEPRESSION

Nurses who derived their living from private duty work in the 1920s had their livelihood shattered by the Depression. As private duty work evaporated, they sought refuge in the hospitals where they could work for survival wages. Remember that up until this time, most hospital nursing care was given by students under the supervision of the instructors who were staff of the hospital. The Federal Emergency Relief Act of 1933 and the Social Security Act of 1935 provided relief programs that enabled the employment of additional nurses. Throughout this period, there was little or no emphasis on documentation, much of which was in narrative form. The predominant model of nursing practice in the hospital setting was **case assignment** of students and paid graduate nurses to individual patients. This period marked the first introduction of large numbers of licensed nurses into the bureaucratic setting of the hospital and the

beginning of nursing's loss of control over its practice (Manthey, 1980). Documentation was done by case, was narrative in format, and was limited in the information it conveyed (see display, Documentation Then . . . and Now).

World War II and Beyond

War again placed a strain on the available supply of registered nurses (RNs). One significant response to this shortage was the creation of two levels of assistive personnel, the licensed practical nurse (LPN) and the nurse aide. LPNs were trained in vocational programs approximately a year in length; nurse aides were prepared in short courses offered by the American Red Cross or hospitals. The inclusion of nursing personnel who had a lower level of educational preparation and a more restricted license created a differentiation in practice and a delineation of separate nursing roles. Multiple nursing personnel with different education and expertise created the need to develop ways of assigning them to appropriate activities within the care enterprise.

 DOCUMENTATION: THEN AND . . . NOW

Then

Florence Nightingale (1859) thought that writing down one's observations about patients was a mental crutch that would diminish the nurse's capacity to observe and remember. She permitted it reluctantly. "But if you cannot get the habit of observation one way or the other, you had better give up being a nurse, for it is not your calling, however kind and anxious you may be" (p. 63).

Now

A breakdown in the clinical information system at the burn unit at Jackson Memorial Hospital left bedside computers inoperable for 4 days. A comparison of the documentation completed during the down period with time sampling just before and after revealed:

▲ The number of progress notes was 13 times greater with the computer than the traditional flow sheet method on the ICU and 4 times greater on the step-down unit.
▲ One in four shifts had errors of commission or omission when flow sheets were used.

The researchers point out that physicians rely on clinical data rather than examination of the patient; timely access to accurate data is essential.

FUNCTIONAL NURSING

Whereas RNs once had total **responsibility** and **accountability** for their cases, they were now assigned to duties of patient care that required complex skills and knowledge *and* the supervision of LPNs and aides who were assigned routine tasks of stabilized patient care. As a result, the need for communication about the patient and appropriate care—now performed by a number of individuals—increased. This **functional nursing** method of assignment in which one caregiver did the patient's bath, another made the bed, and yet another did the treatments and medications created a fragmented system that frustrated patients and caregivers alike. As Manthey (1980) indicates, the functional method also complicated communication among the nursing staff and between nursing and other disciplines. Functional assignments led to bits and pieces of care being documented separately. All accountability in this assignment method was vested in the head nurse or charge nurse who reported on all patients on the unit to physicians and the oncoming shift of nurses. This notion of accountability is a recurrent theme as the occupation of nursing continues to seek professional status.

The Hill-Burton Hospital Construction Program enacted by Congress in 1946 financed the construction of additional hospital space across the country—creating beds that required additional nursing staff and increased access to hospital care for rural populations. The nursing shortage continued after World War II, becoming acute in the 1950s when only 40% of RNs were employed in nursing and turnover for all nursing personnel was high (Levine, 1971). In hindsight, the functional method of assignment of hospital nurses and the effects of the hospital bureaucracy were blamed for the high level of job dissatisfaction and low retention among RNs at this time of real shortage. From a sociologic perspective, nursing functions had evolved over time from primary to secondary relations (nurses no longer worked directly for the patient, but for the hospital); from kinship to professional responsibility; from folk to technical knowledge; and from simple to complex activities and division of labor (Saunders, 1958).

The end of World War II saw the introduction of new technology into the hospital setting and the development of more complex surgical procedures and medications used in the treatment of hospitalized individuals, all of which increased the need for knowledgeable nurses. Nurses continued to assume additional technical tasks traditionally done by physicians and deferred activities deemed nonnursing—such as cleaning the patient's unit and performing pharmacy chores—to other departments. Consider that the thermometer and blood pressure cuff were once the exclusive implements of the physician!

NURSING PROCESS

During the 1950s, the term **nursing process** began to appear in the nursing literature to describe the problem-solving method nurses used to assess and meet patients' needs. By naming what we were doing and specifying the steps in the process *as they relate to patient care*, we made the intellectual nature of nursing care explicit. Bear in mind that the introduction of ancillary nursing personnel in hospitals, which had occurred earlier, created the need for policy and procedure manuals that dictated exactly how specific aspects of care were to be performed. These manuals suggested a cookbook approach to care that, in part, seemed to deny the individuality of the patient as well as the expertise of the nurse. Within the bureaucratic structure of the hospital (organized on an industrial model), any departure from established procedure or policy was considered heresy and an occasion for reprimand.

Early descriptions of the nursing process identified three steps that nurses followed in the course of patient care: they assessed the patient's needs, planned how they would meet the identified needs, and then implemented the plan. As nurses developed the concept of nursing process further, they specified additional steps that more fully explained what nurses were actually doing in practice: assessing, reaching a decision regarding the basic nature of the patient's problem(s), planning care to alleviate the problem(s), implementing the care, and evaluating the effect of that care. It was not until almost 20 years later that nurses began to put formal labels on their problem statements. These labels or *nursing diagnoses* were developed by practitioners to clarify the nature of patient problems within the domain of nursing care. These labels and their definitions allowed nurses to communicate with each other across settings and formed a vocabulary that facilitated patient care, education, and research. The diagnostic labels included terms that defined the etiology or cause of the patient's problem to which the nurse would direct attention to relieve or correct the problem. Before the mid 1970s, however, nursing process was not universally accepted in the United States nor was it applied in most institutions (see display, Nursing Diagnosis Then . . . and Now).

TEAM NURSING

Whereas the functional method of nursing assignment divided patient care by task categories (eg, medications given by the RN, baths and ambulation by the LPN, and bed making by aides), **team nursing** organized care by the physical structure of the nursing unit *and* staff resources. Team nursing was developed to solve some of the problems with the functional method that so dissatisfied both patients and nurses. Staff were organized in

▲ NURSING DIAGNOSIS THEN . . . AND NOW

1973

The First National Conference on Classification of Nursing Diagnosis.

1980

Nursing Diagnosis was delineated as a separate step in the nursing process.

1990

More than 100 separate nursing diagnoses appear on the accepted list.

1992

Additional nursing diagnoses adopted at the 10th NANDA Conference reflect the problems encountered in contemporary nursing practice, for example:

Caregiver Role Strain: a caregiver's felt difficulty in performing the family caregiver role

Dysfunctional Ventilatory Weaning Response: a state in which a client cannot adjust to lowered levels of mechanical ventilator support, which interrupts and prolongs the weaning process

The addition of diagnoses to the accepted list demonstrates the responsiveness of nursing to the changing needs of its clients as technology changes and clients survive acute illness episodes to live with the effects of chronic, disabling conditions.

teams of multilevel personnel led by an RN team leader who assigned them to care for the patients on their team. This team leader bore the ultimate responsibility for the work of the team. At change of shift, the team leader going off duty reported to the oncoming leader. On nights, it was common to have minimal staff, hence a single team. Because some patients were less sick than others, it was possible to assign the total care of selected ambulatory patients to an aide. Formal physical assessment by nurses was minimal. Nursing care was task oriented and driven by the Kardex and medical orders. In a word, nursing did not, for the most part, operate as a profession with an independent contribution to the care of the hospitalized person. Documentation focused on the tasks completed and provided only limited data on the patient's reaction to the illness and care.

One positive outcome of the task orientation of nursing in the 1940s and 1950s was that it helped administrators predict work load and staffing needs. Standardizing the elements of care reduced the need for communica-

tion between shifts and minimized the need for individual nurses to make decisions about patient care (Seward, 1969). In 1958, Coser described the hospital nurse as alienated and powerless to express her identity in the workplace.

EDUCATION RESPONSE

A major innovation in nursing education occurred in 1952 with the development of the associate degree program in nursing at the community college level. Dr. Mildred Montag's original conception of the "technical" nurse mirrored technical education in other fields such as engineering; just as the engineer delegated certain aspects of engineering to the draftsmen, the nurse could develop a similar relationship with a counterpart from the community college. The associate degree was intended by Montag to be a terminal degree because she believed that nursing functions could be differentiated based on educational preparation. As community colleges expanded over the next 20 years, so did nursing programs at that level. Differentiation in practice, however, did not occur. The associate degree nurse sat for the same licensing examination as did the 3-year diploma and the 4- or 5-year baccalaureate graduates. The individual was subsequently hired for similar entry level staff positions on the basis that nursing had but one license to practice nursing and all licensed newcomers to the profession were equal. It is difficult to imagine that a male-dominated group would have been so egalitarian! The concept of licensure as an assurance of *minimal* competency to practice was lost in the translation of education into practice.

1960 to 1980

Access to medical and hospital care continued to increase under the landmark legislation in 1965 that created Medicare and Medicaid, the federally funded medical insurance programs for older Americans and the poor, respectively. These early forms of national health insurance were later extended to persons with selected disabilities, such as black lung disease and end-stage renal failure. Both programs enabled more people to secure a physician's care. Because physicians are the gatekeepers of the health care delivery system in the United States, this increased access to their services increased the use of hospitals and other health services. As hospital admissions increased, so did the need for staff nurses.

THE BIRTH OF THE NURSE PRACTITIONER

Additional federal legislation in 1967 created neighborhood health centers at a time when nurse educators and physicians were collaborating to develop an advanced level of nursing practice. The resulting nurse practitioner role was designed to assist the physician in the practice or serve in areas that had difficulty recruiting physicians. These early nurse practitioner certificate programs provided knowledge and skill acquisition in physical assessment, history taking, diagnostic reasoning, and the management of common health problems in the ambulatory setting according to a medical model, that is, focused on the diagnosis and treatment of disease rather than a nursing model focused on the patient's responses. Attracted by the more independent nature of the practitioner role, some nurses left the hospital setting never to return. The practitioner movement grew, calling attention to the need for *all* nurses to have an education strongly based in the natural sciences and humanities, with good communication skills.

PRIMARY NURSING

A solitary innovation in nursing care delivery in the hospital setting occurred in 1969 at the University of Minnesota, where Manthey and her colleagues wrestled with the deficiencies they perceived in the team method of nursing care (Manthey, 1980). The concept of **primary nursing** as described by Manthey incorporated elements of case assignment with responsibility and accountability for care vested in the RN assigned to a patient for the length of the hospital stay. The primary nurse assessed the patient's needs and planned and evaluated the care throughout the hospitalization. This primary nurse was clearly identified for the patient and communicated directly with the patient's physician. The nurse became thoroughly familiar with patient's care needs and did the planning for discharge, starting at the time of admission. Primary nurses worked with their associate nurses as well as other ancillary personnel who gave direct care to their patients. Primary nursing reduced the multiple channels of communication inherent in team and functional methods, encouraged individualized care, and increased the satisfaction of patients and nursing staff (see display, Four Nursing Care Delivery Systems). Documentation was less fragmented and more cohesive and addressed the patient's problems from a unified perspective.

It is still Manthey's contention that primary nursing can be instituted in any setting and within contemporary budget restraints. Primary nursing requires a change in perspective, a transfer of responsibility and accountability from the head nurse to the staff nurse, and a willingness of nurses to accept the principles on which it is based. A significant element in the model—clinical decision-making by the primary nurse—clearly depends on clinical expertise, skillful communication, and articulate documentation of nurse–patient interactions, nursing

decisions, and patient outcomes. Documentation is the responsibility of the primary nurse.

Variants of primary nursing were implemented in the late 1970s and early 1980s, including all RN staffing. The latter increased the operating costs of hospitals and left primary nurses with a heavy burden of tasks generally thought of as nonnursing, not an intent of Manthey's original model. Continuity of nursing care improved as did patient and nurse satisfaction, but nurses struggled with accountability and the lack of support staff. An additional motivation for hospitals in creating all RN staffing was the notion that the RN was a more flexible worker who could perform a number of different functions under the broad definition of nursing practice contained in most state laws. All RN staffing eventually led to discontent in settings where RNs had to assume responsibility for nonnursing tasks, which they perceived as draining at best, menial at worst.

COLLABORATIVE PRACTICE

In the context of evolving roles for nurses in community settings, the National Joint Practice Commission was established in 1972 to "make recommendations concerning the congruent roles of the physician and the nurse in providing quality health care to the American people" (Hall, 1975). One recommendation dealt specifically with recording. Supported by grants from the W. K. Kellogg Foundation, the American Medical Association (AMA), and the ANA, the Commission issued position statements on the need for flexible nursing and medical practice acts; institutional joint practice committees to promote collaboration among nurses and physicians; joint documentation in progress notes; and nursing staff by-laws. Several teaching medical centers did develop joint or collaborative practice committees in the 1970s, which still exist and are experimenting with collaborative practice in the hospital setting. Where effective collaboration occurs, patients, physicians, and nurses report increased satisfaction with the process of care and its outcomes.

The concept of **joint documentation** in progress notes, that is, allowing nurses to document their care on the "medical progress" pages of the patient record has yet to be universally accepted, particularly in the acute care environment. The benefit of joint documentation is that each member of the health care team contributing to the care of a patient can quickly follow the patient's progress and the activities of other professionals in a central location in the record. Our colleagues in medicine object that joint charting is not appropriate. Colleagues in nursing who object to the practice seem to do so from a lack of confidence and professional self-esteem.

▲	**FOUR NURSING CARE DELIVERY SYSTEMS**				

Elements of Organization	Primary Care*	Case Management*⁺	Total Care*	Teams (Includes Modular)*	Functional
Clinical decision-making	Continuous (24 h/day)	Continuous (24 h/day)	Shift based	Shift based	Shift based
Responsibility and authority	*Personal* responsibility to manage nursing care for small groups of patients	*Personal* responsibility to manage patient care across units and coordinate interdepartmental activities	*Role* responsibility for small groups of patients	*Role* responsibility for large groups of patients	*Role* responsibility for large groups of patients
Work allocation	Patient-based assignments**	Patient-based assignments**	Patient-based assignments**	Task-based assignments	Task-based assignments

*May use skill-mixed staff with mix on acuity or may use all RN staff. The skill mix will vary according to philosophy, acuity and market availability. Assignments should be based on skill mix.

⁺ Some versions of Case are a form of Team Nursing using new language.

** Auxiliary workers may perform delegated activities.

ROLE DEVELOPMENTS

Differentiated Practice Model	Basic entry level competency expectations defined and used to create roles for professional and technical levels. Differentiated levels may function in Team and Primary systems.
Expanded Role Model	Case manager role is based on enhanced collaboration with MD along with multi-unit responsibility. Nurse's role expands to manage hospital experience for patient, based on outcome criteria, known as critical paths.

(Marie Manthey 1990, Creative Nursing Management, Inc. Revised 1/93)

NURSING STANDARDS OF PRACTICE: A PROFESSIONAL RESPONSIBILITY

In 1973, the ANA first published its *Standards of Practice*, which address the responsibilities of nurses for specific aspects of nursing care and are organized according to the steps in the nursing process. The *Standards* make explicit the role of data collection and documentation in nursing practice and specify that data collection is systematic and continuous and that data are accessible, communicated, and recorded (ANA, 1991). The *Patient's Bill of Rights*, published by the American Hospital Association (AHA) that same year, also addresses health communication in that the patient is due respectful care, information about his treatment, and the assurance of privacy and confidentiality (AHA, 1972).

PRACTICE INNOVATIONS

To attract more nurses to the hospital setting in a period of high RN vacancy rates, hospitals adopted the "Baylor shift" concept (named for the Texas medical center where it originated). Nurses were able to complete their work week and earn benefits in two or three 12-hour shifts while the hospitals benefited by using these nurses to provide care in unpopular time slots. Baylor shift options increased staffing and nurse job satisfaction, but little research has been done to document the effects of Baylor work patterns on the continuity of care. Most attempts to optimize the working conditions of nurses were limited to reassignment of the tasks nurses do and had marginal results (Seitz, Donaho, & Kohles, 1991). The explosion of medical technology led to the creation of special care units and staff specialized in the care of patients with high-intensity needs. Nurses in intensive care units developed new ways of recording their observations out of frustration with the traditional narrative form of charting. These **flow sheets** facilitated review of the patient's status over a period of time and tended to be unit specific. One side effect of the development of special nursing care units is the observation that they have created subspecialty interest groups in nursing that tend to become isolated. Isolation decreases communication with those outside a group.

PROGRESS IN ADVANCED NURSING PRACTICE

Graduate programs in nursing began preparing clinical specialists and nurse practitioners at the master's degree level. Clinical nurse specialists were hired by hospitals to act as supervisors and consultants to staff nurses to improve the clinical care of patients with specific problems (eg, diabetes, cardiac disease, ostomies, and cancer). Because clinical specialists were an "add-on" for hospitals, that is, they did not replace other nurses, they increased the nursing costs for the institutions and tended to find work only in teaching medical centers. Nurse practitioners continued to find employment in predominantly community-based practice settings, working one-on-one with individual patients under the supervision of a physician. In an attempt to recognize and control advanced practice in nursing, states began to add a definition of advanced practice to the nurse practice act on a state-by-state basis (see display, Florida Nurse Practice Act).

COLLABORATION—A RECURRENT ISSUE

In 1980, yet another commission was formed to examine nursing issues and develop and implement "action plans for the future" (National Commission on Nursing, 1983, p. 1). Funded by the AHA, the Hospital Research and Education Trust, and the American Hospital Supply Corporation, the National Commission on Nursing made recommendations (see display, Recommendations of the National Commission on Nursing, 1989), which have implications for medical and nursing practice that are based in communication and documentation. **Collaboration** is defined by the ANA Congress on Nursing Practice (1980) as a "true partnership, in which the power on both sides is valued by both, with recognition and acceptance of separate and combined spheres of activity and responsibility, mutual safeguarding of the legitimate interests of each party, and a commonality of goals that is recognized by both parties" (p. 7). The reader will note that the party most involved with the nurse and the

---

▲ FLORIDA NURSE PRACTICE ACT

Definition of Professional Nursing

"Practice of professional nursing" means the performance of those acts requiring substantial specialized knowledge, judgment, and nursing skill based on applied principles of psychological, biologic, physical, and social sciences, which shall include, but not be limited to:

1. The observation, assessment, nursing diagnosis, planning intervention, and evaluation of care; health teaching and counseling of the ill, injured, or infirm; and the promotion of wellness, maintenance of health, and prevention of illness of others.
2. The administration of medications and treatments as prescribed by a duly licensed practitioner authorized by the laws of this state to prescribe such medications and treatments.
3. The supervision and teaching of other personnel in the theory and performance of any of the above acts.

"Practice of practical nursing" means the performance of selected acts, including the administration of treatments and medications, in the care of the ill, injured, or infirm and the promotion of wellness, maintenance of health, and prevention of illness of others under the direction of a registered nurse, a licensed physician, a licensed osteopathic physician, a licensed podiatrist, or a licensed dentist.

The professional nurse and the practical nurse shall be responsible and accountable for making decisions that are based on the individual's educational preparation and experience in nursing.

(Florida DPR, Ch 464.003, Rev. 1989)

---

patient in the hospital setting—the physician—is not represented here, except indirectly.

The Commission's recommendation urging the inclusion of nurse administrators at the top level of hospital management has been realized in many institutions and should facilitate positive structural and procedural changes in the hospital to enhance interprofessional communication. One example of a structural change implemented in many hospitals is the investment in bedside computers for direct data entry during patient care. The efficacy of computers in documentation will be discussed more fully in later chapters. Nurse executives set the tone for nursing services and can support nurse–physician collaboration, clinical decision-making by nurses, and nursing practice models that are grounded in educational preparation and appropriate experience.

RECOMMENDATIONS OF THE NATIONAL COMMISSION ON NURSING, 1989

The Commission's 16 Remedies for the Shortage

1. Providers should strengthen support staff to save the RN's time for patient care.
2. Staffing patterns should take into account RNs' different levels of education and experience.
3. Computers and other labor-saving technologies should be applied to support nursing.
4. To better manage nursing resources, providers, professional groups, and the government should track staffing, costs, and utilization.
5. Nurses' "relative wages" should be increased by a "targeted, one-time increase."
6. Government and private payers should reimburse at levels allowing for recruitment and retention of nurses.
7. Nursing should play a more active role in policy-making in government, regulatory bodies, and employment settings.
8. Employers should ensure active nurse representation in governance.
9. Employers should foster collaboration among all heath care providers.
10. Financial aid to students should increase.
11. Nonfinancial barriers to nursing education should be eliminated for nontraditional students and nurses seeking advanced degrees.
12. Schools should work with employers and state boards to ensure that curricula and clinical learning experiences are kept "relevant."
13. Nursing must actively promote "positive" images of the profession.
14. The Secretary's Commission on Nursing should be extended by at least 5 years.
15. Public and private groups should increase research in the factors influencing nursing supply and demand.
16. The federal government should develop the data needed to assess nurse-power problems.

(National Commission on Nursing. [1989]. Nursing commission urges Congress to hike pay; says RN shortage endangers the nation's health. *American Journal of Nursing, 89*[2], 278–279.)

Contemporary Nursing Practice

Health care and nursing practice in the 1980s and 1990s continue to be influenced by powerful technologic, socioeconomic, and political factors. The development of new technology and drugs supports biomedical procedures we would have thought impossible even 10 years ago. As the complexity of hospital-based treatment increases, so does the complexity of treatment provided in the patient's home and the nursing home. The current emphasis on cost containment and efficient use of finite resources underscores the increasing proportion of the gross national product that is devoted to medical care. As the proportion of the United States population whose medical and hospital care is funded by Medicare increases in an environment of expanding diagnostic and therapeutic technology *and* medical malpractice litigation, the cost of medical care has increased each year significantly more than the annual rate of inflation.

DIAGNOSIS-RELATED GROUPS

In 1983, the Health Care Financing Administration implemented a new system of reimbursement for Medicare beneficiaries. Hospitals were paid on a prospective basis for services "bundled" by diagnosis-related groups (DRGs); physicians were paid according to a schedule of fees. This radical departure from the "reasonable cost basis" of reimbursement has had profound effects on American medicine and health services and will likely be extended to all forms of reimbursement for health care, including private insurance.

One response to increasing regulations has been the expansion of ambulatory diagnostic and surgical services and preadmission testing of elective hospital admissions. A second has been the review of hospital admissions (utilization review) to ensure that the hospitalization was appropriate and therefore should be reimbursed by the third-party payer. These developments have effectively decreased the number of hospital admissions and shortened the average length of stay for hospital patients (see display, AHCPR Research: The Effects of Utilization Review on Length of Stay). Today's typical hospital patient is older, has one or more chronic conditions, is sicker, and may have a weak support network in the community. Because hospital length of stay is dictated by a formula that reflects the needs of an "average" patient in the diagnostic category, an individual patient who has more than "average" problems may be discharged from the acute care setting with multiple needs for services at home or in an extended care facility. Hospital staff must accomplish all aspects of the nursing process in an efficient and expedient manner. As multiple agencies participate in a single patient's care, their ability to communicate verbally and in writing becomes a criterion for successful collaboration and the delivery of quality care.

ACQUIRED IMMUNODEFICIENCY SYNDROME (AIDS)

The reality of the AIDS epidemic in the United States and around the globe has profound implications for nursing and health care. The nature of human immunodeficiency virus (HIV) infection is such that it has affected the level of acuity in the hospitals and nursing homes that care for AIDS patients; it has changed our procedures for infection control. AIDS has raised important legal, ethical, and economic questions for health care professionals, policy makers, and the community at large. The challenge of

---

▲ AHCPR RESEARCH: THE EFFECTS OF UTILIZATION REVIEW ON LENGTH OF STAY

Sixty-five percent (65%) of private group insurance plans in the United States now use utilization review (UR) to examine hospital care for reimbursement. This study reviewed pooled quarterly claims between 1984 and 1986 for patients drawn from 233 private insurance groups.

Findings: Utilization review appeared to reduce admissions by 12%, room and board charges by 14%, hospital ancillary service charges by 10%, and total medical expenditures by 6%.

The main factor appeared to be preadmission screening, which reduced unnecessary admissions.

(Agency for Health Care Policy and Research. [June 1992]. *Research activities*, [154]. Rockville, MD: United States Department of Health and Human Services, Public Health Service.)

---

offering humane and expert care to these brothers and sisters will continue as their numbers increase and new experimental treatments extend the life span of those with AIDS. So complex are the needs of the immunologically compromised person that providers must be expert in the care process and in communication and collaboration with others.

THE NURSING SHORTAGE OF THE 1980S

The shortage of hospital staff nurses experienced in the last decade occurred at a time when hospitals were closing beds to increase their efficiency and most licensed nurses were employed in nursing. A 1987 AHA survey indicated that more than half the responding hospitals were experiencing moderate or severe shortages, with 10% or more of their nursing positions vacant (ANA, 1988), yet most nurses were working in nursing. Shortages were worse in public institutions and large, urban hospitals—the very institutions who carry the lion's share of the burden of caring for persons with AIDS. When it became clear that turnover of nursing staff was costly *and* preventable, nurse researchers began to examine hospitals in the United States that had the reputation for attracting and retaining nurses, later dubbed "magnet" institutions. The objective of the research was to identify characteristics these hospitals shared that might be imitated by others to increase the retention of nurses.

MAGNET HOSPITALS

Magnet hospitals had several common features related to the job satisfaction and low turnover rate of the nurses who staffed them, including:

▲ New nursing care delivery models
▲ Differentiated nursing roles
▲ Collaborative practice
▲ Decentralized decision-making
▲ Increasing use of computers (Kramer & Schmalenberg, 1988)

The magnet hospitals continued to increase their ratio of RNs to occupied beds from 1.2 RNs per bed in 1986 to 1.5 in 1989. Many of the institutions sampled by Kramer had decreased the number of LPN positions on staff in favor of increasing the proportion of RNs who, by law, had a broader scope of practice and were therefore more flexible workers. Remember that the LPN has no independent function by law and must practice under the supervision of a licensed physician, osteopath, dentist, or RN. At the same time that hospitals were experiencing a shortage of nurses, additional employment opportunities for the finite pool of nurses had opened up in fields such as home care and occupational health where nurses experience considerably more professional autonomy and job satisfaction than they do in hospitals. One result of the shortage of nurses was additional stress on those already working and an increased attention to the legal ramifications of documentation—an activity that absorbed a significant amount of the staff nurse's time each day. Nurses continue to have a very high participation in the work force, but many choose to work part-time. The inclusion of a large proportion of part-time nurses on the team increases the complexity of intraprofessional communication.

NURSE MANAGERS

Kramer's (1990) follow-up interviews of nurse executives in the sample of magnet hospitals she studied indicated that these nurse leaders excelled in experimentation, appreciation of the importance of values in the workplace, and autonomy for workers. These qualities of leadership facilitate professional practice and shared governance (see display, Characteristics of a Professional Practice Model of Nursing). The characteristics or traits of nurse leaders identified by Ehrat (1991) in her research include:

▲ Influence
▲ Persuasion
▲ Ability to challenge
▲ Humor
▲ Character and personal presence

CHARACTERISTICS OF A PROFESSIONAL PRACTICE MODEL OF NURSING

The following are characteristics identified as those that facilitate professional practice:

▲ Multidisciplinary and interdisciplinary collaboration
▲ Accountability
▲ Practice based on a sound and discipline-specific foundation of knowledge, theory, and inquiry, ie, scholarship
▲ Autonomy rooted in a clear understanding of the scope and boundaries of the discipline of nursing
▲ Awareness of the socio-political context of practice
▲ Self-motivated professional development, including self-peer evaluation

(Hannah, K.J., & Shamian, J. [1992]. Integrating a nursing professional practice model and nursing informatics in a collective bargaining environment. *Nursing Clinics of North America, 27*[1], 31–45.)

These characteristics clearly rely on the personal communication skills of the individual nurse executive and support the premise that communication and critical thinking are essential components of leadership behavior.

CARE MANAGEMENT

Staff nurses who assume responsibility and accountability for the care process in case management or similar primary-focused forms of nursing practice "need clear, efficient, professional documentation skills; conflict resolution skills; and knowledge about principles of delegation, supervision, collaboration, and accountability [and]... experiences with peer review, ethical decision making, and patient advocacy" (Cronenwett, Clark, Reeves, & Easton, 1991, p. 71). The knowledge and abilities depend on communication theory and skills, both written and oral, and require a fairly sophisticated level of behavior.

Documentation and Communication in Nursing Practice

Legal definitions of nursing practice in the United States vary from state to state but resemble the form and substance of the Florida Nurse Practice Act (see display on page 9). This legislation clearly delineates the responsibility of the RN for implementing the nursing process, exercising clinical judgment, and communicating this to others in the form of documentation, communication, and supervision. For our purposes, **documentation** is defined as written evidence of the interactions between and among health professionals, patients and their families, and health care organizations; the administration of tests, procedures, treatments, and patient education; and the results or patient's responses to them.

Documentation includes all aspects of the nursing process as well as the contributions of all other health team members to the patient's care. Carefully constructed and clearly written descriptions of what we have done and the patient's responses contribute to an individualized verbal picture of the patient, which third-party payers and other disciplines can read and evaluate. Thoughtful communication and documentation provide essential information about the patient and facilitate continuity of care. **Continuity** is defined as an uninterrupted process with appropriate linkages and services to meet a client's needs. Continuity enhances the quality of care, that is, the degree to which patient care services increase the probability of desired outcomes and reduce the probability of undesired outcomes given the current state of knowledge (Fromberg, 1986). Continuity based on careful documentation and verbal reports minimizes the need for health care workers to be repetitious in their queries of the patient and conveys the message that someone is "in charge" and is taking care.

Effective documentation meets the standards or expectations of the various constituencies with a stake in the patient's care: the patient; the nursing department; the hospital; the state agencies that license institutions and health professionals; insurance carriers; the Joint Commission on the Accreditation of Healthcare Organizations (see display, JCAHO Nursing Standards, 1992); various professional associations such as the AMA and ANA; lawyers; and the state and federal agencies who finance the care. Each looks to documentation for evidence that the care given is in keeping with their expectations and affirms the old adage: IF IT'S NOT DOCUMENTED, IT'S NOT DONE!

Interdisciplinary Communication

Communication is "the process of sharing information according to a common set of rules" (Northouse & Northouse, 1992). In health care, it "refers to health-related transactions between individuals who are attempting to maintain health and avoid illness" (p. 19). Like all human communication, it is continuous, dynamic, and multidimensional. Because the health of the client or patient is the focus of health communication *and* health transactions imply a contract between the patient and the professional, it is imperative that health professionals understand communication theory and apply it in a meaningful way in their practice.

Health care is a team effort. As knowledge and technology have expanded, additional specialties have developed; each contributes to the patient's care in a particular area of expertise and depends on the clinical record for past and current information. The record is the primary communication tool for the multidisciplinary health team. For various reasons, the traditional paper record has inherent deficits that interfere with the ability of the health team to function effectively and efficiently, as outlined below.

1. All health team members use the same data but in different ways. To meet the needs of multiple users, multiple entries of the same data are made, leading to a transcription error rate of 3% to 5%.
2. Single sheets are often misfiled or misplaced altogether.
3. It is difficult to identify significant test results quickly.
4. Aggregation of data for research purposes is almost impossible.
5. Time and energy are spent simply trying to locate the record to enter data or retrieve it.
6. Only one person can use the record at a time (Korpman, 1990).

Problems in Documentation

The increasing acuity among hospital patients, the complexity of their care, and the expanding responsibilities of the staff nurse place a heavy burden on the documentation and communication skills of the nurse and present a need for nurses to have timely and accurate data on which to base their clinical judgments. One strategy is the increasing use of computerized records and bedside terminal entry of data at the time an observation is made or an intervention completed. Research indicates that automated data entry enhances the amount *and* accuracy of documentation by nurses (Hammond et al., 1991). Quality care depends on the practitioner's ability to handle a large amount of information about the patient. To demonstrate the contribution nursing makes to patient outcomes, nurses need to integrate all clinical data; this depends on a "single, integrated patient-centered data base" (Mowry, 1992).

Katz and Green (1992) recommend that we discard what they describe as "obsolete" practices: narrative charting, duplication in charting, individualized care plans, and the Kardex and move to a unified, computerized medical record. The potential benefits of computerization and the limitations of the Kardex are discussed in later chapters. Duplication of any effort is time consuming and clearly must be avoided. As professionals, we

---

 JCAHO NURSING STANDARDS, 1992

NC.1.3.4 The patient's medical record includes documentation of
 1.3.4.1 the initial assessments and reassessments;
 1.3.4.2 the nursing diagnoses and/or patient needs;
 1.3.4.3 the interventions identified to meet the patient's nursing care needs;
 1.3.4.4 the nursing care provided;
 1.3.4.5 the patient's response to, and the outcomes of, the care provided; and
 1.3.4.6 the abilities of the patient and/or, as appropriate, his/her significant other(s) to manage continuing care needs after discharge.
NC.1.3.5 Nursing care data related to patient assessments, the nursing care planned, nursing interventions, and patient outcomes are permanently integrated into the clinical information system (eg, the medical record).

will make decisions about what components of practice need to be revised in the light of new knowledge and changing technology; when we do, the first consideration should be the effect(s) on patient care. Narrative charting in and of itself is not a poor methodology; physicians have used it for years and continue to do so. Where nursing has failed in the past is in the quality of the content of what narrative charting we did. We must document the data that represent the patient as an individual, that is, the data that drive our clinical decision-making. *How* we achieve that objective may change over time. We must retain the principles underlying our practice in the process.

Role of Documentation in Research

Nursing and health services research studies in the last decade have not adequately addressed important areas of concern such as the costs and benefits of specific nursing care strategies or models of nursing practice (Ingersoll, Hoffart, & Schultz, 1990). As the profession has responded to societal as well as internal forces, it has moved from one model of nursing care delivery and set of nursing interventions to another or resurrected abandoned practices without establishing their effectiveness or cost. The inability of nursing and health care researchers to quickly and efficiently access large amounts of data on selected groups of clients typifies the inadequacies of the traditional patient chart or clinical record as a source of data for research.

Specific areas of inquiry for nursing research include the explication of concepts such as *involvement* and *distance* in the nurse–patient relationship; how nurses perceive and interpret early warning signs of deterioration in a patient's condition; the character and content of the caring function of nursing (Benner, 1984); the *integrator role* of the nurse who is the continuous presence in the hospital setting (McClure, 1991); and innovative practice at the "edges" of nursing (as we know it), which may redefine professional practice, for example, cardiac clinical specialists who manage caseloads of patients after heart attack. Studies of patient outcomes of specific nursing interventions in large populations describe nursing activities using a common vocabulary that allows comparisons across multiple groups of patients (McCloskey & Bulechek, 1992; Figure 1–1). This is but one effort to define the results of nursing care. To establish the value of specific nursing interventions determined by specific nursing diagnoses, we will need a classification system for nursing interventions. Present nursing practice reflects the use of multiple terms for individual nursing treatments or interventions, which inhibits cross-institutional comparisons of nursing care.

Role of Communication in Quality Management

Quality assessment and improvement activities are an essential part of nursing practice and depend heavily on documentation of nurse–patient interactions and patient outcomes (Katz & Green, 1992). As professionals, we are required to critically examine our services and validate their effectiveness. The blueprint illustrates the relationship among the elements of **quality management** and the essential role of the records of what transpired during care in the overall process of evaluating our practice (Figure 1–2). Evaluation helps to answer the question all professions must ask of themselves: what is the value of our service to society?

Quality management may depend on existing records (retrospective data collection) or the collection of specific data to describe nursing care as it is delivered (concurrent or prospective data collection). The data are then compared to standards of care or predetermined thresholds of acceptable care. When nurses do not record what they do for patients, it is impossible to claim a stake in the positive outcomes of care. More importantly, absence of documentation may associate the nurse with poor outcomes. The 10-step monitoring evaluation model required by JCAHO (see display, JCAHO 10-Step Monitoring and Evaluation Model) delineates data collection as a basis for evaluation and proactive strategies to improve the quality of nursing service.

Current Issues in Documentation and Communication

The incidence of health care malpractice claims in the United States continues to increase. Each and every legal action depends on the patient chart or clinical record for evidence that the clinical judgments and actions of health team members were appropriate and timely. This reliance on the quality of documentation will continue. What has not yet evolved is a substantive body of case law that tests computerized health records or **charting by exception**, a method of documentation that assumes normal parameters and documents only aberrations from normal or what is expected. Flow sheets present observations in a clear, concise check-off format for immediate and quick data entry and reference; only abnormal findings are expanded in a narrative fashion. This method minimizes the time and cost necessary to document care (see display, Researching the Cost of Documentation) and will be explained in greater detail in a later chapter. Bear in mind that the method assumes that all abnormal findings are, in fact, charted. Charting by

Classification of Nursing Interventions

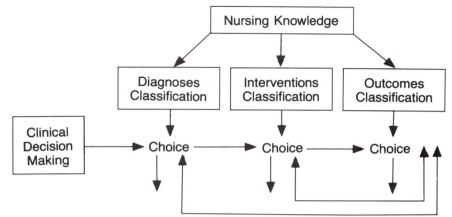

FIG. 1-1A. Relationship of nursing knowledge classifications to nurse's clinical decision-making. (Iowa Intervention Project, McCloskey, J. C. & Bulechek, G. M. [Eds.]. [1992]. *Nursing in Classification [NIC]*, St. Louis: Mosby—Year Book. Reprinted with permission.)

Anticipatory Guidance

DEFINITION: Preparation of patient for an anticipated developmental and/or situational crisis

ACTIVITIES:

Assist the patient to identify possible upcoming, developmental, and/or situational crisis, and the effects the crisis may have on personal and family life

Instruct about normal development and behavior as appropriate

Provide information on realistic expectations related to the patient's behavior

Determine the patient's usual methods of problem-solving

Assist the patient to decide how the problem will be solved

Assist the patient to decide who will solve the problem

Use case examples to enhance the patient's problem-solving skills as appropriate

Assist the patient to identify available resources and options for course of action as appropriate

Rehearse techniques needed to cope with upcoming developmental milestone or situational crisis with the patient as appropriate

Assist the patient to adapt to anticipated role changes

Provide a ready reference for the patient (ie, educational materials/pamphlets) as appropriate

Suggest books/literature for the patient to read as appropriate

Refer the patient to community agencies as appropriate

Schedule visits at strategic developmental/situational points

Schedule extra visits for patient with concerns or difficulties

Schedule follow-up phone calls to evaluate success or reinforcement needs

Provide the patient with a phone number to call for assistance if necessary

Include the family/significant others as appropriate

BACKGROUND READINGS:

Denehy, J. A. (1990). Anticipatory guidance. In M. J. Craft & J. A. Denehy (Eds.), *Nuring interventions for infants and children* (pp. 53–68). Philadelphia: W. B. Saunders.

Rakel, B. A. (1992). Interventions related to patient teaching. In G. M. Bulechek, & J. C. McCloskey (Eds.), Symposium on Nursing Interventions. *Nursing Clinics of North America.* Philadelphia: W. B. Saunders.

Schulman, J. L. & Hanley, K. K. (1987). Anticipatory guidance: An idea whose time has come. Baltimore: Williams and Wilkins.

Smith, C. E. (1987). Using the teaching process to determine what to teach and how to evaluate learning. In C. E. Smith (Ed.), *Patient education: nurses in partnership with other health professionals* (pp. 61–95). Philadelphia: W. B. Saunders.

FIG. 1-1B. Anticipatory guidance. Example of one intervention from NIC. (Iowa Intervention Project, McCloskey, J. C. & Bulechek, G. M. [Eds.]. [1992]. *Nursing in Classification [NIC]*. St. Louis: Mosby-Year Book.)

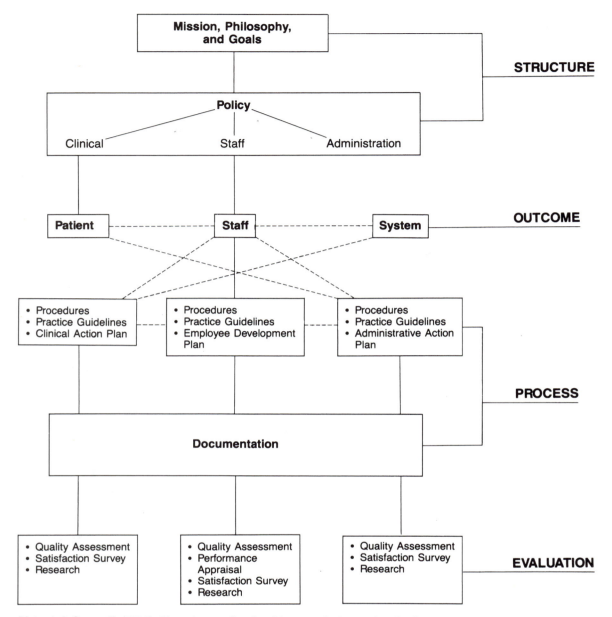

(Katz, J. & Green, E. (1992). *Managing quality. A guide to monitoring and evaluating nursing services*. St. Louis: Mosby–Year Book, p. 20. Reprinted with permission.)

FIG. 1-2. The blueprint for quality management

exception clearly departs from the "not documented, not done" edict of the past.

The Near Future

Events or trends that will continue to place a burden on documentation and communication in health care include:

▲ Increased acuity level of patients in the hospital

▲ Increased community-based services for acute illness

▲ Use of ancillary or cross-trained personnel to carry out nursing tasks

▲ Cross-training of nurses in other nursing specialties, such as respiratory therapy, phlebotomy, and electrocardiography

▲ Decentralized clinical decision-making

▲ Development of easy access to trend data

▲ Short lengths of hospital stay

▲	**JCAHO 10-STEP MONITORING AND EVALUATION MODEL**

1. *Assign responsibility.* Who will do the evaluation?
2. *Delineate the scope of care and practice.* What should the patient expect and how should the professional perform?
3. *Identify important aspects of patient care and service.* What activities or services are important in terms of high volume, high risk for the patient, or are prone to untoward events?
4. *Identify indicators.* What structure, process, or outcome variables will be used to monitor care?
5. *Establish preset levels of expected performance for evaluation.* What proportion of negative results is acceptable?
6. *Collect and organize data.*
7. *Evaluate the data.*
8. *Take action to correct the problem identified in #7.* What can be done to improve the performance on the indicators?
9. *Assess the actions and document improvements in practice.* Did the corrective activity work?
10. *Communicate relevant information within the organization.*

(Adapted from Patterson, C. H. [1988]. Standards of patient care: The Joint Commission focus on nursing quality assurance. *Nursing Clinics of North America, 23*[3], 625–638.)

▲	**RESEARCHING THE COST OF DOCUMENTATION**

Based on data collected at the 962-bed hospital at Abbott Northwestern in Minneapolis, the authors identified four problems with the narrative charting method in use: irrelevant data; redundancy and repetition; inconsistency across units; and the time devoted to documentation.

Method: With input from clinical specialists, staff developed the FACT system composed of four elements:

1. Flow sheets specific to each service
2. Standardized assessments with baseline parameters
3. Concise integrated progress notes and flow sheets
4. Timely entries by nurses at the time care is given.

Narrative notes follow a *Data, Action, Response* format and records are placed at the point of care, the bedside.

Results: RNs reported an increase in time spent with patients. In the 6-month period following the institution of the new charting system, administration calculated savings approaching $500,000, of which $470,000 was in nursing overtime. Despite cutbacks in nursing positions, overtime has not increased, patient days have remained stable, and length of stay has decreased.

▲ Decreasing availability of part-time work
▲ Emphasis on elimination of narrow-focused jobs
▲ Reduction in LPN positions in acute care hospitals
▲ Use of clinical case studies for performance evaluation
▲ Reliance on the nurse as the integrator of services: managed care and case management
▲ Staff nurse preceptorships to ease the transition of nurses from student to practitioner role

KEY POINTS

▲ Health care delivery in the United States is sensitive to social, political, technical, and economic factors in the larger society, which will increase in intensity in the future.

▲ The focus of professional nursing has traditionally been and continues to be the *responses* of people to actual or potential health problems, not just the disease process.

▲ The practice of nursing has moved beyond its traditional roots in the patient's home to the institutional setting of the hospital and nursing home where nursing practice has become increasingly specialized and fragmented.

▲ Whereas the Nightingale era was characterized by a one-on-one relationship between the patient and the nurse, contemporary nursing practice is characterized by multiple caregivers and complex channels of communication.

▲ Nursing care delivery systems directly affect the kinds of communication necessary to deliver nursing care that is continuous and coordinated.

▲ Modern health care is multidimensional and requires the participation of a number of professional and occupational groups that must communicate with each other.

▲ Recording and reporting are the major avenues of communication that health care professionals use to expedite clinical decision-making and care.

▲ The role of nursing leadership is to facilitate nursing practice by creating an environment conducive to nursing clinical decision-making and nursing communication.

REFERENCES

Agency for Health Care Policy and Research. (June 1992). *Research Activities, (154)*. Rockville, MD: USDHHS, PHS.

American Hospital Association. (1972). *A patient's bill of rights*. Chicago: Author.

American Nurses Association. (1991). *Standards of clinical nursing practice*. Washington, DC: Author.

American Nurses Association. (1988). *The nursing shortage. Situations and solutions*. Washington, DC: Author.

American Nurses Association. (1980). *Nursing: A social policy statement*. Washington, DC: Author.

Ashley, J. A. (1976). *Hospitals, paternalism, and the role of the nurse*. New York: Teachers' College Press.

Benner, P. (1984). *From novice to expert. Excellence and power in clinical nursing practice*. Menlo Park, CA: Addison-Wesley.

Bernal, E. W. (1992). The nurse as patient advocate. *Hastings Center Report, 22*(4), 18–32.

Branden, N. (1969). *The psychology of self-esteem*. New York: Bantam Books.

Bulechek, G. M., & McCloskey, J. C. (Eds). (1992). Symposium on nursing interventions. *Nursing Clinics of North America, 27*(2).

Coser, R. L. (1958). Authority and decision-making in a hospital. *American Social Review, 23*(2), 56–63.

Cronenwett, L., Clark, K., Reeves, S., & Easton, L. (1991). Building on shared values: The Dartmouth-Hitchcock Medical Center approach. In I. E. Goertzen (Ed.), *Differentiating nursing practice into the twenty-first century* (pp. 61–71). Kansas City: American Academy of Nursing.

Edelstein, J. (1990). A study of nursing documentation. *Nursing Management, 21*(11), 40–46.

Ehrat, K. S. (1991). An administrator's response to three models of differentiated practice. In I. E. Goertzen (Ed.), *Differentiating nursing practice into the twenty-first century* (pp. 423–428). Kansas City: American Academy of Nursing.

Fitzpatrick, M. L. (1991). Differentiated nursing practice: Historical parallels and paradoxes in public health nursing. In I. E. Goertzen (Ed.), *Differentiating nursing practice into the twenty-first century* (pp. 383–394). Kansas City: American Academy of Nursing.

Fromberg, R. (Ed.). (1986). *Monitoring and evaluation in nursing services*. Chicago: Joint Commission on Accreditation of Hospitals.

Hall, V. C. (1975). *Statutory regulation of the scope of nursing practice—A critical survey*. Chicago: National Joint Practice Commission.

Hammond, J., Johnson, H. M., Varas, R., & Ward, C. G. (1991). A qualitative comparison of paper flowsheets versus a computer-based clinical information system. *Chest, 99*(1), 155–157.

Hannah, K. J., & Shamian, J. (1992). Integrating a nursing professional practice model and nursing informatics in a collective bargaining environment. *Nursing Clinics of North America, 27*(1), 31–45.

Ingersoll, G. L., Hoffart, N., & Schultz, A. W. (1990). Health services research in nursing: Current status and future directions. *Nursing Economics, 8*(4), 229–238.

Ingersoll, G. L., Ryan, S., & Schultz, A. W. (1991). Evaluating the impact of enhanced professional practice on patient outcomes. In I. E. Goertzen (Ed.), *Differentiating nursing practice into the twenty-first century* (pp. 301–314). Kansas City: American Academy of Nursing.

Joint Commission on Accreditation of Healthcare Organizations. (1992). *Accreditation manual for hospitals*. Chicago: Author.

Katz, J., & Green, E. (1992). *Managing quality. A guide to monitoring and evaluating nursing services*. St. Louis: Mosby-Year Book.

Korpman, R. A. (1990). Patient care automation: The future is now. Part 2. The current paper system—can it be made to work? *Nursing Economics, 8*(4), 263–267.

Kramer, M. (1990). The magnet hospitals. Excellence revisited. *Journal of Nursing Administration, 20*(9), 35–44.

Kramer, M., & Schmalenberg, C. (1988a). Magnet hospitals: Institutions of excellence. Part 1. *Journal of Nursing Administration, 18*(1), 13–24.

Kramer, M., & Schmalenberg, C. (1988b). Magnet hospitals: Institutions of excellence. Part 2. *Journal of Nursing Administration, 18*(2), 11–19.

Levine, E. (1969). Nurse manpower: Yesterday, today, and tomorrow. *American Journal of Nursing, 69*(2), 290–296.

Manthey, M. (1980). *The practice of primary nursing*. Boston: Blackwell Scientific.

McCloskey, J. C., & Bulechek, G. M. (Eds). (1992). *Nursing interventions classifications (NIC)*. St. Louis: Mosby-Year Book.

McClure, M. (1991). *Introduction to differentiated nursing practice*. Kansas City: American Academy of Nursing.

Moses, E. R. (1992). RN shortage seen for 21st century. *American Nurse*, July/August, 4.

Mowry, M. (1992). Computerization and quality. In M. Johnson (Ed.), *The delivery of quality health care* (pp. 153–171). St. Louis: Mosby–Year Book.

Mussalem, H. K. (1969). The changing role of the nurse. *American Journal of Nursing, 69*(3), 514–517.

National Commission on Nursing. (1989). Summary report and recommendations: Chicago, The Hospital Research and Educational Trust. *American Journal of Nursing, 89*(2), 1989.

Nightingale, F. (1859). *Notes on nursing: What it is, and what it is not*. Commemorative Edition (1992). Philadelphia: J. B. Lippincott.

Northouse, P. G., & Northouse, L. L. (1992). *Health communication. Strategies for health professionals* (2nd ed.). Norwalk, CT: Appleton & Lange.

Patterson, C. H. (1988). Standards of patient care: The Joint Commission focus on nursing quality assurance. *Nursing Clinics of North America, 23*(3), 625–638.

Saunders, L. (1958). Permanence and change. *American Journal of Nursing, 58*(7), 969–972.

Schuyler, C. B. (1992). Florence Nightingale. In *Notes on nursing: What it is, and what it is not* (pp. 3–17). Commemorative Edition. Philadelphia: J. B. Lippincott.

Seitz, PM, Donaho, BA, & Kohles, MA. (1991). Initiatives to restructure hospital nursing services. In: Aiken, L & Fagin, C. *Charting nursing's future* (pp. 98–107). Philadelphia: J. B. Lippincott.

Seward, J. F. (1969). Professional practice in bureaucratic structure. *Nursing Outlook, 17*(12), 58–61.

Starr, P. (1982). *The transformation of American medicine.* New York: Basic Books.

Warne, M. A., & McWeeny, M. C. (1991). Managing the cost of documentation: The FACT charting system. *Nursing Economics, 9*(3), 181–187.

▌PRACTICE SESSION▐

CHALLENGE FOR CRITICAL THINKING

1. Identify three historical events that had an effect on the practice of nursing in the hospital setting.

2. Discuss the evolution of charting by hospital nurses from the 19th century to the present.

3. Examine the annual index for a selected nursing journal for a 10-year period, using the form below. What proportion of articles address the topic of recording or reporting? How did it change over the decade?

4. Role play an end-of-shift report you create for each of the four nursing care delivery models in the display, Four Nursing Care Delivery Systems. What are the key differences in the role of the caregiver with respect to reporting in each model?

5. Define what you mean by "leader." What are the qualities you admire in leaders you have known? List these qualities. How does a person acquire these qualities?

JOURNAL ARTICLES ON REPORTING/RECORDING: NUMBER AND FOCUS BY YEAR OF PUBLICATION

Year	Number by Subject		Focus
	Reporting	*Recording*	
19__0			
19__1			
19__2			
19__3			
19__4			
19__5			
19__6			
19__7			
19__8			
19__9			

Communication Concepts and Documentation

LEARNING OBJECTIVES

After studying this chapter, the learner should be able to:

▲ Define communication and key terms related to communication.

▲ Describe features of effective communication.

▲ Discuss four barriers to effective communication.

▲ List four strategies to improve communication.

▲ Describe the role of communication in nursing practice.

▲ Discuss the role of communication in conflict resolution.

KEY TERMS

Attending behaviors	Conflict	Negotiation	Self-esteem
Communication	Empathy	Perception	Transactional

Eggland ET, Heinemann DS. NURSING DOCUMENTATION:
CHARTING, RECORDING, AND REPORTING.
© 1994 J.B. Lippincott Company.

Communication is the basis of all relationships. Because documentation is a form of communication, sound communication skills are essential for producing accurate, helpful documentation. In several places in *Notes on Nursing*, Florence Nightingale discusses communication between the nurse and the patient, reflecting concepts consistent with those being taught in contemporary courses and in texts on communication skills. All good documentation begins with effective communication within the nurse–patient relationship. Those concepts that underlie nurse–patient relationships include attending behavior, empathy, verbal and nonverbal communication, and autonomy of the patient.

> Always sit down when a sick person is talking business to you, show no signs of hurry, give complete and full consideration if your advice is wanted, and go away the moment the subject is ended. Always sit within the patient's view . . . Never speak to an invalid from behind, nor from the door, nor from any distance from him, nor when he is doing something (Nightingale, 1859, p. 28).

Communication is also the core of the professional relationship that enables health team members to provide information to each other to administer goal-directed, high quality care to patients.

This chapter discusses specific applications of communication concepts to health care situations and the importance of communication to documentation. Much of nursing practice depends on communication skills, and these skills are critical to patient care and patient care reporting and recording.

Communication Process

Communication is a process of sharing information, either in one transaction, as in giving an order, or in a continuous process of transactions or interactions, as in discussing patient care. All human communication is **transactional**: each participant responds to the content of the message and the context within which it occurs and is, in turn, affected by the responses of the other person(s) involved (Wilmot, 1979). Communication requires at least two people, a sender and a receiver. A message is imparted from the sender to a receiver and is interpreted by the receiver. The message and its delivery can cause the receiver to interpret or misinterpret the information. Feedback to the sender to verify what was transmitted is important to avoid misinterpretation, confusion, or inappropriate actions based on misunderstood information.

Communication is primarily composed of language and symbols, posture, gestures, and silence. It is verbal and nonverbal. Verbal communication includes either written or spoken language, as in documenting care in nurses' notes or giving a report on care provided. Words or phrases can be symbols or have special meaning to a person based on past experiences in relation to the concept of the symbol. For example, although a nurse can be male or female and work in a variety of settings, the word "nurse" usually suggests a caring woman, dressed in white, working in a hospital. If a child remembers getting a painful immunization from a nurse, that child's picture of a nurse may be quite different, causing sudden fear and withdrawal.

Nonverbal communication includes body language such as posture and gestures, facial expressions, gait, eye contact, distance between sender and receiver, touch, silence, physical appearance, and quality of voice and sounds. These variables affect participants' perceptions during transactions and are important components of communication. Slouched posture can suggest lack of energy or disinterest. Avoidance of eye contact can give the impression that someone is not being candid or is fearful or angry. A worker's informality or relaxed clothing in a professional setting can indicate that the person may not take work seriously.

Professional demeanor is conveyed by erect but relaxed posture, minimal hand gestures, eye contact during conversation, appropriate silence when it can enhance communication, a well-groomed appearance, and an appropriate tone of voice and rate of speech. In American culture, persons maintain a distance of approximately 2 feet for conversation, reserving the immediate space (18 to 24 inches) for close personal relationships. When nurses must enter the personal zone of physical contact, permission from and respect for the other person will enhance interactions and contribute to a professional, trusting relationship.

If nonverbal communication is congruent with what is said, the message of the sender is reinforced; if it is incongruent, the message is contradicted or questionable. For example, if a patient complains of severe abdominal pain and is bent at the waist, pressing a hand against the abdomen, and has a facial grimace, the message of pain is reinforced. If, however, a patient complains of severe abdominal pain and is sitting relaxed in a chair, laughing and talking with visitors, the message of pain is somewhat contradictory.

Factors That Affect Communication

Communication is affected by the relationship of the individuals involved. Because human communication involves people, it occurs within the context of relationships that affect the transaction, even to the point of determining how the content of the message is interpreted. For example, a new resident of a busy hospital unit runs the risk of being misunderstood when he casually observes that "This place is a classic example of controlled chaos!" If he has not established a good working relationship with the nurses, his attempt at a humorous compliment may be interpreted as criticism, especially if the nurses feel overworked and underpaid.

Because all participants can interpret information based on their own knowledge, feelings, values, and past experiences, communication is affected by every participant in the interaction. Primary variables that affect the communication process are perception, self-esteem, and attending behaviors. Northouse and Northouse (1992) identify more variables to the communication process: empathy, control, trust, and self-disclosure. It is important to consider these variables because negative influences can result in biased communication, inappropriate care, and inaccurate documentation.

PERCEPTION

During communication and patient care, nurses use the senses of sight, hearing, touch, and smell to collect information about patients, which is a basis for clinical decision-making. The data nurses collect include their own perceptions and measurements of the person's response to real or potential health problems (objective data) and the patient's perceptions and feelings (subjective data). **Perception** is the "complex process by which we [nurses] select, organize and interpret . . . sensory stimuli into a meaningful view . . . " of the patient (Sereno & Bodaken, 1975, p. 24). When nurses organize information into meaningful clusters and evaluate them for their importance, they do so in the context of past experience, attitude, and values. Because no two nurses bring the same background to a situation, it is reasonable to expect that the same situation or communication can be perceived in different ways by two different people.

Perception can be influenced by attitude, "a tendency to evaluate any object or issue or person in a favorable or unfavorable manner" (Sereno & Bodaken, 1975, p. 64). When a nurse receives a message, a meaning is attached, part of which comes from previously formed attitudes. Attitudes help people interpret the environment, protect themselves, and express personal values. To influence or persuade a patient or a colleague to change an attitude, a nurse must know how that particular attitude serves that person. This concept assumes great importance when the goal of a nurse's communication is to motivate a patient or coworker to adopt or change a health care behavior.

SELF-ESTEEM

Two other personality traits with major consequences for sending and receiving communications are **self-esteem**, an individual's sense of self-worth, and dogmatism, closed-minded beliefs or opinions. People with high self-esteem hold themselves in high regard and are likely to perceive themselves as competent. They present themselves with confidence and with the expectation that they will be successful in what they attempt to do. This confidence and expectation is perceived by those receiving their message and generally promotes positive communication and motivation. Many dogmatic or closed-minded people have low self-esteem and protect themselves with strong assertions of their beliefs, opinions, or perceptions. Dogmatic people are generally not open to new ideas unless these are presented by other dogmatic persons. In contrast, open-minded persons are receptive to new ideas and tend to place more credence in the idea than in the characteristics of the person presenting the idea (Sereno & Bodaken, 1975). Nurses need to become conscious of these dynamics to use the communication process effectively as they strive to achieve professional goals.

Confirming or affirming another person during communication reinforces the individual's self-esteem, which has profound effects on how the person will think, handle emotions, set goals, and formulate values (Branden, 1969). The course of a communication transaction and a person's outlook can be improved using this technique of confirmation. When patients are affirmed, they can be motivated to become involved in and improve their health care. By affirming nurse colleagues, a nurse can enhance others' work performance, resiliency, and job satisfaction (Strasen, 1992).

ATTENDING BEHAVIORS

Attending behaviors described in this chapter means the activities a nurse performs to focus on the other participant of a communication transaction (see display, Physical Attending Behaviors). In this context the other participant may be a patient or another caregiver.

During communication, the other participant becomes the focal point of a nurse's attention. The first step in establishing focus is positioning for eye contact. For example, during communication with a patient, the nurse should consider the physical ability and posture of the patient when interviewing a newly admitted person. If the patient is sitting in a chair, the nurse pulls up a second chair to approach the patient at eye level. Preferably a nurse sits to carry on a conversation with someone confined to bed.

Interprofessional communication is also best performed when caregivers are both either sitting or stand-

PHYSICAL ATTENDING BEHAVIORS

S—face the person **squarely**
O—adopt an **open** posture
L—**lean** toward the other person
E—maintain good **eye** contact
R—be at home and relatively **relaxed** in this position

(Egan, G. [1976]. *Interpersonal living. A skills/contract approach to human-relations training in groups* [p. 97]. Monterey, CA: Brooks/Cole Publishing.)

ing. Eye contact and implied dominance of the conversation are factors to consider in positioning oneself before communication begins.

Effective communication includes control of the environment within which transactions occur, particularly with respect to noise. Nurses initiating communication should provide privacy to the extent possible. Focus should center on the conversation and not on mental notes of tasks to be accomplished. A relaxed, professional demeanor puts the patient or other participants at ease and suggests that the transaction is important. A good beginning is to explain the exact purpose of the interview or transaction. Throughout communication with a patient or other participants, a nurse should avoid jargon and frequently validate the other person's response to verbal and nonverbal cues.

Acceptance of what the patient says reinforces the notion that the patient's welfare is the central theme of a nurse's caring. Acceptance of what health care colleagues say during communication reinforces the team concept of sharing information and open communication for the goals of patient care. Within attending behavior, as in all communication, the nonverbal communication nurses exhibit either reinforces or contradicts what is said.

EMPATHY

What most people want and expect from others in human relationships is understanding. **Empathy** is the understanding of another's situations or feelings. "The communication of understanding is a kind of oil that lubricates the entire communication process and makes all kinds of interchanges (transaction) go more smoothly" (Egan, 1976, p. 91). Egan describes the good communicator as an active participant who is perceptive to verbal and nonverbal cues, who clarifies what is sensed, and who builds on that information to develop understanding.

To fully understand, nurses must listen to other participants in a communication transaction. Listening to what the other person is saying, encouraging the person to talk, and using silence and attending behaviors encourages the transaction to continue. The nurse learns the perspective of the other person and can empathize (for more information on listening, see Chapter 10).

Nursing research that addresses aspects of empathy can enlighten nurses about the role of nurses' perceptions of patients' needs and the necessity of validating those assumptions. A study by Reed (1992) was designed to determine why nurses are perceived as cold and indifferent by women who have experienced a miscarriage. Although the study did not answer the question as to why the nurses did not show empathy, it demonstrated factors that influence the nurses' judgment about the patients' need for emotional support (see display, Nursing Research: Nurses' Perceptions of Emotional Care). Other barriers to establishing empathy are listed in the display, Common Barriers to Establishing Empathy.

Empathy in communication with coworkers. Nurses take their profession seriously and want to improve the quality of their practice. "Empathy . . . enables health professionals to improve the accuracy of their communication with clients and to reduce communication problems with other health professionals" (Northouse & Northouse, 1992, p. 26). The current emphasis on cost containment in health care delivery systems throughout the world places severe pressures on all health professionals to deliver complex care to patients in a relatively compressed time frame with fewer resources. The emphasis is on working "smart." Pressured health care providers may give patients and each other mixed verbal and nonverbal messages that impair the development of empathy and a true appreciation of each other's contribution to the health care enterprise. Lack of empathy affects the ability and willingness of caregivers to communicate effectively and to collaborate on patient care issues.

CONTROL

Patients feel a sense of control over their situation when they perceive that health care providers understand their needs. This balances the patient's feeling that the health care provider is controlling, dominant, or more powerful in the health care relationship. It is important for nurses to promote a sense of a shared balance in this relational control or power. This is important because what a person perceives in a communication depends not only on the content of the message but also on the relationship with the sender. Most people can quickly recall at least one instance when what they heard or read was influenced by the quality of the relationship with the person speaking or writing.

▲ NURSING RESEARCH: NURSES' PERCEPTIONS OF EMOTIONAL CARE

Reed, K. S. (1992). The effects of gestational age and pregnancy planning status on obstetrical nurses' perceptions of giving emotional care to women experiencing miscarriage. Image: *Journal of Nursing Scholarship, 24*(2), 107–110.

Although texts stress the need to give psychological support, the research literature suggests that patients perceive nurses and physicians to be cold and indifferent to the miscarriage situation. Reed questioned 396 RNs licensed in North Carolina; 292 usable questionnaires were analyzed, for a response rate of 74%.

Method: RNs responded to a series of questions about a vignette in which a patient miscarried a first pregnancy at 10, 15, or 20 weeks in a planned or unplanned pregnancy. Each respondent received one vignette and a questionnaire. The responses represented all six vignettes and were analyzed in a 3 × 2 factorial design to manipulate the gestational age and planning variables. The questionnaire on care priorities required a scaled response on the importance of the item in the nurse's judgment and dealt with emotional seriousness of the case, priority of care, and emotional support for the patient.

Results: 67% of the responding nurses were diploma or advanced degree graduates; 85% were married; 69% were 25 to 40 years old; 78% worked in hospitals, and 55% had worked in obstetrics 10 years or less. 73% had never had a miscarriage.

As gestational age increased, so did the RN's perception of emotional seriousness and priority of care. Planned pregnancy vignettes also had a higher score on these aspects. Nurses were less willing to give emotional support to women with unplanned pregnancies. Gestational age did not have a significant effect on nurses' responses to support items.

Discussion: Although nurses may be considering the more complex care required by a miscarriage at 20 weeks than at 10 weeks and the fact that the vignette described a *first* pregnancy, the results suggest that the OB nurses sampled respond to specific situational variables when they design care.

▲ COMMON BARRIERS TO ESTABLISHING EMPATHY

- ▲ Responses that imply condescension or manipulation
- ▲ Unsolicited advice
- ▲ Judgmental remarks
- ▲ Defensive responses
- ▲ Responses that ignore what the person has said
- ▲ Closed, inappropriate, or irrelevant questions
- ▲ Clichés
- ▲ Premature confrontation
- ▲ Incomplete or inadequate responses
- ▲ Patronizing or placating responses
- ▲ Responses that reflect disrespect or rejection
- ▲ Longwindedness

(Adapted from Egan, G. [1976]. *Interpersonal living. A skills/ contract approach to human-relations training in groups* [pp. 131–132]. Monterey, CA: Brooks-Cole Publishing.)

Besides relational control, personal control also affects participation in communication. A well-known theory of personal control is called *locus of control* (Rotter, 1954), the personal belief about the role of one's behavior in life. Persons who have an internal locus of control tend to see their behavior as the determining factor in what happens to them. Those who believe that what happens to them is under the control of outside influences, such as fate or luck or deity, are described as having external locus of control. The issue of control has special implications for communication and motivation in patient teaching. The issue of control also has implications for communication and clinical decision-making among health care providers.

TRUST

In any relationship, trust means accepting others as they are, believing the relationship is predictable, dependable, and positive. Trust promotes a feeling of security, reliability, respect, and the reciprocal nature of effective helping relationships. Gibb (1971) addresses the priority of trust in a helping relationship and lists other characteristics that can help or hinder communication transactions that ultimately affect professional relations (see display, Helpful and Hindering Orientations to Professional Relations).

SELF-DISCLOSURE

Self-disclosure of some portions of personal information enhances relationships (Northouse and Northouse, 1992). Although self-disclosure by health care providers should be limited, self-disclosure by a patient is important for nurses to assess effectively the patient's health status and efficacy of treatment. Research by Dawson (1985) suggests that how much a patient is willing to share with a provider may depend, in part, on the patient's perception of the provider's level of empathy (see display, Nursing Research: Perceived Empathy and Patient Self-disclosure). Self-disclosure involves honesty with oneself as well as others (Wennburg & Wilmot, 1973).

GENDER

Because the majority of nurses are women and interpersonal communication plays such an important role in patient care, the unique ways in which women and men communicate deserve serious consideration. Tannen's (1990) linguistic studies reveal that people have styles of communicating that may impair or facilitate how well they are understood by others. Studying the conversational styles of men and women has application in inter-

professional communication and patient teaching. Both the content and relationship aspects of communication are involved.

According to Tannen (1990), men and women view the world from different perspectives and, as a result, use communication to achieve different ends. Men perceive the world as a "hierarchical social order" in which they are "either one-up or one-down" (p. 24). The purpose of conversation in such an ordered world is to negotiate one's position, the preferred end being one-up. For men, "life is a contest, a struggle to preserve independence and avoid failure" (p. 25). This perception stratifies communication so that it is not symmetrical, that is, the participants do not have equality because the concept of status is always operative.

Women, on the other hand, tend to view the world as a "network of connections" . . . in which "conversations are negotiations for closeness in which people try to seek and give confirmation and support, and to reach consensus" (Tannen, 1990, p. 25). Women actively seek to achieve intimacy in their communication style, which establishes symmetry rather than asymmetry among the participants. This connectedness is consistent with Jean Watson's theory of caring (Bennett, Porter, & Sloan, 1989) and the interpersonal transaction in the goal attainment theory of Imogene King (Ackermann et al., 1989). Although all human beings need both intimacy and independence, women tend to focus on the first and men on the second (Tannen, p. 26).

Gender and the helping relationship. The notion of symmetry in communications plays a significant role in professional relationships wherein the professional seeks to give information and advice to the patient. Giving advice presumes an asymmetry, at least in the arena of knowledge in which the advice is offered; advice can create a distance between the parties to an interpersonal communication (Tannen, 1990). For men, independence means doing it alone and is associated with self-respect. Most women, however, freely seek out or offer help because helping establishes or reinforces connections. In view of this, it is important to discern how an individual perceives help or advice to be able to offer it in an acceptable way; for example, for a man to value, accept, and participate in an intervention, he may need to see that a particular nursing strategy will enable him to regain his independence. Helping behavior can reinforce connectedness, or it can emphasize the status differences between the patient and the professional involved.

Gender and intraprofessional issues. The nuances of gender in communication influence peer relationships between nurses and among nurses and other health professionals. Sovie (1989) identifies leadership skills

---

▲	**HELPFUL AND HINDERING ORIENTATIONS TO PROFESSIONAL RELATIONS**

Helpful	**Hindering**
Reciprocal trust	Mutual distrust
Cooperative learning	Indoctrinating
Mutual growth	Evaluating
Reciprocal openness	One-way helping
Shared problem-solving	Paternalism
Encouraging autonomy	Control
Experimentation	Standard setting

(Lassey, W. R. [Ed.] [1983], *Leadership and social change.* San Diego, CA: Pfeiffer and Company.)

▲	**NURSING RESEARCH: PERCEIVED EMPATHY AND PATIENT SELF-DISCLOSURE**

Dawson, C. (1985). Hypertension, perceived clinician empathy, and patient self-disclosure. *Research in nursing and health, 8*, 191–198.

Patient self-reports are crucial data. This study compared 54 hypertensive and 47 diabetic outpatients with 115 controls who had no known illness on their perceptions of clinician empathy and the importance and perceived difficulty of disclosing personal information to health care providers. They received their care at either a health cooperative or a university clinic. The sample, both men and women, was caucasian and well-educated (30% had postbaccalaureate degrees). Diabetics were significantly older, followed by the hypertensives, and the controls. The diabetics and hypertensives were seen by male providers; the controls, by both men and women.

Method: Volunteers from each group completed a questionnaire in the clinic or at home. The questionnaire included the empathy scale of the Barrett-Lennard Relationship Inventory; a 21-item patient self-disclosure questionnaire developed by the author and colleagues; general information items; and a self-rating item on present health status. Response was greater from university clinic patients; specific subgroup response rates are not reported.

Results: The study subjects reported low to moderate levels of perceived empathy. Among the nonchronically ill controls, those seeing female providers perceived more clinician empathy than those seeing male providers *and* perceived more clinician empathy than the hypertensives or diabetics. Analysis revealed that the gender effect of the provider was consistent for nurse and physician providers. Diabetics perceived more empathy than hypertensives who had very low mean empathy scores, which accounted for the difference in perceived empathy between the chronically ill subjects and those who had no known chronic illness.

There were no observed group differences on self-disclosure. Different disclosure categories were affected by subject age, perceived health status, perceived clinician empathy, and mental condition.

Discussion: The research raises questions about the role of perceived clinician empathy and its role in patient self-management of hypertension.

---

that nurses must use in contemporary health care to cope with change. These skills include planning and leading meetings, leading staff in brainstorming sessions, and resolving conflict at various levels. These activities find their root in solid communication skills.

As specialization in health care has increased, so has our reliance on communication among different providers. Whereas men and women have been observed to have similar leadership ability, they practice the leader role in ways that reflect gender differences in communication (Edwards & Lenz, 1990). Female nurse leaders focus on interpersonal aspects of the role; men focus on task completion. Women tend to consider their intuition in their decision-making and value decision by consensus (Helgesen, 1990). Men leaders tend to be less democratic than women, to give more direction, and to not focus on the needs of the specific individuals. The price women may pay for this person orientation to leadership is that they may be perceived as less powerful

or less competent than men in the same position because they are less directive (Tannen, 1990).

CULTURE

The foregoing discussion presumes an American cultural orientation in an environment that is rapidly becoming multicultural. All aspects of verbal and nonverbal communication have cultural variants. The gender role is only one aspect of daily life that is culturally determined. *Acculturation* is the process of acquiring or changing our perceived identity, language, and ethnic orientation as we are continuously exposed to a particular culture or tradition (Keefe & Padilla, 1980). Culture influences our perception of reality, which, in turn, affects our interpersonal communication. We come to know ourselves through others (Sereno & Bodaken, 1979). How we create meaning from our perceptions is determined, in part, by the cultural lens through which we view ourselves and the world. Although we may regard particular cultural groups as closely related—for example, we may think of Mexican-Americans, Cuban-Americans, and Puerto Ricans as *Hispanic*—research indicates that each group experiences different realities, particularly with respect to access to health care (Solis, Marks, Garcia, & Shelton, 1990).

For example, the Hispanic Health and Nutrition Examination Survey conducted by the federal government indicates that:

▲ The Hispanic cultural group is not homogeneous.
▲ The ability to speak English is the strongest predictor of recent use of health services.
▲ A larger proportion of mainland Puerto Ricans receive Medicaid and receive Aid for Dependent Children because they consist of more single female heads of households with children.
▲ Mexican-Americans tend to fall among the "working poor" who are employed in jobs with no health insurance benefits and, as a result, report less utilization of health services than either Cuban-Americans or mainland Puerto Ricans.

What had previously been thought to be health behavior influenced primarily by culture has been shown to be health behavior influenced by the person's ability to use the language of the system. In a separate study of pregnant black women, which compared their prepregnancy nutritional state, prenatal health practices, and the intrauterine growth of their babies, those born in the United States had poorer outcomes than black women born outside the United States (Cabral, Fried, Levenson, Amaro, & Zuckerman, 1990). These results suggest that life-style and factors other than cultural orientation played a role in the health of the subjects.

The complexity of the cultural influence on an individual's behavior and expectations of others is magnified by the sheer number of different cultures represented in the world and the fact that we are a global society. The patient population in any given institution in the United States will reflect the multinational origins of our country and the ease of access to world travel existing today. Although we cannot become expert in all cultures and their mores, we can study those of the groups we encounter frequently to be able to communicate effectively with them and minimize problems arising from cultural differences by using recommended techniques (see display, Avoiding Culture-based Errors in Communication). The *Standards of Clinical Nursing Practice* (American Nurses Association, 1991) stipulate that the nurse will consider the patient's cultural, racial, and ethnic background in planning and providing nursing services.

▲ **AVOIDING CULTURE-BASED ERRORS IN COMMUNICATION**

▲ Accept all human beings for who they are.
▲ Remember that health beliefs and health behaviors are culturally defined and may include faith in nontraditional health practices and healers.
▲ Ask patients how they would like to be addressed. Oriental names usually place the surname before the given name.
▲ Maintain an appropriate distance from the person (2–4 feet) until you have established some rapport and have the person's permission to touch specific areas of the body. For example, Hmong people believe the spirit resides in the head and would regard unwarranted touching there an affront.
▲ Enunciate clearly, but do not raise your voice unless the person is hard of hearing.
▲ Consider the content of your message; information related to sexuality should be obtained in the utmost privacy and by a provider of the same sex.
▲ Make one point at a time, but do not point. Use your open hand to gesture. Use visual aids and demonstration, but consider the content.
▲ Avoid jargon, colloquialisms, slang, and contractions.
▲ Avoid attempts at humor unless you know the person's culture well. Humor is learned and culture specific.
▲ Evaluate facial responses in the eyes. Many cultures will smile and nod to avoid saying no so as not to offend you.
▲ Accept gifts appropriate to the situation; to refuse can be interpreted as an insult.
▲ Follow the patient's lead!

(Adapted from Axtell, R. E. [Ed.]. [1990]. *Do's and taboos around the world.* New York: John Wiley & Sons.)

Role of Communication in Nursing Theory and Its Impact on Documentation

Nursing theory communicates a particular view of what nursing practice is. A common thread of communication is evident in each theory or view of the practice of nursing. As nursing theories continue to evolve, it is unlikely that any nursing theory would exclude this vital component of interaction among nurses and patients.

The work of nursing theorists guides the daily practice of many nurses by giving them an organizing framework for their practice. If a hospital uses a particular nursing theory, the design of documentation forms reflects that theory. For example, admission assessments based on the theory by Sister Callista Roy would include specific reference to the stimuli that have been identified for particular patients and nursing diagnoses that describe the person's level of adaptation. As nurses in that hospital discuss patient care, they would communicate in terms consistent with Roy's view of nursing. The result is communication with a common set of ideals and an established vocabulary.

Role of Communication and Documentation in the Nursing Process

The nursing process is transactional and involves the nurse, patient, and other health care providers in the nurse's effort to diagnose and treat the patient's responses to actual or potential health problems (American Nurses Association, 1980). Communication skills are essential for the nurse to effectively use the nursing process (see Chapter 3 for more information on documentation based on the nursing process).

Assessment

Nurses communicate to collect data about the patient to identify needs, problems, concerns, and reactions or responses to existing or potential health problems. The nurse's responsibility for assessment and assessment documentation has increased over the last century to the point that a nurse must build the nursing data base on a firm knowledge of physical and psychosocial sciences (see display, Documenting Assessment Then . . . and Now). Assessment of the newly admitted hospital patient or home care patient begins with a complete *nursing history* and *physical assessment*. In this phase the nurse uses verbal and nonverbal communication skills and powers of observation to establish a beginning relationship and collect information about the patient as a person

and in what areas the nurse may help (see Chapter 4 for more information about assessment).

Interviewing is a special kind of communication that focuses on the content of the transaction rather than the relationship (Northouse & Northouse, 1992). The nurse, however, sets the tone for the interview and must give attention to the patient's perception of the nurse's role in overall care (see Chapter 4 for more information about interviewing).

To complete the assessment of the patient's health status, the nurse also consults laboratory and test reports, reviews the patient's record of previous hospitalizations, and communicates with previous health care providers or facilities.

Nursing Diagnosis

After compiling the data, the nurse interprets the information and then arrives at a tentative hypothesis about the patient's problems that may be amenable to nursing intervention. The hypothesis is documented as a *nursing diagnosis* (see Chapter 5 for further information about documentation of nursing diagnoses). The nurse validates the hypothesis by corroborating the data and conclusions with the client and family, other professionals, the records, and references such as nursing literature. Nursing diagnoses are tentative, that is, they are always subject to revision as new information is communicated. The nurse continually evaluates the validity of the diagnoses by asking a number of questions:

▲ Has the nurse collected all of the required data?
▲ Are the data accurate?
▲ Are the related factors that the nurse identified consistent with the diagnosis?
▲ Is the nurse knowledgeable about the problem area?

The validity of any nursing diagnosis depends on the nurse's communication skill, assessment expertise, and the quality—depth and breadth—of the assessment, which is the core of the nursing process.

Nursing diagnoses are communicated to all caregivers for continuity of care. Nursing diagnosis language allows communication to become standard from nurse to nurse, which enhances clarity and facilitates continuity of care.

Planning Care

Planning is transactional and relies on effective communication techniques. The nurse and patient discuss and agree on the outcomes they would like to achieve as a result of the caring process. The plan includes nurse and patient behaviors or strategies designed to achieve the

▲	**DOCUMENTING ASSESSMENT THEN . . . AND NOW**

1930s

In admitting a patient to the hospital, the nurse was required to:

▲ Record the patient's name, hospital number, and doctor's name on all chart sheets in blue ink, whether the patient is admitted day or night.
▲ Complete the date column for the week on the Graphic Sheet, recording the day that the patient enters the hospital as "Admitted."
▲ Record TPR on both the Graphic Sheet and the Nurses' Notes.
▲ Chart on the Nurses' Notes how the patient was admitted: walking, by wheelchair, by stretcher, or carried.
▲ Chart the presence of dressings, appliances, splints; of bruises, burns, swelling, discharges; or any symptoms presented or that you have observed (Salt Lake City Hospital School of Nursing, 1932, p. 38).

1990s

According to *Practice Standards*, the nurse will collect health status data including, but not limited to:

▲ The patient's perceptions and expectations related to health services
▲ Current and previous medical diagnosis and therapy
▲ Environmental, occupational, recreational, and spiritual information related to health status
▲ Growth and development, mental and emotional responses and patterns of coping and interaction
▲ Performance of activities of daily living
▲ Function and status of the major body systems
▲ Sleep, rest, activity, and comfort
▲ Education and discharge planning needs

(Department of Nursing, Naples Community Hospital, 1991)

goals they have outlined. The notion that the patient takes an active and interactive part in this aspect of the nursing process recognizes the patient's autonomy and particular priorities, which may or may not agree with the nurse's. In the case of disagreement, the patient and nurse negotiate mutually acceptable goals for care. Goals should be stated in terms of observable and measurable patient behaviors and should include a reasonable time line for achievement.

The written care plan becomes part of the patient record and demonstrates the relationship between the assessment data, the nursing diagnosis, and the rationale for nursing action. Care plan communication promotes coordination and continuity of care (see Chapter 5 for more information about communication and documentation of care planning).

Nursing Intervention

The nurse practice acts of every state in the United States define the scope of nursing practice to include both delegated activities that the registered nurse performs under the direction of a physician, dentist, or osteopath and independent activities that the nurse defines. All nursing activities require clear communication and feedback to prevent patient care errors. Oral and written communication of nursing interventions enable each nurse to know what is being done for the patient, how often it is being done, when it is being done, and why it is being done.

Evaluation

To evaluate is to establish worth. In nursing care, evaluation determines the effectiveness of care by examining outcomes or responses to nursing interventions. Communication of evaluations enable nurses to know what interventions were effective and what interventions were not. This communication facilitates determining what changes are necessary to document in the plan of care. This evaluation process also promotes coordination and continuity of care because all caregivers learn the results of interventions and take direction from information learned.

Communication and Documentation in the Helping and Teaching Roles of Nursing Practice

Deeply ingrained in the activities of the *helping* and *teaching* domains of nursing practice (see display, The Helping Role and the Teaching–Coaching Role) are the knowledge and skills of human communication (Benner, 1984).

The helping role includes specific tasks such as comfort measures and the administration of pain medication, but the essence of both helping and teaching domains is the relationship between the nurse and the patient, the one-on-one interactions or transactions that must occur for the nurse to assess and meet the patient's need for care. Although the verbal and nonverbal aspects of the transactions between nurse and patient may be straightforward in these domains, the role of documentation may be less clear. When it comes to documenting what nurses do, these activities are much more elusive than

tasks or procedures and are part of what has been referred to as the "hidden work" of nurses (Wolf, 1989).

As nurses administer and monitor therapeutic interventions and regimens, they exhibit a helping role by explaining treatments and procedures to patients and by monitoring their responses. Nurses also explain treatments and procedures to ancillary staff, delegate selected treatments to other caregivers, and collaborate with other caregivers in planning, implementing, and evaluating care.

A nursing strategy that deserves specific attention with respect to health-related communication is that of teaching. It has been said that one cannot *not communicate*. Everything nurses do—even being silent—sends a message or communicates. In the same way, it is difficult to imagine a nurse who does not teach—by what the nurse says and does not say to a patient, family, and staff, and by what the nurse teaches, both formally and by example. The principles of communication theory apply here with special emphasis on the content of the transaction.

Anderson (1990) outlines principles that maximize learning (Figure 2–1). Teaching is a specific type of

 THE HELPING ROLE AND THE TEACHING-COACHING ROLE

The Helping Role

- ▲ The healing relationship: Creating a climate for and establishing a commitment to healing
- ▲ Providing comfort measures and preserving personhood in the face of pain and extreme breakdown
- ▲ Presencing: Being with the patient
- ▲ Maximizing the patient's participation and control in his or her own recovery
- ▲ Interpreting kinds of pain and selecting appropriate strategies for pain management and control
- ▲ Providing comfort and communication through touch
- ▲ Providing emotional and informational support to patients' families
- ▲ Guiding a patient through emotional and developmental change: Providing new options, closing off old ones by channeling, teaching, and mediating
  - Acting as a psychological and cultural mediator
  - Using goals therapeutically
  - Working to build and maintain a therapeutic community

The Teaching-Coaching Role

- ▲ Timing: Capturing a patient's readiness to learn
- ▲ Assisting patients to integrate the implications of illness and recovery into their lifestyles
- ▲ Eliciting and understanding the patient's interpretation of the illness
- ▲ Providing an interpretation of the patient's condition and giving a rationale for procedures
- ▲ The coaching function: Making culturally avoided aspects of an illness approachable and understandable

(Benner, P. [1984]. *From novice to expert: Excellence and power in clinical nursing practice.* Menlo Park, CA: Addison-Wesley, pp. 50, 79. Reprinted with permission.)

Effective Learning

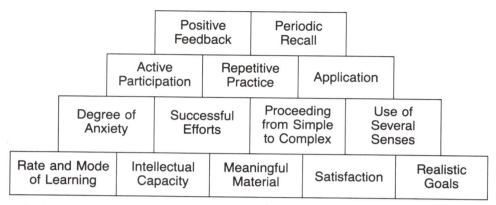

FIG. 2-1. Building Blocks of Effective Learning. (Anderson, C. (1990). *Patient teaching and communicating in an information age* [p. 109]. Albany, NY: Delmar Publishers)

communication that starts from simple to complex information, uses several senses, requires active participation, and uses positive feedback and periodic recall. All patients have learning needs related to their health status and health care. When the nurse assesses the patient's need for teaching, the plan, objectives, and accomplishments should be documented to reinforce what learning has occurred and to facilitate continuity of care from all caregivers (for more information on teaching, see Chapter 8).

Role of Communication and Documentation in Referrals

Health care today is a multidisciplinary endeavor; even within the walls of a single institution, a patient receives services from many departments and on more than one nursing unit. This is one effect of continuing specialization in health services. The referral process facilitates communication among departments and institutions and promotes continuity of care, an essential element of quality. Because nurses cannot be all things to all people, it is an ethical responsibility to direct patients to services that can meet needs for information, direct care, social services, counseling, and other assistance.

Referrals depend on accurate verbal and written communication. The referral should prepare the agency for what to expect with regard to the patient's condition and individual concerns. For example, a referral to another unit in the hospital or a home care agency might address the patient's and family's reaction to the illness episode, the condition of the patient's wound, and what dressing technique the staff has been using successfully. Referrals are particularly important if the patient has a newly diagnosed chronic condition that requires self-care and

any extenuating personal circumstances that might interfere with the ability to provide self-care. A quality referral describes the patient as an individual and gives the receiving professional a head start on establishing a positive relationship with the new patient.

Communication in Reporting and Recording

Communication activities of the nurse include *recording* the care the nurse has planned, given, and evaluated, and *reporting* to others the health status of the patient and the response to care. These activities should be guided by several straightforward principles: clarity of thought, simplicity, truthfulness, and confidentiality. Verbal and written reports must be organized and concise and convey the essential information other caregivers need to provide continuity of care stipulated in the standards of practice. Regardless of the type of nursing care delivery system used in an agency, all nurses must process a great deal of information about the patients for whom they are responsible. Reports should convey a summary statement of the patient's overall status, with specific information on deviations from the norm or the expected rate of progress.

Florence Nightingale (1859) admonished nurses to give the physician facts, not opinions about the patient, particularly for cases unusual in their presenting signs and symptoms. Central to this process of recording and reporting is a clear understanding of what the goals of care are for that person and an evaluation of movement toward those goals. Reporting and recording are purposeful and should help the listener or reader focus on the crucial elements of care to which the caregiver must attend. Reporting and recording should present a clear picture of the individual patient and priority needs (see display, Documenting Nursing Care Then . . . and Now).

What is reported and recorded for a patient must be consistent. Departures in the record from what was said at the change-of-shift report can create confusion and errors. If the practice is to use tape-recorded shift reports, the quality of the machine and tape, the diction and clarity of the speaker, and the hearing ability of the listener are variables that affect the sending and receiving of the message. Walking rounds, on the other hand, provide an opportunity for both sets of caregivers to observe each patient who is the subject of report and confirm, firsthand, the essential elements of the report. Although this method may take more time initially, it leaves less to chance and provides a unique opportunity to include the patient in evaluation and planning. Walking rounds also place full accountability on the departing caregiver for the condition of the unit and its occupant (for more information on shift reports, see Chapter 10).

All forms of communication about patients and their care must be truthful and within the bounds of confidentiality. The reader must remember that all patient information is confidential. The record is for the eyes of qualified employees who have a "need to know," and oral conversations about the patient should be restricted to the appropriate places and circumstances, such as change-of-shift report.

DOCUMENTING NURSING CARE THEN . . . AND NOW

Mr. Simms is a patient who had an appendectomy yesterday. The nurse's note might read:

1950s

"Patient OOB after AM care. Sitting in chair × 2. Tolerated it well. Complained of incisional pain. Medicated. Resting comfortably.

1990s

Focus: Pain

0700/Data: Patient states he spent a sleepless night due to incisional pain, which he rates as a 9 on a scale of 1–10. Incision dry, not reddened. Bowel sounds moderately active in all quadrants.

0710/Action: Demerol 100 mg IM.

0750/Response: Rates pain at 3 on a scale of 1–10. (Each functional area is addressed in a timely manner. Data, actions, and responses are noted separately in relation to a single focus.)

Communication in Nursing Management

Expertise in communication skills is essential to the success of the nurse who is acting in the role of manager (Marquis & Huston, 1992). Florence Nightingale (1859) wrote that

> . . . whoever is in charge keep this simple question in her head (*not*, how can I always do this right thing myself, but) how can I provide for this right thing to be always done? . . . To be "in charge" is certainly not only to carry out the proper measures yourself but to see that every one else does so too . . . (p. 24).

A manager with effective communication skills facilitates this continuity and organization of care.

Benner (1984) describes the activities of the nurse in the domain of *organizing and work-role competencies*. This domain includes activities related to setting priorities for care and communicating these to others, building and maintaining the therapeutic team, and coping with shortages and staff turnover. Enter the nurse of the 1990s who may preside over several units or a "superunit" of related services and who has a number of subordinate personnel. However, all nurses who set priorities, delegate, and communicate patient care needs to others act as managers of care.

Managing the Practice Environment

The nurse manager has the responsibility to provide an environment in which other nurses can give care according to the standards established by the nursing profession. These standards are communicated to the staff in the philosophy and standards of the institution. The nurse manager uses communication in problem-solving to collect data, identify problems, develop strategies, document evaluation of outcomes, and communicate the information to the staff and administration. The nurse manager is a communication link among team members and between the team and the organization. Workers need to understand the goals and objectives of the organization, and the organization needs to hear the concerns and ideas of the staff.

Communication as Power

Communication skills are a source of power and an expression of leadership. These strategies relate to the behavior of the nurse as an individual practitioner and as a member of the community and the profession. Formal and informal networking depends on effective verbal and nonverbal communication. Using these skills to contact experts and seek counsel are important to building one's power base as a professional (see display, Power-Building and Political Strategies). Using communication to acquire information and communicating astutely are priority functions in building political strategies.

Porter-O'Grady (1986) describes the behavior of nurses in the work setting as "vocational" or "professional," referring to the job or career orientation of the individual nurse. Porter-O'Grady emphasizes that lateral communication among staff is essential to professional practice. Communication establishes and reinforces the trust that professionals perceive for one another. Nurses who view their work from a job perspective tend to operate as individuals rather than team players and communicate less with their peers. Modern health care has a multidisciplinary nature. When communication within the care team or organization breaks down, the group process fails and there is less likelihood that the group or organization will achieve its goals for the care of individuals or the community.

Employee Feedback

The nurse manager's communication skills play an important role in appraisal of employee performance. Most employees seek feedback to confirm self-esteem; employees with low self-esteem may react defensively to even constructive criticism. Texts on leadership and management can provide the nurse manager with principles and techniques to implement performance appraisal in a fair and objective manner, but the success of the

process will depend on the manager's ability to communicate effectively with the staff on a daily basis and their ability to communicate with the nurse manager.

Managing Conflict

The nurse manager is often challenged to resolve interpersonal conflict within the staff and the organization. Northouse and Northouse (1992) point out that conflict occurs within the transactions of communication and reflects both the content of communication and the relationships among the parties involved. "**Conflict** is a felt struggle between two or more interdependent individuals over perceived incompatible differences in beliefs, values, goals, or over differences in desires for control, status, and affection" (p. 218). Nursing clearly encounters conflicts in both the content and relationship aspects of communications in the health care setting where issues of control or territoriality, self-esteem, goals, and values arise every day. "Effective communication is the pivotal element that prevents differences among individuals from escalating and that facilitates constructive resolution to conflict situations" (p. 239). The nurse manager can orchestrate the communications on the unit to facilitate early recognition of conflict and encourage its prompt resolution.

The art of **negotiation** is the communication process of coming to terms or compromise. Successful negotiation depends on excellent communication skills. Through communication, one can identify the personal concerns,

---

 POWER-BUILDING AND POLITICAL STRATEGIES

Power-Building Strategies
Expand personal resources
Present a powerful persona
Pay the entry fee
Determine the powerful
Learn the organizational culture
Use organizational priorities
Increase skills and knowledge
Have a broad vision
Use experts and seek counsel
Be flexible
Be visible and have a voice
Toot your own horn
Maintain a sense of humor
Empower others

Political Strategies
Use information acquisition
Communicate astutely
Become proactive
Assume authority
Network
Expand personal resources
Maintain maneuverability
Develop conflict management and negotiation
skills
situations
Remain sensitive to people, timing, and situations
Promote subordinate's identity
Meet organizational needs
Expand personal wellness

(Marquis, B. L., & Huston, C. J. [1992]. *Leadership roles and management functions in nursing. Theory and application* [p. 132]. Philadelphia: J. B. Lippincott.)

needs, and wants that fuel conflict and reach a satisfactory conclusion (Ury, 1991). Ury suggests the following strategies:

▲ Treat the other person the way you want to be treated.
▲ Ask clarifying questions.
▲ Listen and acknowledge what the person is saying.
▲ Agree where you can.
▲ Paraphrase what you have heard and ask for correction.
▲ Acknowledge the person's feelings.
▲ Respect the other person.
▲ Read the nonverbal behavior.
▲ Use "I" statements.
▲ Ask open-ended questions to reframe the problem.

Skillful negotiation requires time and attention to the interests of the other person. Impasses between individuals develop when the transaction is based on the notion that what one person wins, the other loses. The object of negotiation is to allow both parties to come away with a sense of satisfaction at what has been achieved.

Effective negotiating, like high quality nursing practice, depends on effective communication skills. Communication skills are critical to patient care and patient care reporting and recording.

KEY POINTS

▲ Communication has two components: the content of the message and the relationship of the individuals involved.

▲ All human communication is transactional; each participant responds to the content of the message and the context within which it takes place and is, in turn, affected by the responses of the other person(s) involved.

▲ All communication is filtered through the perception of the person receiving the message and is affected by personal variables such as gender, attitudes, and self-esteem.

▲ Verbal communication is affected by the relationship between the parties and depends on symbols, which may have different meaning for different people.

▲ Nonverbal communication in the form of body language, distance, silences, appearance, and voice may send a message that contradicts or reinforces what is actually said.

▲ Empathic responses reinforce communication by attending to the relationship aspect of communication.

▲ Appropriate self-disclosure reinforces human connectedness.

▲ Nursing process and clinical practice are transactional and are grounded in communication.

▲ Communication forms the basis for data gathering, clinical decision-making, teaching, referral, and evaluation.

▲ Reporting and recording enhance continuity of care and provide a foundation for quality management and research.

▲ Communication among professionals enhances relationships and professional collaboration.

▲ Effective leadership and management depend on clinical expertise and communication skills.

REFERENCES

Ackermann, M. L., Brink, S. A., Clanton, J. A., Jones, C. G., Moody, S. L., Perlich, G. L., Price, D. L., & Prusinski, B. B. (1989). Imogene King. Theory of goal attainment. In A. Marriner-Tomey (Ed.), *Nursing theorists and their work* (2nd ed., pp. 345–360). St. Louis: C. V. Mosby.

American Nurses Association. (1991). *Standards of clinical nursing practice*. Washington, DC: Author.

American Nurses Association Congress on Nursing Practice. (1980). *Nursing. A social policy statement*. Washington, DC: Author.

Anderson, C. (1990). *Patient teaching and communicating in an information age*. Albany, NY: Delmar Publishers.

Axtell, R. E. (Ed.). (1990). *Do's and taboos around the world*. New York: John Wiley & Sons.

Benner, P. (1984). *From novice to expert. Excellence and power in clinical nursing practice*. Menlo Park, CA: Addison-Wesley.

Bennett, P. M., Porter, B. D., & Sloan, R. S. (1989). Jean Watson. Philosophy and science of caring. In A. Marriner-Tomey (Ed.), *Nursing theorists and their work* (2nd ed., pp. 164–173). St. Louis: C. V. Mosby.

Branden, N. (1969). *The psychology of self-esteem*. New York: Bantam Books.

Cabral, H., Fried, L. E., Levenson, S., Amaro, H., & Zuckerman, B. (1990). Foreign-born and US-born black women: Differences in health behaviors and birth outcomes. *American Journal of Public Health*, 80(1), 70–71.

Dawson, C. (1985). Hypertension, perceived clinician empathy, and patient self-disclosure. *Research in Nursing and Health*, 8, 191–198.

Edwards, J. B., & Lenz, C. L. (1990). The influence of gender on communication for nurse leaders. *Nursing Administration Quarterly*, 1, 49–55.

Egan, G. (1976). *Interpersonal living. A skills/contract approach to human-relations training in groups*. Monterey, CA: Brooks/Cole Publishing.

Gibb, J. R. (1971). Is help helpful? In W. R. Lassey (Ed.), *Leadership and social change* (pp. 11–17). La Jolla, CA: University Associates.

Helgesen, S. (1990). *The female advantage: Women's ways of leadership.* New York: Doubleday.

Keefe, S. E., & Padilla, A. M. (Eds.). (1980). *Acculturation theory, models and some new findings.* Boulder, CO: Westview Press.

Marquis, B. L., & Huston, C. J. (1992). *Leadership roles and management functions in nursing. Theory and application.* Philadelphia: J. B. Lippincott.

Nightingale, F. (1859). *Notes on nursing: What it is, and what it is not.* Commemorative Edition (1992). Philadelphia: J. B. Lippincott.

Northouse, P. G., & Northouse, L. L. (1992). *Health communication strategies for health professionals* (2nd ed.). Norwalk, CT: Appleton & Lange.

Porter-O'Grady, T. (1986). *Creative nursing administration. Participative management into the 21st century.* Rockville, MD: Aspen Systems.

Reed, K. S. (1992). The effects of gestational age and pregnancy planning status on obstetrical nurses' perceptions of giving emotional care to women experiencing miscarriage. *Image: Journal of Nursing Scholarship, 24(2), 107–110.*

Rotter, J. B. (1954). *Social learning and clinical psychology.* Englewood Cliffs, NJ: Prentice-Hall.

Sereno, K. K., & Bodaken, E. M. (1975). **Trans-Per** *understanding human communication.* Boston: Houghton Mifflin.

Solis, J. M., Marks, G., Garcia, M., & Shelton, D. (1990). II. Acculturation, access to care, and the use of preventive services by Hispanics: Findings from HHANES 1982–84. *American Journal of Public Health*, 80(Suppl.), 11–19.

Sovie, M. (1989). Clinical nursing practices and patient outcomes: Evaluation, evolution, and revolution (legitimizing radical change to maximize nurses' time for quality care). *Nursing Economics*, 7(2), 79–85.

Strasen, L. L. (1992). *The image of professional nursing. Strategies for action.* Philadelphia: J. B. Lippincott.

Tannen, D. (1990). *You just don't understand. Women and men in conversation.* New York: Ballantine Books.

Ury, W. (1991). *Getting past no. Negotiations with difficult people.* New York: Bantam Books.

Wennburg, J. R., & Wilmot, W. W. (1973). *The personal communication process.* New York: John Wiley & Sons.

Wilmot, W. W. (1979). *Dyadic communication: A transactional perspective* (2nd ed.). Reading, MA: Addison-Wesley.

Wolf, Z. R. (1989). Uncovering the hidden work of nursing. *Nursing and Health Care*, 10(8), 463–467.

PRACTICE SESSION

FILL-IN

1. Some personal variables that affect communication include:

   _____ , _____ ,

   _____ , and _____ .

2. Gestures and posture are categorized as _____

   _____ .

3. Verbal communication means _____

   _____ .

4. In communicating, women generally focus on _____

   _____ .

   and men focus on _____ .

5. Culture influences perception of reality, which affects _____

   _____ .

6. Communication among professionals enhances _____

   _____ .

7. Types of communication include _____

   _____ .

8. A nurse manager uses communication skills to _____

   _____

   _____ .

9. Communication involves two key components: _____

   _____ and

   _____ .

10. Nursing practice is transactional and is based on _____

    _____ .

CHALLENGE FOR CRITICAL THINKING

1. During the next week, begin a journal. Record one conversation each day and identify the communicators, the message, the relationship between the parties, and the outcome of the transaction.

2. Go to the library and choose one annual volume of *Nursing Research, Nursing and Health Care, The American Journal of Nursing, Nursing,* or *Image*, and list the titles of articles that address any aspect of communication in health care or nursing. Examine the article and identify the aspect of communication each article addresses.

3. Write a critical review (1–2 pages) of the portrayal of a nurse in a movie, fictional work, play, or television in terms of the verbal and nonverbal communication of the nurse and the image it creates.

4. Interview two nurses to ascertain their personal philosophy of nursing.

5. Read the Philosophy of Nursing of your educational program. What questions does it address? What questions about nursing does it not address?

6. During your clinical laboratory hours, ask your patients to share with you what they expect of nurses. List their responses and identify those responses that include aspects of communication.

7. During the course of 1 day, monitor your conversations for "I" messages. Do you use "I" messages to express yourself? If not, make a conscious effort to do so for 1 day. Record your reactions to the effort. How do "I" messages affect the outcome of the communication?

The Clinical Record

LEARNING OBJECTIVES

After studying this chapter, the learner should be able to:

▲ Identify and describe the content of a patient clinical record.

▲ Define key terms as applied to the clinical record.

▲ Describe the key components and purpose of accurate, concise nursing documentation.

▲ Explain the difference between the types of forms: standardized forms, flow sheets, and graphs.

▲ Explain the use, advantages, and disadvantages of a computerized clinical record.

KEY TERMS

Admission form
Advance directives
Clinical record
Consent for treatment forms
Discharge summary
Flow sheets
Graphs
Intake record
Kardex

Medical orders
Medication administration record (MAR)
Multidisciplinary care plan
Nursing assessment
Nursing care plan
Nursing documentation
Nursing history
Nursing orders

Nursing information system (NIS)
Nursing minimum data set (NMDS)
Progress notes (also called nursing notes or clinical notes)
Standardized forms
Teaching plans
Transfer summary

Eggland ET, Heinemann DS. NURSING DOCUMENTATION: CHARTING, RECORDING, AND REPORTING. © 1994 J.B. Lippincott Company.

A patient's **clinical record** is the comprehensive collection of data that describes a patient's condition, health care needs, health care services received, and response to care. The traditional manual clinical record usually takes the form of the patient's chart composed of handwritten entries by multidisciplinary providers, who are individuals from the different disciplines providing care. These professional providers include physicians, nurses, physical therapists, occupational therapists, speech and language pathologists, respiratory therapists, nutritionists, and social workers.

In contrast to a traditional manual clinical record, a computerized clinical record can be created by health care professionals entering data into the computer. Because most health care services are not computerized, the data in computerized systems are printed on paper to create a traditional, but typewritten, paper chart. Futurists forecast, however, that with progressive technology paperless charts will communicate data through a network of computer screens.

Contents of a Clinical Record

A clinical record is maintained for each patient in accordance with accepted professional standards, regulatory requirements, and accrediting guidelines. Although different health care organizations use different forms and form designs (formats), the clinical record generally contains the following generic information:

▲ Patient identifying information
▲ Past and current diagnoses
▲ Health care history
▲ Reason for admission
▲ Known allergies
▲ Consent for treatment
▲ Treatment goals and expected outcomes
▲ Medical, nursing, and other professional assessments, orders, and plans for care
▲ Current medications
▲ Dietary patterns and restrictions
▲ Patient teaching plans and summaries
▲ Clinical progress notes
▲ Laboratory, radiology, and other diagnostic test results
▲ Release of information forms
▲ Consultation reports
▲ Progress summary reports
▲ Transfer summary
▲ Discharge summary

Although clinical record forms used by all disciplines

are briefly described in this chapter, only nursing documentation will be explained and demonstrated.

Nursing Documentation

Nursing documentation is that part of the clinical record written by nurses and is the total written information concerning a patient's health status, nursing needs, nursing care, and response to care. Key components of nursing documentation include assessments, nursing diagnoses, planned care, nursing interventions, patient teaching, patient outcomes, and interdisciplinary communication. Because nurses coordinate different aspects of care with other professionals for total patient care, nursing documentation should include interdisciplinary communication involving nurses (see display, Key Components of Nursing Documentation).

Nursing documentation communicates that certain factors or situations occurred during the time a health care organization provided care. Because nursing is a major portion of health care, nursing documentation is a major portion of a patient's clinical record. Documentation of care is written by nurses in all health care organizations such as hospitals, long-term care facilities, home health care agencies, clinics, and other settings where nurses provide care.

Nursing Documentation and the Nursing Process

The nursing process is a dynamic interrelated sequence of activities performed by nurses. A nurse determines a patient's problem or need, decides on expected outcomes or goals related to the need, chooses alternatives to solve the problem, takes or coordinates action to solve the problem, and then determines how effective the plan is in resolving the need. Nursing documentation should be based on the nursing process. Therefore, forms on which nurses document should parallel or relate to each step of the nursing process.

Nursing documentation facilitates effective care because a patient need can be tracked from assessment, through identification of problems, care plan, implementation, and evaluation in correlation with the nursing process (Figure 3–1).

MAKING THE ASSESSMENT

On a day-to-day basis, documentation is used as a source for ongoing assessment of patient needs. Assessment information is received from all caregivers to present a composite view of the whole patient with various needs.

▲	**KEY COMPONENTS OF NURSING DOCUMENTATION**

Component	Description
Assessments	Include assessments and reassessments that are ongoing. Routine frequency is determined by health care organization policy.
Identified patient needs or nursing diagnoses	Include needs documented on a problem list or on a care plan and sometimes on an assessment. Health care organizations are increasingly using standardized diagnoses.
Planned care	Includes a separate care plan or planned care documented in progress notes or separate guidelines for care.
Revisions of planned care	Includes reasons for change, supporting evidence, and agreement from patient or family for the revised plan of care.
Nursing interventions	Include patient observations, treatment interventions, teaching, clinical judgments. Documented on flow sheets and progress notes.
Patient teaching	Includes learning needs, teaching plan content, mode of instruction, who was taught, patient response and comprehension.
Patient outcomes	Include the following: Patient progress toward goals (expected outcomes) Patient response to tests, treatments, nursing interventions Patient/family response to significant events Questions, statements, complaints voiced by the patient or family
Interdisciplinary communication and team conferences	Include communication with physician and other disciplines and outcomes of that communication

Nurses use the information from other disciplines and the information in the nursing history and physical examination to perform and document a nursing assessment. Information gathered in the assessment is clustered to support clinical judgments the nurse makes about identified problems or needs and nursing diagnoses.

IDENTIFYING NEEDS AND NURSING DIAGNOSES

Appropriate clinical judgment using accurate assessment documentation leads to correct nursing diagnoses, patient teaching needs, prevention of potential or high-risk problems, better and earlier discharge planning, and effective plans for care. Documenting patient care needs allows all nurses to focus on the same priorities of care.

PLANNING CARE

Care plans include patient goals, termed expected outcomes. Each expected outcome has a target date, which establishes the time when the nurse anticipates the expected outcome will be accomplished. These expected outcome statements reflect the planning process of nursing care.

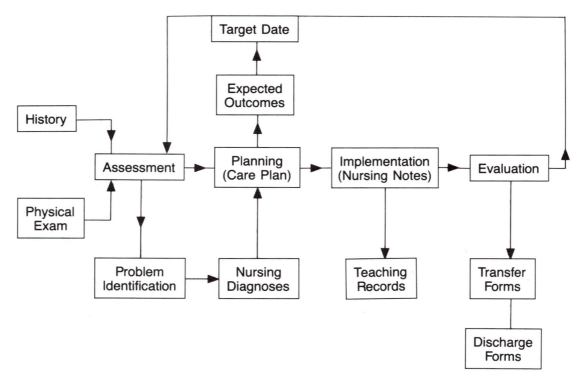

The nursing process is the foundation for nursing documentation. Relevant information is moved through the process and reenters into reassessment to form a dynamic continuum.

Copyright © Ellen Thomas Eggland, 1990.

FIG. 3-1. Documentation based on the nursing process.

IMPLEMENTING CARE

As the plan for care is followed, nursing notes document the dates of implementation of the nursing care and the condition of the patient. Implementation of the nursing process includes documentation of observations, treatments, and teaching. In many organizations teaching is documented in nursing notes, with plans for teaching documented in the patient's care plan. But some organizations have teaching documented on separate teaching records, which may also be called teaching plans or teaching summaries.

EVALUATING CARE

By analyzing the nursing care documented in progress notes, a nurse can determine what approaches and interventions continue to be effective for the patient, which long- and short-term goals remain realistic, and what progress is being made by the patient. Maintaining goal-directed care is a characteristic of quality care.

Evaluation of a patient's care is documented on outcome reports and progress summaries. These forms indicate the progress the patient made in meeting goals for care and the patient's continued needs. This evaluation information is also documented on transfer and discharge forms, where the information contributes to the continuity of care. Continuity of care maintains goals and effective interventions and is important when a patient is transferred to another level of care or discharged to another organization for care.

Purpose of Documentation

Although providing nursing care is the action that affects a patient's condition, writing nursing documentation supports and reports that nursing action was performed and indicates the patient's resulting condition. "If it isn't documented, it wasn't done" is an accepted nursing axiom.

Because of the not documented/not done guideline, a common dilemma in nursing documentation is determining how much documentation is necessary and how frequently a nurse should chart. To help resolve this concern, a nurse should consider the general purpose of documentation. In high-risk situations a nurse should also consider the potential consequences if documentation is omitted or incomplete, which can include health care reimbursement denial, ineffective defense in malpractice or civil law suits, and deficiencies in surveys investigating quality of care.

In the last 5 years, documentation formats have become more detailed in the attempt to capture pertinent nursing information and prevent critical consequences for inadequate or inconsistent documentation.

The positive reasons for frequent, accurate and complete, pertinent, and concise documentation have not changed. The purposes of documentation include communication, legal protection, reimbursement, education, quality assurance, and research.

COMMUNICATION

Documentation is *the primary communication tool* to keep all caregivers current about the needs, care, and progress of a patient. Nursing documentation allows a patient's nurse to keep nursing colleagues and other health care professionals informed, so that each caregiver knows what everyone else is doing for a patient. Effective communication facilitates consistent care and a consistent approach that best meets the patient's needs. Communication and subsequent continuity of care among caregivers depends on careful documentation, so information is easily retrievable and correctly understood.

Accurate documentation facilitates communication among health care professionals who do not provide direct patient care but are involved in various aspects of a patient's care. With current, accurate, documented data, other staff nurses, supervisors, or case managers can effectively collaborate with a patient's physician and therapists, when a primary caregiver is not available to discuss care. With accurate documentation, nurses can help a patient to contact and use appropriate community resources for continuity of care.

LEGAL PROTECTION

Accurate documentation provides legal protection and is an important defense in a lawsuit. Documentation provides a description of the patient condition, significant occurrences including details of how an event occurred, and direct results of an occurrence or therapy intervention. As a data base for investigation of legal concerns, accurate documentation protects nurses, patients, and health care organizations.

REIMBURSEMENT

Reimbursement is determined by documentation when government-reimbursed care or private insurance companies are the payers or when one health care organization contracts with another to provide services. Documentation then becomes a data base for reimbursement decisions for Medicare, Medicaid, third-party insurance coverage, worker's compensation, and pension payments to a patient for health-related expenses.

Documentation also provides a data base for determination of health care costs for an individual patient. Patients are charged for services received that are documented as being provided. If services are not documented as being provided or assessment data do not show the need for the service, reimbursement can be denied.

PATIENT TEACHING

Documentation is a source for determining educational needs of the patient and the patient's response to teaching. Documented teaching and patient knowledge, learned skills, and attitude toward disease and treatment can be factors that affect a patient's compliance to treatment. Similar to a care plan, goals or teaching outcomes are established in the teaching plan. If actual outcomes of teaching do not indicate progress toward goals, teaching plan interventions or goals are revised.

EDUCATION

Nursing documentation is used as an educational resource for health care students. Although patients with the same diagnoses, symptoms, or treatments do not all respond in the same way, some similarities in diagnoses, treatment, care, test results, and behavior can be determined. The similarities help the student to know what signs, symptoms, complications, or expected treatments to look for in particular patients. Students can judge the effect of care, based on similar or different care given to other patients.

QUALITY ASSURANCE

Quality of care is formally measured by quality assurance or quality improvement programs. Nursing audits are documentation surveys to measure quality. Audits are performed by a nurse who compares patient information that was documented in a chart to standards that state what nursing care should have been provided and what patient outcomes should have resulted.

Quality assurance audits help determine if minimum standards of care have been met. If minimum standards are not met, other action is taken to improve the adherence to standards. Quality assurance then becomes part of a quality improvement program. Quality assurance or quality improvement cannot be performed without continuous, accurate, routine documentation of care because such documentation reflects quality of care.

Using documentation in quality assurance programs is a usual requirement for licensure and certification by state or federal health care programs such as Medicare and Medicaid. Accrediting organizations such as the Joint Commission on the Accreditation of Healthcare Organizations (JCAHO) also require quality assurance programs using documentation. Licensing or accrediting organizations conduct audits in which nursing documentation is investigated to determine if care meets minimum standards and the health care organization meets standards for accreditation.

Another aspect of quality is efficiency. Nurse managers scrutinize documentation to determine how efficiently health care is provided, if policies and procedures are being followed, and what patient needs are on a unit to determine appropriate staffing.

RESEARCH

Nurse researchers use documentation to determine if patients meet their research requirements to enter into a study. Researchers collect information from the clinical record in the course of the research study. Information may be about patient symptoms, behavior, or patient outcomes such as the effect of medication to relieve pain. Nurses must document accurate information because nursing documentation can affect outcomes of research studies.

Documentation can also be a source for determining research needs. For example, if documentation shows that a high percentage of patients with catheters have urinary tract infections, research can investigate types of patients or specific variables of patient care that may contribute to the incidence of infection.

Finally, documentation provides statistics for public health care information, health care analysis, and future health care plans or investigative research for specific populations.

Categories of Documentation Forms in a Clinical Record System

Patient information in a clinical record is documented within four basic categories of forms:

▲ Assessment and data base forms
▲ Care plan forms
▲ Nursing or progress note and outcome forms
▲ Continuity of care forms

Nursing documentation occurs on all of these forms; other multidisciplinary caregivers document on a few of these forms (see display, A Summary of Clinical Record Forms).

Assessment and Data Base Forms

Assessment and data base forms in the clinical record include the intake or admission record, the nursing his-

tory, the nursing assessment, medical history, and physical examination and test results data.

INTAKE OR ADMISSION RECORD

Assessment and data base forms include an intake or admission record. On admission to an inpatient facility such as a hospital or long-term care facility, several forms will be initially completed, including the intake or admission form, consent for treatment forms, and advance directives documents.

An **intake record** is the first form completed by an organization when the patient is admitted for care; it becomes the first page documented in the clinical record. Usually a clerical person completes this form. An intake record includes demographic data; billing, family caregiving, and emergency information; chief complaint or purpose of admission to care; who referred the patient; and name of primary physician.

When the patient is admitted, the quantity and accuracy of information systematically collected saves time for the nurse, who then performs and documents a patient assessment. For example, if the clerical intake person can document a patient's chief complaint, a nurse has a starting point to determine patient care needs and patient expectations of care.

Communicating information among clerical and health care providers at the beginning of care has another benefit. Documenting pertinent information so that a patient is not asked the same questions by different caregivers has a positive influence on the patient and family. It prevents frustration and reduces anxiety. Patients learn that information is communicated in an efficient, patient-focused manner, which gives them a feeling of confidence that caregivers are concerned about them and will make clinical decisions based on current, accurate information.

An **admission form** is a form completed by nursing personnel when a patient is admitted and includes basic data concerning the patient's current health status and past health problems. It includes cues or reminders to document an abbreviated nursing history and physical examination.

Consent for treatment forms are separate forms on which the patient agrees to allow physicians and other professionals in the health care organization to provide treatment, surgery, or potential treatment in emergency situations.

Advance directives are legal forms on which the patient documents what treatments are desired or not desired in the event that a condition makes the patient incapable of communicating. One type of directive is commonly called a living will. Durable power of attorney for health care or health care surrogate forms are signed by patients to state who will make decisions for care if a

---

▲ **A SUMMARY OF CLINICAL RECORD FORMS**

Patient information in a clinical record is documented in basic categories of forms, including assessment or data base forms, plan of care forms, clinical progress notes, and continuity of care forms.

I. Assessment and data base forms
  1. Intake or admission record
  2. Nursing history and assessment
  3. Medical history and physical examination
  4. Test results
    a. Lab
    b. X-ray
    c. ECG
    d. MRI
    e. CT scan reports
    f. Diagnostic test result data

II. Plan of care forms
  1. Medical orders
  2. Nursing care plan including nursing orders
  3. Multidisciplinary care plan or discipline-specific plans documented on assessment/care plan or progress notes
  4. Teaching plans, which may be separate or may be incorporated into a care plan
  5. Kardex

III. Progress notes forms
  1. Clinical progress notes documented by all disciplines providing care
  2. Medication administration record (MAR)
  3. Outcome reports
    a. Weekly narrative outcome summary note
    b. Nursing plan outcome record
    c. Criteria-based outcome record

IV. Continuity of care forms
  1. Teaching records
  2. Progress summary
  3. Transfer form
  4. Discharge summary

---

living will is not executed or further decisions are needed. Many times these forms are prepared in advance and are brought to the facility.

The next part of the clinical record to be completed is usually the nursing history and assessment. The nurse performs a history and assessment on the day of admission, and the physician completes a medical history and physical examination.

NURSING HISTORY

A **nursing history** usually includes the following components:

▲ Patient's past hospitalizations
▲ Surgical history
▲ Past and present health problems
▲ Allergies
▲ Functional capabilities and limitations
▲ Perception of illness
▲ Care received at home
▲ Expectation of treatments/nursing care

Documenting a review of body systems or health care functions during a nursing history helps the nurse identify problems, learning needs, psychosocial needs, assistance needed in activities of daily living, and adaptation to changes in life-style due to illness.

Effective listening and interviewing techniques are important in obtaining an accurate and pertinent nursing history. Knowing when to pause, be silent, redirect a question, or not probe further are skills generally developed over time. A nurse should observe how other nurses, physicians, and therapists communicate with patients. It is helpful to listen to verbal responses given by patients and family members to questions asked by others. By observing body language, a nurse can see how some patients express more nonverbally than verbally. Effective communication skills will elicit complete, accurate, and comprehensive information regarding a patient and past needs. An accurate nursing history and nursing assessment best determine a patient's present needs and successful nursing approaches to meet those needs.

NURSING ASSESSMENT

Another assessment or data base form is the **nursing assessment**. In some organizations the nursing assessment is a combination of a nursing history and a physical assessment. When a nurse clusters related assessment information and analyzes the data, past and present needs are identified along with possible future complications.

MEDICAL HISTORY AND PHYSICAL EXAMINATION

The medical portion of the admission data base is a history and physical examination performed by a patient's physician. This information is often documented on a medical progress note and written in a narrative format. Topics begin with a patient history of the primary health-related complaint and progress through physical examination categories from head to toe, addressing each body system.

TEST RESULTS

Diagnostic test results report information from many departments; for example, laboratory, radiology, electrocardiography (ECG), magnetic resonance imaging (MRI), and computed tomography (CT) scanning. This part of the clinical record is used by caregivers to verify diagnoses, plan effective interventions, and monitor therapeutic doses of medication. A nurse uses the information for ongoing assessment of nursing diagnoses and for determination of therapeutic progress toward goals. Keeping current test results filed in the clinical record is important for correct diagnoses and appropriate plans of care.

Plan of Care Forms

Plan of care forms in the clinical record include medical orders, nursing orders, care plans, and the Kardex.

MEDICAL ORDERS

Medical orders are orders written by a physician for a nurse or other care provider to perform; most often they are treatments and medication administration. In home

health care, medical orders can also include drawing blood for diagnostic tests.

Medical orders are written on a separate sheet in the clinical record and are signed and dated by the physician. Orders usually provide details regarding medication administration (dose, route, frequency) or nonroutine treatment.

Verbal orders are later written and signed within a time frame specified by health care organization policy. The time frame must comply with governmental or accrediting regulations. No medical treatment may be given without a written or verbal medical order.

NURSING ORDERS

Nursing orders are nurse-initiated, planned interventions that do not require a physician's order. Nursing orders are intended actions by a nurse to remedy or alleviate a patient's health care needs.

In some nursing documentation formats, such as charting by exception, nursing orders are written and identified as orders. In traditional nursing documentation, some nursing orders can be found in the intervention portion of the care plan and may be called nursing actions, interventions, or nursing approach. In the new *Nursing Intervention Classification* (McCloskey & Bulechek, 1992), nursing orders are labeled nurse-initiated treatments.

CARE PLANS

The *care plan* is an outline of care that the nurse intends to provide to the patient. After the assessment data are collected, verified, clustered, and analyzed, a nursing diagnosis or nursing need is identified. A care plan is then formulated on the basis of the identified nursing diagnoses. Identified goals called expected outcomes are a part of the care plan and are formulated based on the identified needs. Nursing orders or interventions are documented on the care plan and are formulated based on expected outcomes, as steps to achieve expected outcomes (see display, Sample Nursing Care Plan).

Types of care plans include a nursing care plan or a multidisciplinary care plan. A **nursing care plan** contains the identified nursing diagnoses, expected outcomes or goals, and nursing orders or interventions for a particular patient. A **multidisciplinary care plan** includes all of a patient's identified problems, diagnostic orders from all disciplines of caregivers, proposed therapy from all members of the health care team, and expected goals related to all types of therapy. Depending on a patient's need, contributors to a multidisciplinary plan of care may include the physician, nurse, physical therapist, occupational therapist, speech therapist, nutri-

SAMPLE NURSING CARE PLAN

Long-Term Expected Outcome: *Maintain effective airway clearance and efficient breathing pattern by discharge*

Date	Resolution		Nursing Diagnosis	Expected Outcome	Nursing Intervention	Revision	
	Init.	Date				Init./Date	
1/21			Ineffective airway clearance R/T tracheobronchial secretions	Reduced hypoxemia c̄ maintenance of PCO_2 and PO_2 WNL c̄ in 1 hr of acute episode	Administer O_2 via nasal cannula 2-3 l as ordered.	EE	1/21
					Assess resp rate, depth & pattern, breath sounds, for s/s resp. dysfunction		
				Maintain VS within	Monitor VS q 1 h till stable then q 4 h	EE	1/21
				Produce by C & DB clear/white sputum			
				Discard sputum per infection control	Perform percussion, postural drainage, suction.	EE	1/21
					Instruct cough & deep breathing.		
					Monitor sputum characteristics.		
					Teach infection control.		
					Encourage fluids 2-3 l q 24 h	AN	1/22
					Monitor I & O, s/s infection.		
1/22	EE	1/23	Knowledge deficit R/T disease process and treatment of asthma	Verbalize understanding of asthma, its tx and rationale	Instruct per asthma teaching plan and pt education brochure.	—	—
				Exhibit compliance	Demonstrate and get return demo of C & DB		

Review Dates

Date	Signature	In.	Date	Signature	In.	Date	Signature	In.	Date	Signature	In.
1/21	Ellen Eggland, RN	EE									
1/23	Ann Nagle, RN	AN									

tionist, medical social worker, respiratory therapist, and enterostomal therapist.

KARDEX

A Kardex is a traditional documentation form still used in many health care organizations. Originally a summary worksheet reference that never became a part of the retained chart, the **Kardex** is a concise source of patient care information kept at the nurses' station in a Kardex book. At a flip of a card, basic patient care information is available, including:

▲ Patient data
  • Name, address, and marital status
  • Date of birth and Social Security number
  • Religious preference
▲ Medical diagnoses
  • Listed in priority order
▲ Nursing diagnoses
  • Listed in priority order
▲ Current medical orders
  • Medication and treatments
  • Diet
  • Intravenous therapy
  • Consultations
▲ Diagnostic tests
  • Tests scheduled
  • Tests completed, with results
▲ Activities permitted
  • Functional limitations
  • Assistance needed in transfers or activities of daily living
  • Safety precautions required

When not a part of the permanent clinical record, the Kardex is written in pencil. Nurses use this working Kardex by including information helpful for details of daily interventions. Helpful, practical information includes the time a patient prefers a bath or an effective approach to encourage a patient toward managing self-care.

Many organizations do not use a Kardex. In those that do, the Kardex can be a temporary worksheet but more often is a permanent part of a patient's clinical record. When it is permanent, nurses document in ink. In some organizations the nurse also documents a care plan on the Kardex, so practical daily information for care is in a concise format for fast reference.

Types of kardex. There are different types of Kardex, with different names and different sizes. The Kardex can come in various shapes and sizes, from a 3-inch by 6-inch card to a 10-inch by 12-inch folder. An acute care Kardex is often technology oriented to provide quick access to task-oriented interventions, for example, intra-venous solutions, medications, and treatments (see display, Sample Kardex). This format results in an efficient use of time in areas where many skilled interventions are performed. A long-term care Kardex, on the other hand, includes functional topics: activities of daily living, the patient's ability or inability to provide self-care in those activities, level of assistance needed, quick patient status notes, therapy and socialization needs, and basic nursing care needed. Finally, a home health care Kardex includes additional home care, community, and emergency procedure information: local family contacts, other community services providing care, and emergency phone numbers. This helps a nurse accomplish effective care management and quality home health care.

No matter how a Kardex is used or its format, four situations decrease its effective use.

1. The Kardex is not filled out completely.
2. The Kardex does not have adequate space for the amount of entry necessary.
3. The Kardex is not updated in a timely manner.
4. The Kardex is not read by nurses before they render care.

Combining kardex and care plan. This is a creative and space-saving innovation for the Kardex. Nursing diagnoses can be incorporated into the Kardex format, with room beside diagnoses to document nursing orders. When the care plan is included on the Kardex, it should include basic components of:

▲ Brief, applicable assessment data
▲ Nursing diagnoses, listed in priority order
▲ Expected outcomes
▲ Nursing orders
▲ Family involvement in care and discharge planning
▲ Patient outcomes and response to care

Kardex medication and treatment orders. In some organizations a Kardex includes medication and treatment orders; other organizations use a separate medication order record kept on the medication cart or in a medication room, and treatment order record kept on the treatment cart or in a treatment room. Some medication and treatment forms include both orders and columns where a nurse documents administration of each order.

Although many hospitals have a separate medication form, some have medications listed at the top of a Kardex. An example of this practice is in pediatric areas where medication carts are not used for safety reasons. Without a medication cart, it is not necessary to have a medication order sheet separate from the Kardex or other plan of care form.

If medication orders are included in the Kardex,

SAMPLE KARDEX

Vital Signs
   Temp O R AX
   B/P
   Pulse & Resp
		Respiratory care	

Resuscitation Status—CPR? Living Will?		Diet Fluids	
Notify physician if . . .		Weight	
Sensory deficit		Treatments	
Communication method and barriers		I & O	
Safety Measures		Consult/Regarding Date	
Activity		Referrals Date	
Hygiene care Time preference		Isolation	Date order: Date stop:
Bowel Continence		Bladder Continence	
Assistance Needed in ADL		Skin Care	

DIAGNOSTIC TESTS

Date Ordered	Test	Schedule Date	Preparation

Allergies _____

Diagnoses _____

Physician _____   Phone _____

Name _____   Room _____ Bed _____

medication information includes the name of the drug, dosage, frequency, administration route, injection site if parenteral, date and time medication was ordered, duration of therapy if applicable, and date and time to discontinue regimen.

In some health care organizations, the Kardex is used for nonnursing information. Nursing information is not written on a Kardex to avoid duplicating nursing orders and care plans. Especially organizations using computers for care planning use a paper Kardex for a unit manager to record lab work, x-rays, tests to be scheduled, and patients transported. Information on this type of Kardex includes basic identifying information, medical orders, interdisciplinary referrals and consults, activity, precautions, diet, vital signs, special tests, lab work, x-rays, and specimen cultures.

Progress Note Forms

Progress note forms in a clinical record include medical, nursing, and multidisciplinary progress notes and medication administration records.

PROGRESS NOTES

Progress notes include those forms labeled nursing notes, medication administration sheets, personal care flow sheets, teaching records, intake and output forms, vital sign record, and specialty forms. Examples of specialty forms are a neurologic assessment checklist or a diabetic intervention flow sheet. A neurologic assessment checklist has columns to document neurologic responses for fast comparison. Diabetic flow sheets include columns to document blood test results and insulin administration.

Although type and design of documentation forms vary with each organization, all **progress notes** include patient condition, complaints, identified problems, interventions, and patient response to care. Progress notes can be completely narrative or can be in a standardized flow sheet format with an area to document narrative for further description.

MEDICATION ADMINISTRATION RECORD

The **medication administration record** (MAR) is an ongoing patient record on which the nurse documents medication administered to a patient. Each administration is recorded by date, time, medication name, dose, route, and frequency. Most acute care settings have a medication record that remains on a medication cart, which is rolled from room to room as a nurse administers prepackaged doses of medication. When a medication is omitted, the nurse must document what dose was omitted by circling the time it was scheduled and the reason the medication was not given (eg, a patient refuses a medication, or a patient misses a dose while off the unit for diagnostic tests).

OUTCOME FORMS

Patient outcomes are the results from care provided to a patient. Outcomes indicate progress a patient made in meeting goals for care. Requiring health care organizations to document outcomes is one of many attempts by accreditation groups to halt rising health care costs. Outcomes facilitate analysis of direction and effectiveness of health care services. Documenting outcomes enhances quality of care by focusing on expected outcomes as goals of care and revising care plans to achieve those outcomes.

Some organizations use progress notes or weekly outcome summary notes to document outcomes. In this way nurses use actual patient outcome information to focus on resolution of unmet expected outcomes. Other organizations do not document outcomes until the end of care, at which time the information is documented on a discharge summary or an outcome flow sheet.

Continuity of Care Forms

As a patient's condition improves or deteriorates, the patient may need more intense or less intense nursing care. A patient may move from a rehabilitation unit to home care or from a medical floor to intensive care. Documentation accompanies a patient between departments or between organizations and plays a key role in communication to provide a smooth transition between services. Continuity of care forms usually include:

▲ Identified problems
▲ Established goals developed with the patient
▲ Interventions implemented (successful and unsuccessful)
▲ Progress made toward expected outcomes
▲ Problems, complications, or barriers to progress or continuity of care
▲ Revisions made to planned care
▲ Actual outcomes of care
▲ Continued needs and plans for care

Care and attention to these aspects will greatly influence the next phase of health care delivered. For example, an elderly patient became confused and combative at night unless a night light was on. Communication of that information is important in correctly determining patient needs and providing appropriate interventions for patient comfort and care.

TEACHING RECORDS

Patient teaching is an important intervention and must be planned for effectiveness. Most teaching is used to assist the patient and family to learn to manage care independently or assist effectively with care provided by professionals. In teaching a patient, a nurse participates with other disciplines to assess learning needs, outline knowledge a patient or caregiver needs, and demonstrate skills caregivers need to manage care and maintain continuity of care. For example, a patient and caregiver should be able to:

▲ Verbalize signs and symptoms of problems related to each prescribed medication or treatment
▲ Appropriately return demonstrate procedures required to manage care, such as a dressing change or insulin injection

In essence, **teaching plans** are a type of care plan in which a patient's knowledge deficit is identified as a need. A goal of what should occur as a result of teaching is documented as an expected outcome, and learning objectives used in the teaching process are outlined in a step-by-step progression. Teaching records are maintained to document outcomes of teaching, the patient's response to teaching, and level of learning. Teaching a patient contributes to continuity of care after discharge from a health care service. Consequently, developing a teaching plan that reaches the goal of making a patient and caregiver knowledgeable and more independent about their health care empowers them to be self-sufficient and accountable for their own well-being.

PROGRESS SUMMARIES

Progress summaries are brief narrative reports routinely sent to a patient's physician for home care or routinely documented on a patient's record to communicate a patient's condition and progress. These summaries provide a picture of the patient's status so that a physician can determine continued medical orders for treatment. Occasionally progress summaries are sent to multi-disciplinary caregivers who are also involved in a patient's care.

TRANSFER FORM

Decades ago, a transfer form was used when a patient was transferred from a hospital to a long-term care facility or from a long-term care facility to a home health care agency. To meet contemporary health care documentation requirements, organizations now complete a discharge summary instead of a transfer form.

Transfer forms are still used in some hospitals when a patient is moved from one unit to another, but more often when a patient is sent from one hospital to another. Consider the situation in which a pediatric burn patient is taken to a community hospital emergency room, and the hospital personnel determine they do not have the facilities nor staff to provide appropriate care. Emergency room personnel may call another hospital for permission to send the patient there and will complete a transfer form to send with the patient. A **transfer summary** provides transition of care information as a patient moves from one level of care to another within the same health care organization or from a short-stay health care setting such as an emergency department to another hospital.

When a transfer form is used, information usually includes patient identifying information and:

▲ Diagnosis
▲ Physician who provided care
▲ Person contacted in the receiving organization
▲ Dates of care (admission to and discharge from unit)
▲ Reasons for care
▲ Services provided
▲ Reason for transfer (can be patient preference or unavailability of necessary treatment)
▲ Type of reimbursement (such as Medicare or insurance)
▲ Allergies
▲ Current medications
▲ Current therapies with regimen schedule including last administration time
▲ Patient status at departure from originating point of service
▲ Needs and goals achieved

▲ Needs and goals still unmet
▲ Time and method of transportation

As noted previously, attention and care aimed at communicating accurate and complete information affects the quality of health care delivered.

DISCHARGE FORM

The documentation form used when a patient is discharged from a health care organization is the discharge summary. The **discharge summary** provides patient condition and information regarding services received for the purpose of assisting the next health care providers in determining patient needs, effective treatment, and continuity of care.

The discharge summary includes:

▲ A summary of services provided before discharge
▲ Plans developed with the patient or recommended by the nurse
  • The setting to which a patient is going
  • Caregivers available and capable to provide care
  • Community resources contacted or recommended
▲ Goals achieved and progress made toward still unmet goals
▲ Equipment or supplies needed or obtained

Discharge planning should begin at patient admission. Documentation of assessment of discharge needs and discharge plans should also begin at admission. Discharge planning documentation is required by standard-setting organizations, such as JCAHO.

Special Types of Forms

Standardized forms, flow sheets, and graphs are the designs of forms included in a clinical record. The purpose of these formats is quick documentation, fast retrievability, and easy data comparison.

Standardized Forms

A **standardized form** includes key words, phrases, or questions as cues to gather certain information. A standardized form is usually designed for easy inclusion of data using one or two words or a symbol (check mark). A flow sheet lists standardized cues in columns with a column for dated data entry of yes, no, time designation, check mark, or codes that represent specific information. Standardized forms are often used for 24-hour assessments or for clinical notes in which a column of preprinted data is listed down one side of a page and times and dates are printed across the top of the page.

Standardized care plans and standardized progress notes have been both hailed as a wonderful timesaver and condemned as a "cookbook" approach to nursing. Opponents of standardized care plans say these forms depersonalize care. With the volume of specific data that must be documented in today's health care, however, more nurses are realizing the need for standardized forms.

Proponents say that with room for individualization of standardized forms, care is individualized, not depersonalized. Further, standardization assists the nurse in decreasing documentation time, allowing an opportunity to increase productivity and patient care time at the bedside. Nurses further state that standardization of care plans eliminates the "trial and error" approach to nursing care and instead includes in a plan what are commonly determined to be effective interventions for particular nursing diagnoses. Standardized care plans include detailed information that can be easily overlooked and could potentially be a problem for a patient. Standardized care plans are goal directed and ensure that all nurses are assessing in a standard way and are providing consistent care.

Flow Sheets

Standardized forms refer to the actual content of forms, whereas **flow sheets** refer to the columned format that allows key data to be documented concisely for easy accessibility and comparison. Flow sheets have regulated vertical or horizontal columns of date(s) and times in which the nurse can insert data quickly and concisely, usually at the time information is observed or care is given.

NURSING NOTES FLOW SHEETS

Standardized nursing notes are becoming more common in hospital settings, especially within a 24-hour flow sheet format. Traditionally these standardized forms were common only in the intensive care units, where most of the data included were monitoring elements such as blood gases. With the advent of audits, which look for specific information in progress notes, accompanied by a contemporary focus on actual patient outcomes, standardized forms eliminate the step of looking in an extensive narrative text to be assured of documentation of all interventions and all outcomes appropriate to care. Standardized nursing notes save time and ensure the inclusion of information required or desired.

For example, a quality improvement auditor must read through pages of narrative progress notes to learn if information such as teaching the patient to take a pulse count before taking digoxin is included. Instead, this standardized intervention can be placed on a nursing notes flow sheet with other planned nursing activities based on the standardized care plan. Standardized information can aid in quality assurance (see display, Quality Assurance and Documentation). A separate standardized teaching sheet can be developed to meet another need for documentation as well.

QUALITY ASSURANCE AND DOCUMENTATION

Step 4 of the Joint Commission on Accreditation of Healthcare Organizations (JCAHO) 10-Step Model for Quality Assurance calls for auditors to evaluate the care given. The data that indicate what care was given must be easily retrievable to determine quality assurance or quality improvement programs.

Step 4. Identify indicators (and appropriate clinical criteria) for monitoring the important aspects of care.

For each aspect of care, an indicator, which can be set up as a standard, is identified to measure that aspect of care. For example:

For all patients with alteration in myocardial tissue perfusion requiring thrombolytic therapies, the following are monitored and documented according to protocol:

Heart rate   _____

Blood pressure _____

Chest pain   _____

This information can be easily identified and retrievable if on a standardized form or flow sheet, particularly if included on a 24-hour flow sheet.

FLOW SHEET ADVANTAGES

Using flow sheets has many advantages. They allow the nurse to document information quickly, often at the patient bedside for greater accuracy. Flow sheets are faster to use than narrative formats because of the brevity of entry. Flow sheets make it easier to locate specific measurement or intervention information, eliminating looking through pages of purely narrative notes in a clinical chart. Further, flow sheets give a fast comparison of information within the past 24, 48, or 72 hours, whatever time review desired. Finally, these forms provide proof of regulated, intermittent observation or intervention with a patient—an area particularly scrutinized by accrediting agencies or prosecuting attorneys.

Documentation that proves the frequency of observation can be a deciding factor in legal cases such as *Collins v. Westlake Community Hospital* (1974). When no documentation was in the record for a 7-hour period, the jury assumed no observations were made of the condition of a boy's casted leg. Nurses stated circulation in the toes was normal, so no information was charted. The jury decided against the nurses and the hospital when the boy's leg required amputation because of a circulation problem. Providing a circulatory assessment on a flow sheet could have successfully addressed this problem and avoided or resolved the circulatory complication.

FLOW SHEET DISADVANTAGES AND PRECAUTIONS

There are disadvantages and precautions to using flow sheets, however. The use of flow sheets does not exempt the nurse from narrative charting, which further describes what cannot be explained in a flow sheet format. Descriptive observations, patient teaching, patient responses, detailed interventions, and unusual circumstances should be documented in a narrative portion of the flow sheet. If allotted space for documentation is too small for the explanatory narrative needed, the nurse should asterisk the section with an initialed note to "*see additional information on 5-11 narrative note." On flow sheets, nurses should not write outside of the lines nor repeat information already documented on the flow sheet. Instead, the narrative should describe, clarify, and provide additional information, in the order (chronological order and sometimes subject order) as presented on the flow sheet.

TYPES OF FLOW SHEETS

The many types of flow sheets can be categorized into specialty flow sheets, activity flow sheets, measurement flow sheets, and intervention flow sheets.

Specialty flow sheets. These forms focus on one, usually primary, aspect or area of care. For example, a cardiovascular flow sheet outlines patient status measurements and nursing interventions implemented in caring for a patient with cardiovascular problems.

Activity flow sheets. These reflect a broad range of daily patient function topics, such as positioning and level of mobility, nutrition, elimination, respiratory status, mental status, and hygiene.

Measurement and intervention flow sheets. In contemporary documentation, flow sheets can be entirely measurement flow sheets used to assess or monitor a patient's condition. Or, flow sheets can be entirely interventions to record nursing activities. Intervention flow sheets, like a medication administration sheet and an intravenous therapy record, give the opportunity to document repetitious procedures for quick verification of completed interventions.

Sometimes the two functions of measurement and intervention are combined to make a flow sheet. For example, on a hyperalimentation sheet, a nurse measures and documents daily weight, temperature, apical pulse, and blood sugar level. After hyperalimentation, a nurse documents specifics about the intervention including time begun and the amount, type, and rate of hyperalimentation.

Specialty or activity flow sheets can include descriptive codes or categories to check off beside each topic. For example, an activity flow sheet that lists bathing can include cues to check or a code to write to indicate the type of bath and amount of assistance received in bathing. Another example is a measurement neurologic flow sheet that defines limb movement as normal power or levels of mild to severe weakness. Further cues are extension and flexion ability, spasticity, coma scales of verbal and pain response, vital signs, and pupil size with response. An example of a combined specialty assessment and intervention flow sheet is a diabetic record on which a nurse documents blood glucose test results and amount of insulin administered.

With flow sheets, observations, measurements, or interventions are presented in a concise format for easy comparison and retrieval. Flow sheets with room for narratives on the back are sometimes the primary or only documentation form used for charting on each shift.

Each type of flow sheet described (specialty, activity, and measurement and intervention) has advantages and disadvantages. Flow sheet design and use is determined by the patient population needs on a particular nursing unit and the nursing and documentation needs. Form design and use will continue to be revised as nursing technology and documentation needs change.

Graphs

Graphs are flow sheets that create a pictorial comparison of data beyond just numerical comparison as seen in category flow sheets. Most hospitals use a vital sign graph sheet for daily comparisons of blood pressure, temperature, pulse, and respiration (See display, Sample Vital Signs Graph).

With the incorporation of the unit secretary in most health care facilities, nonnursing personnel may be responsible for transferring the collected data and transforming the numbers into a graph. Today's computers electronically graph vital signs data entered into the patient's data base. In intensive care units, computers are able to directly monitor, record, and graph vital signs, blood gases, and other values captured by electronic monitoring. Whether manual or computerized collection and graphing are available, the registered nurse responsible for patient care is still accountable for documented graph accuracy of status measurements.

Computerized Documentation

Computerization is not new for billing, payroll, and management functions in health care organizations. The health care industry has learned from other industries that computers facilitate speed in communication, accuracy in information, capability of information storage, data retrieval, and data revision. These assets are essential in patient care documentation now as standards and progressive health care technology are increasing documentation demands and accountability of nurses.

Leaders in nursing and the health care industry are developing computerized clinical record systems as a means to manage the huge volume of clinical, adminis-

SAMPLE VITAL SIGNS GRAPH

Date																									
TEMP. F° C°		0400	0800	1200	1600	2000	2400	0400	0800	1200	1600	2000	2400	0400	0800	1200	1600	2000	2400	0400	0800	1200	1600	2000	2400
105.8° 41°																									
104° 40°																									
102.2° 39°																									
100.4° 38°																									
98.6° 37°																									
96.8° 36°																									
95° 35°																									
Pulse																									
Respirations																									
Blood Pressure																									

▲	A COMPUTERIZED CLINICAL RECORD

This is an example of a computerized, integrated clinical record system, nursing designed, based on the nursing process, with the patient as the center focus.

Types of Information Stored in the Computerized Clinical Record

- ▲ Intake record
- ▲ Assessment
- ▲ Care plan
- ▲ Nursing clinical visit notes
- ▲ Physician orders request
- ▲ Patient care summary
- ▲ Discharge summary
- ▲ Laboratory results
- ▲ Therapies (PT, OT) clinical documentation

Information Used in Integrated Programs With a Computerized Record

- ▲ Medication data base
  With medication history, patient education medication sheets, current medication profile (including dose, route, frequency, status, side effects, medication allergies alert, drug incompatibility alert)
- ▲ Nursing management
  Statistical data collection and reports, medical orders tracking, quality assurance clinical record review flow sheet, patient outcome monitor flow sheet, electronic mail
- ▲ Employee requirements tracking
- ▲ Financial reporting
- ▲ Electronic claims processing

(Adapted with permission of MedPad, Atlanta, GA.)

---

trative, and regulatory information required in contemporary health care (see display, A Computerized Clinical Record). With computerized documentation, nursing administrators seek to make a large volume of documentation more manageable. Although computerized documentation cannot alone guarantee improvement in patient care or nursing practice, it can definitely facilitate nursing documentation and its use in quality assurance, patient acuity programs, and patient statistics reports. Many people believe computerized documentation may help especially when nurses are in short supply (see display, Government Influence on Computerized Documentation).

To actually learn about computerized system(s), it is best to experience hands-on practice.

Information Systems

Hospital information systems (HIS) is a computer network that processes and transmits data for patient admission, billing, pharmacy, diet orders, and other activities. Some large HIS systems have a nursing data base compo-

nent. In recent years, however, development has focused on separate nursing information systems that can be interfaced (share the other system's data) with a larger traditional HIS.

A **nursing information system** (NIS) is defined as "... a computer system that collects, stores, processes,

▲	GOVERNMENT INFLUENCE ON COMPUTERIZED DOCUMENTATION

Secretary Otis Bowen's Commission on the Nursing Shortage in 1989 provided an impetus to computerized nursing documentation by recommending computerized information systems to support nurses in the cost-effective use of their time, to help decrease health care costs, and to help minimize the effects of the nursing shortage.

retrieves, displays, and communicates timely information needed to do the following:

▲ Administer the nursing services and resources in a health care facility
▲ Manage standardized patient care information for the delivery of nursing care
▲ Link the research resources and the educational applications to nursing practice" (Saba & McCormick, 1986)

Five types of information systems are generally available:

▲ A nursing system for general acute (hospital) care
▲ A medical/nursing system for critical (intensive) care
▲ An interfaced HIS with a nursing component
▲ Home health care clinical record system(s)
▲ Long-term care clinical record systems

Some computer software companies have developed systems that can effectively computerize and integrate some or all of the following:

▲ Admission data
▲ Nursing history
▲ Medical records abstract
▲ Nursing diagnosis
▲ Patient acuity
▲ Diagnosis-related group (DRG) assignment
▲ Nursing orders
▲ Individualized nursing care plans
▲ Automated Kardex
▲ Nursing goals
▲ Measurable patient outcomes
▲ Nursing intervention
▲ DRG monitoring and reporting
▲ Quality assurance (American Nurses Association, 1989)

Each NIS program is customized for the needs and requests of each health care organization. The hardware and software computer system is tailored to present patient care information in the facility's own prescribed care model, documentation format, and function and application desired for the data.

Advantages of Computerized Documentation

General and practical advantages of computerized documentation are reported in the literature. General advantages of computerization include:

▲ Enhanced data management and communication
▲ Enhanced teaching of patient care management
▲ Enhanced development of protocols

▲ Increased systematic approach to patient care (Cox, Harsanyi, & Dean, 1987)

Specific practical advantages of computerization have been studied and reported in literature focused on computerization in nursing. Advantages include legibility, accuracy, timely data, rapid communication, definite documentation accountability, and potential for enhanced patient education and reduction in medication errors.

Legibility. A conspicuous advantage to computerization is legibility. With computers typing output on printers, the time, frustration, and risk of incorrectly deciphering patient care information is decreased.

Accuracy. The quality of data collection is improved for two reasons. First, if a bedside terminal is used, the nurse records observations at the time seen and interventions when completed. Such timeliness has an end result of increased accuracy of charting detail. Second, with protocols or cue phrases prompting for information, data entered are more complete, thorough, concise, and organized, resulting in a more systematic approach to patient care documentation.

The accuracy of data is further enhanced when the computer system includes shared elements and a programmed check on information entered. For example, in shared elements, medication is entered on an assessment and at the same time is electronically entered on a physician's order form and a patient care form for Medicare. Computerization ensures all lists of medication will be the same. A programmed check on a computer can indicate when all spaces in a form are not filled out, or will not let a user continue entering data until a particular required function such as reviewing a care plan is performed.

Standard nursing terminology and documentation process are advantages that facilitate data collection and accurate comparison of data in quality assurance, research, and statistical analysis.

Timely data. Timely information is electronically possible because current information is easily added and information needing updating is easily retrieved and revised. Information is quickly coordinated and integrated with other collected data so that decision-making is based on current data.

Rapid communication. Rapid interdepartmental communication is a nursing timesaver, using computer linkages (networks) and direct input by all departments, lessening telephone calls and patient file courier transfers. In addition, even when the patient's chart is with the patient in radiology, access to that file information for reference is always available to any authorized department or nurse clinician, even when the chart is not on the unit.

Definite documentation accountability. Accountability of the nurse is increased for detailed documentation because definite standardized phrases are used for computer data input. Definite data require nursing judgment, which in turn commands accountability. The traditional, indecisive, narrative phrases such as "appears to be . . ." are replaced with computerized clear, decisive, and concise key words, especially in assessment documentation. The nurse is responsible and accountable for more definite and detailed documentation (Zielstorff, 1979).

Enhanced patient education. Patient education is enhanced through learning needs assessment, a customized teaching plan, actual teaching possible by computer, evaluation of actual learning achieved, and subsequent discharge planning (Cox et al., 1987).

Reduced medication errors. Medication errors can be reduced. If physicians use a computer system to directly input medical orders, nurses can save time by eliminating transcription and transmission of orders. Dosage and administration time errors can be decreased because the pharmacy receives the order at preestablished computer-acceptable doses and routes, and the Kardex and patient medication sheet are immediately updated for the nurse (Scholes, Bryant, & Barber, 1983).

Disadvantages of Computerized Documentation

Disadvantages of computerized documentation include computer malfunction, impersonal effect on the nurse–patient relationship, concern for privacy, dissemination of information, limitations of standard vocabulary, paper storage of printouts, and cost.

Malfunction. The biggest concern about using a computerized system is what to do when the computer is "down" (not working). Some systems are planned to go down for 1 to 3 hours during the night shift to input new programs or process data. At any time, computers can malfunction to scramble information, lose information, or simply not accept, process, or output information.

Impersonal effect. Using a computer is impersonal and could affect the nurse–patient relationship when interaction involves putting patient data into a computer device. A patient may not be as open to giving complete and accurate personal information if a patient thinks

disclosures are being entered into a big data bank accessible by anyone.

Concern for privacy. There is an added concern for privacy, confidentiality, and security of computerized patient information because information can conceivably be accessed or destroyed by unauthorized persons.

Dissemination of inaccurate information. If inaccurate or inappropriate information is entered into the computer, it is disseminated quickly. Additional entries based on inaccurate or inappropriate information can promote further errors and further problems in health care delivery and documentation of care.

Limitation of standard vocabulary. Standardized and limited vocabulary or phrase structure in computer formats can be a restriction on accuracy or completeness of charting. The computer systems that allow only two or three word entries are especially confining and do not allow adequate information to describe patient condition or individualized nursing intervention, with patient response.

Paper storage of printouts. Paper accumulation and storage can be a problem, depending on the organization's policy on how frequently printed output is done for signature and patient record filing (every shift or every 24 hours). It will be many years until health care organizations can move to a paperless chart. Until then, storage of data can be on computer diskette, but because most organizations are not completely computerized, paper charts are still standard and necessary.

Cost. Last, but not least important, is the problem of cost: cost of the hardware and software; cost of the training, including keyboard skills training; and cost of supervisory involvement during the transitional period of change, with accompanying work pace and procedure disruption.

Response to Issues and Concerns: Some Proposed Standards

In response to the computerization concerns, computer technologists, information specialists, and nurses have proposed standards to eliminate current and potential documentation problems inherent in computerized documentation.

SECURITY AND CONFIDENTIALITY

Suggestions to secure privacy of information revolve around a single or double security coding system for entry into the computer system, in which each nurse would have a personal identification code as well as passwords for access to different levels of patient information. When entered into the computer, passwords are not visible on the computer screen. Many hospitals with computerized clinical records change each caregiver's identification code every 6 months to enhance data security. At some hospitals, these codes are permanent employee identifying numbers, and passwords are routinely changed so that access security is ensured. On most computer systems, the identification code is automatically recorded when any documentation is entered, revised, or deleted, so that users know who made a patient entry.

Only essential patient information should be computerized with a provision for separation of information from identities for audit or research purposes. A monitoring system should check for accuracy of information and detect any violation of the security system. Only an authorized administrative person, who is also responsible for information backup (ie, more permanent storage), may delete patient files.

DOWNTIME PROCEDURE

Backup plans, systems, and equipment must be available to function during computer downtimes. If a backup generator or backup computer cannot maintain the automated system, then at least authorized documentation forms must be available for manual documentation use during computer downtimes. These forms and keyboard input reentry of manually documented information would be a facility-specific policy addressing duration of downtime, time requirement for reentry, who would reenter information (nurse or clerical worker with nurse supervision), and backup disk rotation.

A monitoring system should be able to notify users immediately of any input, transmission, or storage problems, or other malfunctions of the computer software or hardware systems, to preclude information being lost, especially unknowingly lost. Most health care organizations maintain a 3- to 5-day backup plan where each day's data are backed up to a separate diskette for data storage. These three to five diskettes are rotated then with the oldest data diskette erased by backing up the most recent data onto it. This generally ensures that the most data that may be lost would be data entered in the most recent 24 hours.

COMPUTERIZED DOCUMENTATION POLICIES AND PROCEDURES

Overall, every organization that is computerized needs "policies and procedures (for) daily operations, charting, error documentation, planned computer downtime, unscheduled computer downtime, backup systems, computer system operations, and certification and/or confirmation of order entry accuracy" (Cox et al., 1987). This process involves an entire policy and procedure manual, specific to the organization's system, needs, and functions.

Using a Computerized Documentation System

DATA INPUT DEVICES

Typical data input devices are the keyboard, touch screen, light pens, and bar code readers. The most recent development in input devices is the pen and tablet computer (using handwriting technology) and speech recognition systems (entering data or ordering input by voice).

COMPUTER INPUT METHODS

Actual input of patient or nursing data is done in different ways:

▲ Keyboard input of word(s) or narrative phrases
▲ Touching the screen with a mouse or light pen
▲ Entering a phrase selected by cursor, underline, or highlight

Specific methods are determined by the hardware and software package. Systems like the MedPad Clinical Record System (Atlanta, GA) also have a variety of coded, window entries that call up selected lists from which coordinated text narrative can be chosen for entry. In the same way, ICD9 codes can be electronically entered when nursing diagnoses are chosen.

Data input is accomplished through different procedures depending on the software used. A nurse can fill in the blank in a form; can answer yes or no (entering y or n) to standardized questions; can keyboard in a word or phrase to individualize documentation on standardized phrases; or can keyboard complete sentences to elaborate on a problem or patient response in the comment section of a form. Further, a nurse can make a menu selection from a pathway that guides or cues topics or specific data that should be reported. Then, a nurse can choose needs, symptoms, interventions, comprehension, or outcomes from multiple choice standard phrases.

The most efficient and comprehensive computer systems are those with standardized assessments, standardized care plans with outcome and intervention phrases, and standardized nursing notes composed of phrases that can be individualized.

Different systems have different methods of computerizing nursing documentation forms. The following examples of those different methods are categorized under basic forms of history/assessment, care plan, and nursing notes. Examples are described step by step, beginning with gaining access to the system.

ACCESS TO THE DATA

To gain access to data and to be able to process data, a nurse must sign on with an individual number, code, or password. As a result of entering one's identification code, the computer will document who is making a computerized entry and the date and time a nurse enters the system. If a password is programmed into the system, the nurse can enter the system only at those levels of information permitted by the password.

Types of Computerized Records

At the present time, most health care organizations have a computer system for various organizational functions, but many organizations do not yet have a system for clinical documentation. Computerized clinical documentation systems in use often have only care plans and sometimes automated Kardexes. Early programs do not include nursing notes, but some use a system in which nurses type in a narrative or fill-in-the-blank text. However, more and more health care facilities are moving toward computerized patient records that include all documentation.

THE HISTORY AND ASSESSMENT

In one type of computerized assessment, the nurse keys in patient identification information, then scrolls through the nursing history and assessment and touches the light pen to either "no problem" or to each symptom listed in a body system format that is a problem for the patient. For example, under the altered gastrointestinal category the nurse points to diarrhea, then keys in 4 to fill in the blank of (4) X/day. The nurse continues through the form, answering every question or filling in every blank, keying in narrative as necessary under "comments."

A different assessment procedure is followed in another type of software program. In this program a nurse keys in basic (well) assessment and enters applicable assessment phrases, such as alert and oriented, skin warm and dry, breath sounds clear. If the patient has an abnormal basic symptom, such as a breath sound problem, then the nurse keys in the system involved, such as the respiratory system, and chooses in sequence standard phrases such as congested, all lung fields. These short phrases are numbered for ease of entry and printed in sequence on a printout.

Progressive computer systems attempt to link certain assessment data to characteristics of a specific nursing diagnosis. Based on assessment data collected, a computer will list potential nursing diagnoses for a nurse to accept or reject for that patient's care plan. Often these expert systems, which help the nurse make decisions, are stand-alone programs, not integrated with nursing documentation application systems.

THE CARE PLAN

Some software programs for care planning use a functional format such as Gordon's functional model with associated nursing diagnoses. For this system, after entering the care plan menu, a nurse chooses the function category of activity, rest, sleep. The next step is to choose from the listed North American Nursing Diagnosis Association (NANDA) diagnoses the diagnosis that applies to a patient, such as Alteration in Mobility related to. . . .

In most systems, when a nurse enters a nursing diagnosis, the computer generates standardized expected outcomes and standardized interventions. Then a nurse chooses what is to be documented on the care plan. The nurse creates a care plan from a patient's nursing diagnoses, individualizing by choosing, modifying, or adding various computer-generated expected outcomes and interventions.

Some common basic care plan systems in current use have standardized care plans for each specific medical diagnosis. A nurse can individualize the care plan by modifying these standardized care plans, thus eliminating the manual accumulation of various standardized care plans, with crossed out interventions and goals.

Some computerized care plan systems use a combination of standard patient guidelines and an individualized standardized patient care plan. The guideline is a printout of care, which is applicable to a patient with a particular medical diagnosis, including criteria of nursing process of care. The second component is a shortened care plan, which is standardized on the computer screen, then individualized to the patient by a nurse before printout. Guidelines are indicated on a care plan for fast reference, and nursing diagnoses, expected outcomes, and nursing orders are presented on the same screen. M/G indicates that mutual goals were established by the care planning nurse and patient. Initials in parentheses are of the primary and other nurses who wrote each related problem and expected outcome of the nursing order (see display, Computerized Plan of Care).

Regardless of the format, computerized care plans become a part of the patient's permanent record. Care plans can be updated at any time, but all entries, changes, or deletions are permanently recorded, including the date and name or identifying code of the nurse making the computerized entry. At any given point in time, a caregiver can see what the care plan included on any day and shift and when further additions, revisions, or deletions were made.

Some software programs incorporate an automatic

▲ **COMPUTERIZED PLAN OF CARE**

```
                        ACTIVE PLAN OF CARE
                        CC  5111A  IP                        10/23/92    1444
PRIMARY NURSE:

GUIDELINES IMPLEMENTED FOR PATIENTS WITH:
URINARY TRACT INFECTION/UTI                           (JL)
-------------------
    RELATED TO:              M/G EXPECTED OUTCOME:       NURSING ORDERS:
    01.INFECTION.(JL)        Y 01.ABSENCE OF SKIN        01.ENCOURAGE CRANBERRY
    02.PARAPLEGIC FROM            IRRITATION/BREAKDOWN      JUICE. (JL)
       WAIST DOWN (JL)           THROUGHOUT             02.I&O Q 8 HR(S). (JL)
                                 HOSPITALIZATION. (JL)  03.MONITOR ELECTROLYTE,
                            Y 02.MAINTAINS PROPER           BUN, AND CREATININE
                                 FUNCTIONING OF             VALUES. (JL)
                                 CATHETER THROUGHOUT    04.OBSERVE COLOR,
                                 HOSPITALIZATION. (JL)      TURBIDITY, AND ODOR OF
                                                            URINE. (JL)
                                                        05.OBSERVE FOR PATENCY OF
                                                            CATHETER. (JL)
                                                        06.PROVIDE SUPPLIES FOR PT
                                                            TO CHANGE OWN CONDOM
                                                            CATH QD. HE NEEDS SIZE
                                                            MEDIUM CATH, SKIN PREP
                                                            AND UNISOLVE.HE DOES
                                                            THIS HIMSELF (JL)
```

(Courtesy of Lee Memorial Hospital, Ft. Myers, FL.)

care plan review into their system, so that every 48 hours (or whatever time frame is designated), the computer will not allow a nurse to enter nursing notes until a review is documented in the care plan. This cues the nurse to remember the review, to meet hospital and JCAHO standards of care plan review. JCAHO requires that a review of the care plan be documented at least every 72 hours. By policy and procedure, some hospitals require nurses to review care plans every 24 hours.

Standardized care plans, especially with nursing diagnoses, facilitate the development of computerized documentation with minimum narrative entry. The literature contains a variety of nursing care plan manuals, and health care organizations have frequently developed their own. The profession continues to classify nursing knowledge in this area and in the areas of nursing diagnoses, nursing interventions, and nursing-related patient outcomes. A recent addition to the literature is *Nursing Interventions Classification* by McCloskey and Bulechek (1992), a standardized comprehensive list of nursing interventions, used to describe nursing actions (as components of interventions) to facilitate documentation of care. Standardization of the next step of documentation, standardizing nursing notes for computerization, however, is more complex because of patient individualization.

NURSING NOTES

A more difficult problem, not yet tackled by most organizations, is standardization of nursing phrases of patient condition and response, nursing interventions, and activities to compile computerized nursing notes. This author has developed home health care clinical text for computer in the form of standardized phrases. When linked together by a nurse via computer, these phrases form complete and concise statements or phrases. For example, a computerized note is created by progressively entering data by touching phrases represented between slash marks in the following example. The slash marks do not actually appear on the computer or on the printed note.

Clinical data:/Respirations labored./Pt complains of /increased fatigue, decreased endurance/weather exacerbates SOB./Pt exhibits/audible wheezing on inspiration and expiration./Nonproductive cough./ Lung sounds clear.

Assessed:/C-P irregularities/asthma management.

Treatment & Interventions:/Instructed pt and family in inhal Rx, aerosol medication regimen, use of inhaler/Instructed in/Dx of asthma, its causes and tx/planned rest schedule to increase endurance.

Pt outcome: Pt verbalized relief from /respiratory distress./ Resp 14, reg, non-labored./ No wheezing nor coughing; lung sounds clear.

In this computer system, vital signs, basic data such as fasting blood sugar or wound sizes, and phrases from various visit notes can be clustered and extracted by computer for use in formulating a narrative summary of patient progress.

MEDICATION SHEETS

In a computerized documentation program, patients have a medication profile that includes current medications, dosage and acceptable dosage range, side effects, limits for each drug, drug allergies, and drug incompatibilities. When a medication is ordered, the computer checks the dosage and incompatibilities, prints the medications to be given during a shift, checks that a nurse enters the medication as given, and displays or prints a message if there are any discrepancies in the above data. Most systems even print a medication information sheet for patient education and compliance at discharge.

In medication systems, it is important that a medication history be maintained so that at any point, the nurse can see what medication a patient was taking at a particular time.

Types of Computers for Documentation

BEDSIDE TERMINALS

Some hospitals not only have a computer in the nursing station but also have terminals at each patient's bedside. These systems are called point-of-care systems because documentation is done at the site where care is given. Before providing care, the nurse can call up a patient's care plan, list of diagnoses, expected outcomes and goals, and interventions.

For fast entry, some bedside input devices have a mouse or have a small keyboard with labeled keys, such as care plan, vital signs, safety, and diet. On these small keyboards, entries and changes that are standard in these areas can be made at the bedside. Narrative comments, however, can only be made at the nurses station where a full keyboard is available for typing in text.

MICROPROCESSORS

Most hand-held microprocessor computers have an approximate 2-inch by 3-inch screen, with coded keys programmed to display diagnoses, outcomes, interventions, and so forth. The advantage of microprocessors is that the nurse can carry the unit in a pocket for immediate entry of medications, treatments, assessments, and evaluations. A disadvantage is that the nurse cannot see more than a few inches of text at a time. Storage for data is limited, and data from most microprocessors must be more frequently transferred into the computer to revise the care plan or add data to a patient's chart.

A new type of microprocessor is called a palmtop or pad. Many new models of pads will be available for use in 1993. Some models weigh only 1.2 lb and are held securely on the palm with an elastic strap. The screen is half the size of the first pen-based computers but large enough to conveniently view narrative text as data are reviewed or entered by pen.

PORTABLE COMPUTERS

The March 1992 issues of *Business Week* and *Fortune* magazines state that the portable pen and tablet computer would be the leading type of computer sales in the 1990s. The new notebook-size laptop computers are also becoming increasingly popular in business and health care settings.

The portable computer may revolutionize how nurses document patient care. Portable computers are used in home health care settings and in the acute care settings. Although the principle use is the same, portable computer systems in home care emphasize the benefits of data transmission over significant distances.

Portable computers in home health care. A progressive innovation in home care is the application of point-of-care computerized documentation. Small, handheld portable computers, laptop portable computers, and pen-based computers are three different types of hardware used in home care systems. Pen-based computers accept touch entry by pen of standard phrases, or the nurse can print with the pen right on the computer screen. Assessments, care plans, nursing notes, and Health Care Financing Administration (HCFA) forms 485, 486, and 487 are all computerized. Standardized text is windowed into the appropriate area on the required forms, and standardized care plans provide fast yet individualized care plans.

An exciting feature for home health care is the fast and easy modem transmission from agency to home and back, to relay information concerning the patient and updating the patient's files immediately. In addition, the nurse can modem information without travel time to come into the office, allowing time for another patient visit.

In home care, a portable computer system works in the following way. A nurse carries a portable computer in the visit bag. From the patient's home the nurse can immediately access the complete patient file from the home health agency office. The nurse can access past patient history and current patient information; obtain past visits and current visit instructions and medical orders; view other staff documentation for additional information; develop or update assessments, care plans, and interventions; and document visit notes according to agency format. Then the nurse can transmit the visit record and other current information to the agency office from the patient's home to immediately update the office patient file. The nurse can also transmit the information from home after all visits are made and documented into the portable computer.

Additionally, with an integrated system, the visit information is electronically transferred through the clinical management information system into a coordinated financial computer system without reentering information. An increasing number of systems have a management software program that interfaces with the clinical record system and generates statistics used in surveys, quality assurance, and research.

Home health care computerized clinical record systems attempt to alleviate five major problems in home health care documentation:

1. Amount of paperwork (time and effort) faced by staff nurses during their work day and after hours
2. Required content and phraseology for regulatory requirements, reimbursement, certification, accreditation, and legal protection
3. Evidence in the documentation system of a parallel to the nursing process, which supports clinical judgments that affect ultimate patient outcome(s)
4. Continuous access to updated patient data for coordination of care, for nursing judgments in patient care, and for judgments in eligibility of care
5. Electronic transmission of data to fiscal intermediaries for more timely Medicare reimbursement, with fewer denials for payment

Portable computers in acute care or long-term care settings. Portable computers can be implemented at a lesser cost than bedside terminals. A bedside computer requires wiring in the hospital, a place in each patient's room where it can be built in or bolted down so it will not be knocked over, and a computer for each bed. In comparison, a portable computer requires no wiring, takes up no space in a crowded patient room, and the number of portable computers purchased can be according to the number of nurses working on the floor during any one shift.

In the hospital or nursing home setting the staff nurse can load data on a portable computer during nursing rounds and can download the information to the mainframe in one of three ways: by wireless LAN (radio waves), by a smart card reader, or by a direct cable. In the mainframe, that patient information can then be accessible to all appropriate departments within the facility.

Some proponents of bedside terminals versus portable computers are concerned about the ease of carrying the portable computer and potential for cross infection as the nurse goes from one room to the next. Further concerns include the potential for theft or damage by dropping the device or getting it wet.

Nursing Minimum Data Set

With computerization of the clinical record and the ability to transmit information from one care setting to another, questions arise as to what data should be included in the nursing portion of the patient clinical record. The nursing minimum data set (NMDS) is an effort to establish standards for the collection of uniform, minimum, essential nursing data. The precedent for national health data standards is set by the uniform minimum health data set (UMHDS), and the NMDS is patterned after the UMHDS with an emphasis on nursing data.

> A **nursing minimum data set** may be defined as a minimum set of items of information, with uniform definitions and categories concerning the specific dimension of professional nursing, which meets the information needs of multiple data users in the health care system. . . . The primary purpose of the NMDS is to establish comparability of nursing data across clinical populations, settings, geographic areas, and time. . . . Reliable, timely and comparable data are needed a) to describe the health status of various populations in reference to nursing care needs; b) to investigate the nursing diagnosis and treatment of human responses to health problems; and c) to investigate the outcomes and management of nursing care, as well as the use and costs of nursing resources. Improved quality of care will be possible with the availability of better, more precise data. (Werley, Lang, & Westlake, 1986)

With a carefully defined and standardized system of data collection, large groups of data from various sources and health delivery settings can be compared and analyzed (see display, Elements of the Nursing Minimum Data Set). This possibility contributes to progress in assessing and diagnosing patient status and planning, managing, and evaluating patient care.

According to Werley, Devine, and Zorn (1988), NMDS has many benefits.

1. Insights and knowledge derived from the accumulated data will contribute to the development of the profession and improve the provision of health care.
2. Accurate and standardized comparisons of daily care from different settings contribute toward the data base for research.

ELEMENTS OF THE NURSING MINIMUM DATA SET

Nursing Care Elements

Nursing Diagnosis
Nursing Intervention
Nursing Outcome
Intensity of Nursing Care

Patient or Client Demographic Elements

Personal Identification*
Date of Birth*
Sex*
Race and Ethnicity*
Residence*

Service Elements

Unique Facility or Service Agency Number*
Unique Health Record Number of Patient or Client
Unique Number of Principal Registered Nurse Provider
Episode Admission or Encounter Date*
Discharge or Termination Date*
Disposition of Patient or Client*
Expected Payor for Most of this Bill (anticipated financial guarantor for services)*

*Elements comparable to those in the Uniform Hospital Discharge Data Set
(Reprinted with permission from Harriet Werley, PhD, RN, and from Leski, JS & Werley, HH. (1992). Use of nursing minimum data set, *Computers in Nursing* (November–December 1992) p. 260.

3. Staffing and costing nursing services can be a result of analyzing associations of intensity of care, nursing interventions, and outcomes.
4. The data base can be used in health care issues, shaping health care policies and laws.
5. Evaluation of data in different settings can lead to new and innovative models of practice.
6. Quality assurance endeavors will be enhanced with the result of improved patient care.

Learning a Computerized Nursing Information System

A nurse can begin by looking at an overview of the system, what forms are included in the clinical record, what is the flow of data, and where data are shared into another part of the clinical record. The nurse should read how to care for the hardware; learn the software screen progression and how to move from one screen to another; learn what the icons or processing buttons mean; learn how to avoid common errors; and watch a demonstration of what to do or whom to call when an error is made or a problem occurs. The best method of learning how to use a computerized information system is to participate in a formal training program followed by supervised practice, before using the NIS on the nursing unit.

KEY POINTS

▲ The clinical record is an integrated set of component forms on which multidisciplinary caregivers document patient needs, problems, plans of care, interventions, teaching, and outcomes.

▲ Nursing-related patient information in a clinical record is documented within basic categories of forms of assessment or data base forms, care plan forms, nursing or progress note forms, and continuity of care forms.

▲ Standardized forms, especially in a flow sheet format, allow for more frequent documentation of assessments and interventions in a format in which data are more easily compared and retrieved than traditional narrative charting.

▲ Computerization of the clinical data has the advantages of legibility, improved quality of data collection, accuracy and timeliness of data entry, consistency of data assessment and intervention, standardized terminology and protocols, ease of data retrieval, and fast interdepartmental communication.

▲ Nursing involvement in the design and development of standards in nursing information systems is essential.

▲ The physician and multidisciplinary caregivers provide and document care in their specialty areas. The nurse in nursing documentation records the response of the patient to disease and treatment and the outcomes of care provided.

REFERENCES

American Nurses Association (1989). Nurses resource directory. *American Nurse* (suppl.), June.

Collins, v. Westlake Community Hospital, 57Ill-2d388, 312 N.E. 2d614. (1974). In Guido, Ginny, JD, MSN, RN. *Legal issues in nursing*. Norwalk, CN: Appleton & Lange, 1988. p. 99.

Cox, H., Harsanyi, B., Dean, L. (1987). *Computers in nursing* (pp. 140, 144–146). Norwalk, CT: Appleton & Lange, citing

J. L. Manzano, J. Villalobos, A. Church, & J. J. Manzano (1980). Computerized information system for ICU patient management. *Critical Care Medicine, 8*, 745–747.

McCloskey, J. C., & Bulechek, G. M. (Eds.). (1992). *Nursing Interventions Classifications* (*NIC*). St. Louis: Mosby-Year Book.

Saba, V., & McCormick, K. (1986). *Essentials of computers for nurses* (p. 120). Philadelphia: J. B. Lippincott.

Scholes, M., Bryant, Y., & Barber, B. (1983). *The impact of computers in nursing: An international review* (p. 87). New York: Elsevier Science Publishing.

Werley, H. H., Devine, E. C., & Zorn, C. R. (1988). Nursing needs its own minimum data set. *American Journal of Nursing, 88*, 1652–1653.

Werley, H. H., Lang, N. M., & Westlake, S. K. (1986). Brief summary of the nursing minimum data set conference. *Nursing Management, 17*(7), 42.

Zielstorff, R. 143, citing J. Gluck (1979). The computerized medical system: Meeting the challenge for nursing. *Journal of Nursing Administration, 9*(12), 17–24.

BIBLIOGRAPHY

Abrami, P., & Johnson, J. E. (1990). *Bringing computers to the hospital bedside*. New York: Springer.

Albarado, R. S., McCall, V., & Thrane, J. M. (1990). Computerized nursing documentation. *Nursing Management, 21*(7), 64–65.

Arnold, J. M., & Pearson, G. A. (1992). *Computer applications in nursing and practice*. New York: National League for Nursing.

Brennan, M. V. (1991). Computerization is possible in rural hospitals! *Nursing Management, 22*(5), 56–60.

Faaoso, N. (1990). Automated patient care systems: The ethical impact. *Nursing Management, 21*(7), 46–48.

Lower, M., & Nauert, L. (1990). Charting: The impact of bedside computers. *Nursing Management, 21*(7), 40–44.

Meyer, C. (1992). Bedside computer charting: Inching toward tomorrow. *American Journal of Nursing, 92*, 38–44.

Perry, W., & Mornhinweg, G. C. (1990). Nursing practice: Promoting computer literacy. *Nursing Management, 21*(7), 49–52.

Schlehofer, G. B. (1990). Informatics: Managing clinical operations data. *Nursing Management, 21*(7), 36–38.

Simpson, R. L. (1992). What nursing leaders are saying about technology. *Nursing Management, 23*(7), 28–32.

Sinclair, V. (1991). The impact of information systems on nursing performance and productivity. *Journal of Nursing Administration, 21*(2), 46–50.

▬ PRACTICE SESSION ▬

FILL IN

1. A basic "snapshot" of a nursing care plan is a _____ .

2. As patients sometimes move quickly among levels of care, which form greatly enhances the next phase of care? _____ .

3. The newest type of nursing documentation form is an _____ .

4. Key components of nursing documentation include assessments, nursing diagnoses, planned care, nursing interventions, patient teaching, patient outcomes, and _____ .

5. Six purposes of documentation include _____

_____

_____

6. Progress notes can be documented as narrative nursing notes or can be documented on

_____ .

7. Vital signs or other measurements can be plotted on a graph to show _____ .

8. _____ can be included in the care plan, or it can be a separate document.

9. Standardized forms include key words, phrases, or questions for the purpose of

_____ .

10. The abbreviation NIS stands for _____ .

MATCHING

For each item in Column A, identify what form(s) of a clinical record in Column B an item would be found:

1. ____ initial vital signs	**a.** Kardex
2. ____ prescribed daily medications	**b.** medication order record, and MAR
3. ____ physical therapy progress notes	**c.** nursing care plan
4. ____ diet	**d.** admission record
5. ____ CAT scan findings	**e.** medical history, nursing history
6. ____ history of allergies	**f.** Kardex, plan of care medical orders
7. ____ chief complaint	**g.** nursing assessment
8. ____ teaching plans	**h.** test results data
9. ____ ECG findings	**i.** specialty progress notes
10. ____ pattern of vital signs	**j.** medical history, nursing history
11. ____ altered respiratory status	**k.** test results data
12. ____ advanced directives	**l.** intake record
13. ____ speech therapy goals	**m.** specialty care plan and progress notes
14. ____ functional limitations	**n.** graph flow sheet
15. ____ past illnesses	**o.** plan of care

MULTIPLE CHOICE

1. _____ Medical orders for how a dressing change should be done will be noted on the
   a) Kardex
   b) teaching plan
   c) progress notes
   d) all of the above

2. _____ The key document that indicates the current medication ordered for a patient is the
   a) medical order record
   b) medication administration record
   c) nursing history
   d) progress notes

3. _____ Evaluation of a patient's care is documented on
   a) outcome reports and progress summaries
   b) transfer forms and discharge summaries
   c) a & b
   d) revised care plans

4. _____ To begin making discharge plans for a patient who cannot manage care, a nurse should first
   a) refer to social service
   b) look on the intake form to see if the patient lives alone or has had someone to give care in the past
   c) ask the doctor who will care for the patient at home
   d) watch and see who comes to visit the patient

5. _____ Progress notes include
   a) patient condition and complaints
   b) identified problems
   c) nursing interventions and patient response to care
   d) all of the above

CHALLENGE FOR CRITICAL THINKING

1. Discuss three advantages and three disadvantages of flow sheets. How would you work to minimize the disadvantages you have cited?

2. Discuss four advantages and four disadvantages of computerized documentation. If appropriate, cite personal experience(s) to support your advantages/disadvantages. In your discussion of disadvantages, identify methods that could be used to change them into advantages.

3. You can safely assume that computers will become standard equipment in health care settings. If you are not currently "comfortable" using computers, what steps can you take to learn how to use a computerized clinical record system?

4. Is nursing documentation just another nursing task or is it an area of responsibility and accountability? How is nursing documentation related to the nursing process? Why is that important for effective care?

5. Now that you have completed this chapter, what purpose of nursing documentation in the clinical record appears to be of primary importance in terms of administering quality care?

LEARNING TO DOCUMENT

Case Study

Mrs. Cora Andrews, aged 45, was found on the floor by her husband when he arrived home from work at 6:45 pm. She could not tell him how she fell to the floor. He called their family internist, Dr. John Morris (telephone 100-1111) who recommended calling a rescue squad to take her to the hospital. On arrival at 8:00 pm, her blood pressure is 80/50, apical pulse 62, respirations 14, and temperature 39°C. Her blood sugar was 54.

She has a 10-year history of diabetes mellitus (DM) and has been insulin dependent the last 4 years; before that, she was controlled by diet, then Diabenase. Lately she has been very anxious about money matters because her husband might lose his job. Her anxiety has caused her to lose interest in eating; thus, she has lost 20 lbs over the last 2 months, and now weighs 145 lb. Mrs. A. has no problems with communication, sensory deficits, bowel or bladder elimination, or respiration. She has no known allergies (NKA).

She is admitted to room 234 bed 2 on an endocrinology division. Over the next 3 days, her a.m. vital signs have been the following: blood pressure readings: 90/60, 96/64, and 100/66; oral temperature: 37, 38, and 36; pulse: 72, 80, 68; respirations: 14, 16, 18. FBS for each day has been 124, 136, and 100, that was below 200 at which her doctor wanted to be notified. She maintained her preadmission insulin dosage of 25 U humulin insulin. She remained on a 1600 ADA diet, and was ordered to drink 64 oz fluids per day. Her primary nurse discussed the importance of eating regular meals every day and told her that increased fluids would even help her dry skin.

Mrs. A. does not have a living will, but her condition is not terminal. Her doctor ordered FBS everyday with no eating (NPO) after midnight. He told her she could be out of bed (OOB) as much as she could tolerate but should walk with someone so she doesn't fall (faint) again. He said she could take a shower if she sits on a shower stool and waits till after breakfast. A social worker came 3/25 to discuss sources of anxiety, and a referral to a home health agency was made. Following an uneventful 3 days, she was discharged.

1. Based on this situation, what data should be included in the nursing history?

2. Using the above patient data, fill out the sample Kardex on page 68 with as much information as you can gather, analyze, and synthesize. A negative response can be documented -0- and N/A can be used for not applicable.

3. Document the above patient's vital signs on the sample vital sign graph on page 69. Graph the temperature to determine if she is febrile or afebrile on the third day.

SAMPLE KARDEX

Vital signs
  Temp O R AX
  B/P
  Pulse & resp
		Respiratory care	

Resuscitation Status—CPR? Living Will?		Diet Fluids	
Notify physician if...		Weight	
Sensory deficit		Treatments	
Communication method and barriers		I & O	
Safety measures		Consult/Regarding Date	
Activity		Referrals Date	
Hygiene care Time preference		Isolation	Date order: Date stop:
Bowel continence		Bladder continence	
Assistance needed in ADL		Skin care	

DIAGNOSTIC TESTS

Date Ordered	Test	Schedule Date	Preparation

Allergies _____

Diagnoses _____

Physician _____ Phone _____

Name _____ Room _____ Bed _____

SAMPLE VITAL SIGNS GRAPH

Date																									
TEMP. F° C°	0400	0800	1200	1600	2000	2400	0400	0800	1200	1600	2000	2400	0400	0800	1200	1600	2000	2400	0400	0800	1200	1600	2000	2400
105.8° 41°																								
104° 40°																								
102.2° 39°																								
100.4° 38°																								
98.6° 37°																								
96.8° 36°																								
95° 35°																								
Pulse																								
Respirations																								
Blood Pressure																								

Documenting Assessments

LEARNING OBJECTIVES

After studying this chapter, the learner should be able to:

▲ Explain documented assessment as the first step in documentation of the nursing process.

▲ Explain the importance of the collection of accurate data in clinical decision-making.

▲ Identify components of a nursing assessment: nursing history and physical assessment.

▲ List sources of data used in documenting assessments.

▲ Define key terms as applied to nursing assessments.

▲ Describe the characteristics and purpose(s) of an accurate, concise assessment.

▲ List specific data to collect for assessments in specialty area situations, assessments of certain types of patients, and assessments for high risk of falls and pressure sores.

KEY TERMS

Clustering data
Individualize
Nursing assessment
Nursing history

Nursing model
Objective data
Patient population

Physical examination
Subjective data
Verification of data

Eggland ET, Heinemann DS. NURSING DOCUMENTATION:
CHARTING, RECORDING, AND REPORTING.
© 1994 J.B. Lippincott Company.

The assessment phase of the nursing process is the first step in the problem-solving process for identifying patient and family needs and providing care to eliminate or resolve those needs. During assessment, clinical decision-making based on a nurse's knowledge and expertise guides data investigation by simultaneously clustering similar data. Analysis of assessment data, then, is the basis for determining a nursing diagnosis. A nursing diagnosis determines direction and provision of care by means of a care plan. If accurate, pertinent assessment data are collected and documented, a patient receives appropriate care. If assessment data are not verified, documented, or sufficient, patient care is compromised.

The importance of the initial assessment as a basis for providing care is evident in that most health care organizations require an assessment to be completed within a specific time following admission. Depending on the *acuity* of the patient, how acutely ill a person is, that time limit can be as little as 15 minutes in a recovery room or as long as 24 hours in home health care.

Nursing assessment is the process of collecting all pertinent data regarding the condition of a patient and patient-identified problems and needs. Assessment also includes collecting data regarding the related strengths of a patient, such as coping ability and problem-solving or self-care skills. Finally, the assessment includes current and past health care management information regarding a patient during an episode of illness or injury or during a period of wellness. Data are collected from a patient's previous health record, current health history, during a physical examination, and by examining test results. Data are also received from interviews with the patient, family, and caregivers.

An initial assessment is documented when a patient is admitted for care at a health care organization. Because assessment is ongoing, information will be added to a patient record as more data are collected. A nurse will gather and document more information as the nurse–patient relationship develops, as contact with the patient increases over a period of time, and as new needs and problems arise.

Purpose and Use of Assessment

The purpose of a documented assessment is to provide a pertinent collection of patient data to determine nursing diagnoses and patient strengths to plan effective nursing care. In addition, an assessment may be used as:

- A core of reference information regarding a patient and family
- A basis for determining patient diagnoses

- A source of information to help diagnose new problems as they arise
- Support for clinical decisions in establishing expected outcomes and proposed interventions
- A basis for determining learning needs of the patient, family, and caregivers
- A basis for determining discharge needs
- A basis for determining eligibility for care and reimbursement
- Support for protection of legal rights
- A component of patient acuity systems

Determining discharge needs. Assessment data provide information to the nurse or social service agency to determine patient resources to manage care after discharge. Financial resources, caregiver's availability, past coping skills, and environmental and equipment needs are a few of the topics included in assessments that will be used for discharge planning.

Eligibility for care and reimbursement. Assessment information is also used as a basis for determining eligibility for care and sometimes reimbursement for care. For example, if assessment data do not support the need for skilled nursing care, Medicare will not pay reimbursement. In care reimbursed by Medicare or insurance, when a "no skilled care" determination is made before care is provided, a patient is determined ineligible for care. If that determination is made after care has begun, then reimbursement is denied and the health care organization receives no remuneration for service provided. To avoid reimbursement denials and disrupted care of a patient, documented assessments and reassessments are important in determining and supporting initial and continued needs for care.

Protection of legal rights. Assessment information is used for legal protection or liability. Documented assessments can be used in a court of law to show that all appropriate data were collected and considered in diagnosis, care planning, and care evaluation, and that assessment data were available or communicated to all caregivers. Assessments are important in legal protection for a nurse and health care organization. The following case shows how the omission of reassessment documentation protects the right of the patient to appropriate care.

A woman was admitted to the hospital for delivery of her 13th child. Pitocin was administered. The mother testified that no one monitored her contractions for 2 hours. She experienced a sharp pain in her abdomen, the child's oxygen supply was compromised, and the child was born with cerebral palsy. The chart did not reflect any observation or assessment during that time. The jury awarded $350,000 to the child. (*Long v. Johnson*, 1978)

If the contractions had been monitored and so documented in the chart, the nurses would have been legally protected. Lack of assessment documentation in this case determined liability.

An assessment provides a documentation source to investigate if the condition of a patient justified cause for concern for high-risk injuries or health complications. The following case points out a problem.

A woman was admitted to the hospital with bursitis in her right knee. She put her call light on to obtain assistance in walking to the bathroom. When no one responded, she attempted to walk alone, fell, and injured her back. It was foreseeable that the patient, when no one answered her call, might fall while walking. The patient received an award of $30,594. (*Newhall v. Central Vermont Hospital*, 1975)

Assessment information in this case supported the potential for injury caused by pain and altered mobility. Nurses were accountable to respond for help and should have done so. But if a nurse had documented in the assessment that instruction had been given to the patient to avoid ambulating alone, the outcome may have been different.

Patient acuity use. Finally, assessment forms can be designed for patient acuity determination, by assigning numerical values to certain levels of care needed for activities of daily living. By determining patient acuity, nurse managers can determine staffing and cost of nursing care. With staffing shortage and nursing interest in establishing costs for nursing, the use of assessment data for patient acuity will become more widely used in practice.

Components of a Nursing Assessment

In the American Nurses Association (ANA) *Standards of Clinical Nursing Practice*, the first standard states that "The priority of data collection is determined by the client's immediate condition or needs" (American Nurses Association, 1991, p. 9).

In determining what to assess, a nurse should note:

▲ Patient health care needs, problems, and complaints
▲ Potential complications related to physical condition or psychological state

▲ Patient and family learning needs
▲ Family relationships, caregiving capability, and willingness to provide care
▲ Patient and family resources
▲ Pertinent factors to consider for discharge planning

Almost every health care organization has a slightly different method for documenting an assessment. In any method, however, usually two components are required: a *nursing history* and a *physical examination*. The **nursing history** is information obtained by interview from a patient or family; it includes past and present health problems and health care and current symptoms. Data recorded in the nursing history focus on issues related to nursing care. The **physical examination** component includes objective data recorded as a direct result of nurse observation, auscultation, and palpation during assessment. Some organizations have separate history and physical examination documentation forms, whereas some organizations combine the history and physical examination components into a single assessment form.

Nursing History Data Base

A nursing history is a means of gathering information about a patient's health status, health care history, and past coping related to self-care and changes in life-style. A nursing history conducted by a professional nurse usually includes the following information:

▲ Patient's past hospitalizations
▲ Surgical history
▲ Past and present health problems
▲ Allergies
▲ Review of systems to identify problems, learning needs, psychosocial needs
▲ Functional limitations and capabilities in assisted or independent activities of daily living
▲ Changes in life-style due to illness or treatment regimen
▲ Alcohol, drug, and tobacco use
▲ Perception of illness
▲ Information regarding care and caregivers at home
▲ Expectation of treatments and medical/nursing care
▲ Perception of patient self-involvement and responsibility in care

Most assessment forms cue for documentation of subjective and objective data. **Subjective data** is information a patient tells a nurse, which cannot be verified easily. For example, a patient complains of pain and describes it. A nurse cannot measure the pain. **Objective data** is information that can be measured, seen, heard, touched, or smelled by a nurse and is verified easily.

Subjective data can sometimes be verified by objective data. For example, a complaint of pain around a surgical wound can be potentially verified by observing and feeling the surrounding wound area, which is red, has drainage, and is warm to the touch. The **verification of data** is accomplished by first **clustering data**, putting similar types of information together. A nurse collects and determines its relationship to see if it fits together to support a conclusion. In this case, subjective and objective data point to an actual infection, which indeed can cause pain. Verification of data also includes obtaining consistent information from more than one source of information. A family caregiver can describe the past appearance of the wound, and a lab report can indicate the presence of infection following a culture of the drainage.

Subjective data need to be documented as such. Statements should begin with "Patient (or family) states . . . "; data should be as measurably descriptive as possible. For example, when documenting pain, report what a patient states the pain level is, on a scale from 1 to 10. Even objective data must be documented on the assessment in measurable terms. For example, instead of "patient voiding frequently," a nurse should document "voided × 4 from 4:00 to 4:30, 200 mL light amber foul-smelling urine, no evidence of sediment. Pt c/o burning on urination." Accurate and detailed documentation provides more information, which contributes to diagnoses and clinical judgments.

A meaningful history can shape a subsequent assessment, care plan, and the care itself. It is also important in evaluating effectiveness of care. The history does not work alone, however. A physical examination includes nursing inspection (seen, smelled), auscultation (heard), and palpation/percussion (felt). A nursing history followed by a physical examination will verify assessment data to determine health or illness.

Physical Examination

When nursing physical examination records are separate, they are written in either a head-to-toe format or a systems format, some with front and back torsos pictured for illustrative drawing. If a nurse completing an assessment has limited time, or a patient tires easily, start with the system involved with the diagnosis, such as cardiovascular, then go to related systems such as respiratory, then mobility if arthritis is a secondary diagnosis. When documenting physical examination findings, as in the assessment, make important notes for reminders, then complete the form, or write the complete form away from the patient. Write both positive and negative findings, but avoid general, relative terms such as normal, abnormal, good, fair, satisfactory, and poor. Be specific about what is observed, inspected, palpated, auscultated, and percussed.

The Complement of History and Physical Examination

By obtaining a history before the physical examination, a nurse can seek specific signs and symptoms that should be investigated during the physical examination. This sequence aids the subsequent diagnostic process as well as care planning and discharge planning. An accurate, complete history of a patient with cardiac disease, coupled with a physical examination, may lead a nurse to an assessment that learning needs are evident to prevent pending congestive heart failure. Also, history interview questions followed by pertinent physical examination data may indicate a previously undiagnosed or unexpected problem. Consider the following example.

Mrs. M, a 35-year-old woman with rheumatoid arthritis, complains of dizziness, fatigue, and joint pain. From comments about feeling inadequate to care for two preschool children and feeling like a burden on family members, a nurse considers the possibility that Mrs. M is also depressed.

Fatigue, joint pain, and depression are common symptoms of rheumatoid arthritis, but dizziness is not. What then, is its cause? In this case a nurse can quickly rule out medication, which is a frequent cause; the patient was taking only small amounts of aspirin and daily multivitamins. Other possible causes include a psychogenic cause such as anxiety, hyperventilation, hypochondriasis, and depression. Dizziness can also be caused by metabolic disorders such as hypoxia, hyperglycemia or hypoglycemia, anemia, uremia, and hepatic encephalopathy. Cardiovascular problems, too, are a major source of dizziness—postural hypotension, arrhythmias, congestive heart failure, or aortic stenosis. Mrs. M had no history of heart, circulatory, liver, or kidney problems, or of a hereditary link with diabetes. Nor did current information from her physician mention any of these.

Still, when documenting a nursing history, a nurse tries to establish what initiated this feeling of dizziness. Did it occur after a position change? Before or after meals? In response to an anxious situation? A nurse should ask questions about chronology, setting, aggravating or alleviating factors, and associated manifestations. The conversation before documentation may resemble the following example.

Nurse: Mrs. M, what does this dizziness feel like?

Patient: Lightheadedness. Then I lose my balance.

Nurse: How often do you experience this feeling?

Patient: Four or five times a day.

Nurse: When was the first episode?

Patient: About 2 years ago, after I delivered my

last child. I just never felt right again—tired, achy, and occasionally dizzy.

Nurse: You started having the dizziness 2 years ago?

Patient: Yes, and ever since then.

Nurse: Any particular time of the day or week?

Patient: No, not that I've noticed.

Nurse: Does there seem to be any activity that sets off this dizziness?

Patient: No.

Nurse: What were you doing when you had the last dizzy spell?

Patient: Playing with my 2-year-old daughter on the bed.

Nurse: Had you just sat up or in any way changed position?

Patient: No, I don't think so. (Pause.) I was sitting with her, cutting out paper dolls.

Nurse: How were you feeling emotionally at the time?

Patient: Happy, contented, and engrossed in play.

Nurse: What time was it?

Patient: About 3 pm.

Nurse: What had you done during the hour before your play–eaten or taken any medication?

Patient: No, I ate at noon and took my aspirin then.

Nurse: And what did you do when you felt dizzy?

Patient: I lay down and ate a candy bar that I kept in my bedstand for snacking.

Nurse: Then how did you feel?

Patient: A lot better after the candy bar.

Nurse: Do you feel hunger or any other symptoms along with the dizziness?

Patient: Yes, now that you mention it. The dizziness seems to occur after I haven't eaten for a few hours. I feel a little hungry, then very weak, and I seem to shake all over. (Pause.) It seems to be relieved when I eat crackers or candy.

Now the interview is pointing to the possibility of a new diagnosis (which the physician will have to make)—hypoglycemia. Until the physician can examine a patient and order lab tests, a nursing physical examination should include blood pressures in both arms in supine and standing positions, a cardiopulmonary auscultation with focus on the heart rate and rhythm, and a check for any sign of respiratory insufficiency.

The nurse would record the previous information on a nursing history (see display, Applied Nursing History Excerpt).

One month later, the patient reported no dizziness, but she had gained 5 pounds. The physician had indeed diagnosed hypoglycemia. Mrs. M was counseled by a nutritionist and instructed in a dietary regimen with good results and weight control.

General Assessment Forms

Many types of assessment forms are available. The format or design used for documenting an assessment is determined by the health care organization. Sometimes different assessment forms are used within a single hospital. The need for different forms is due to special assessment needs in specialty areas such as intensive care units and pediatrics or in short-term care areas such as the emergency department and day surgery.

An initial assessment form is sometimes called a nursing admission form, a data base, initial nursing assessment, or admission assessment. Depending on an organization's documentation procedure, a nurse will also record assessment information on a reassessment form, ongoing assessment flow sheet, or in nursing progress notes. Another tool for collecting assessment data is a patient questionnaire, on which a patient completes checklists and comment areas regarding past and present health status.

A reassessment form is an abbreviated form cued so the nurse can gather data that may have changed since an initial assessment. Daily flow sheets can be used for a frequent assessment, and data can be compared quickly for ease in assessing patient changes. An example is a neurologic assessment flow sheet that shows documentation of neurologic status, such as change in level of consciousness and response. Another example is a reassessment form in home health care. Completed every 30 days, the assessment shows a change in functional ability, such as urinary incontinence or mobility.

Assessment data can be multidimensional because of the holistic nature and needs of a patient and family. With some nursing assessment forms, collection of initial assessment data is a broad spectrum of general, multidimensional topics. This method results in a general holistic view of the patient and family, their strengths, weaknesses, or barriers in adjusting to illness or a change in life-style. Nursing assessment forms can use the framework of general multidimensional areas; can be focused on health care problems, body systems, or functional abilities; or can be oriented to a particular health care setting, type of patient, or patients at risk for injury.

Different from a general initial assessment, another type of nursing assessment focuses on a specific type of

APPLIED NURSING HISTORY EXCERPT

Chief complaint:

☑ dizziness ☐ joint pain ☐ fatigue

Tremors 2-1/2 to 3 hrs after eating 4 to 5 times a day. Possibility of hypoglycemia. Will see doctor on Thursday 11/26

Further in the nursing history, it would be important to check systems:

Circulatory: ✓

No diff. ____✓____   Edema _____

Numbness _____   Cyanosis _____

Anemia _____   Bruising _____

Chest pain _____   Palpitations _____

Cong. defect _____

Comments: _____

Neurologic: ✓

No diff. ____✓____   Incoordination _____

Convulsions _____   Paralysis _____

Paresthesia _____

Comments: _____

Gastrointestinal:

Nutrition:

No diff. ____✓____   Appetite *good*

Adeq. food ____✓____   Adeq. fluid *6-7 glasses*

Diet *Reg c̄ ↑ carbohydrate*

Meal pattern *3 bal. meals, 4 snacks*

Comments: *No history of malabsorption*

Elimination:

No diff. ✓   Stool *q 2-3 days, brown, formed*

Comments: _____

(Information interpreted from the assessment would be incorporated into the patient's care plan.)

Patient Problems or Needs

dizziness

Approach

Encourage Mrs. M to report dizziness to MD, noting times, duration and pre-activity to dizziness, and if symptom was relieved by eating, sitting or lying down. Instruct Mrs. M in ambulation with assistance to prevent falls, and to lower self slowly to floor if dizzy while standing. Encourage high protein rather than high carbohydrate meals with snacks q2h. RN to contact MD for special diet.

(Reprinted with permission from the July issue of *Nursing 77.* © 1977, Springhouse Corp., 1111 Bethlehem Pike, Springhouse, PA. 1977. All rights reserved.)

data. This specific type of assessment uses a form with a particular primary focus, for example, related-symptom data grouped to coordinate with common nursing diagnoses listed in the same section. This facilitates choosing nursing diagnoses. Some forms list body systems and symptoms in a traditional format, which coordinates with medical and anatomy and physiology separation of function. Functional assessment formats present fast reference for what assistance patients need in activities of daily living. Specialty area formats designed for a particular health care setting are generally used only in that area. For example, if a patient is being admitted to day surgery, an initial assessment form will only include information staff need to know to provide safe care during and after surgery, to assess learning needs, and to provide discharge planning for home care. A shorter assessment for day care surgery is a cost-effective way to collect information to plan short-term care. Specific patient population-oriented forms can focus on a particular type of patient, such as a pediatric, geriatric, or psychiatric patient. In an assessment for injury format, a form can be used to document the risk of a complication for a patient population. Examples are an assessment for falls for geriatric patients or assessment for skin pressure areas for bedbound patients.

Types of Assessment Forms

Regulations requiring certain content in documentation and assessment data have resulted in assessment forms becoming specifically standardized. Pertinent content is defined for faster and more thorough data collection.

OPEN-ENDED FORM

Assessment forms traditionally have been open-ended, in which a nurse writes original narrative to describe the medical and nursing history of a patient. Most open-ended assessment forms list a topic of information to collect, followed by lines to write a free-form narrative. Open-ended forms have the advantage of being able to quickly individualize information by writing specific complaints and symptoms in the patient's own words.

Disadvantages are that each nurse asks different questions so questions are not standardized, pertinent questions are often omitted, and writing narrative takes more time than using a checklist or cued format.

CUED OR CHECKLIST FORM

The cued or checklist format is a contemporary standardized format in which a nurse writes a check mark beside symptoms or fills in one or two words in answer to a cue or question. Cued or checklist assessment forms provide not only the category of information to be collected but also list common problems or symptoms that should be asked of a patient. For example, in a body systems model the respiratory category on an assessment can have space to check off the following symptoms: no difficulty; pain; dyspnea; cough; sputum; sinusitis; epistaxis; frequent colds; last chest x-ray with results.

Advantages of cued or checklist forms are that assessments are standardized. Each patient is asked the same questions, and pertinent questions are not inadvertently omitted. A checklist format lists common problems to be considered. Data entry is fast, as only a check mark is needed beside a symptom, instead of writing narrative. Finally, a comment section after each category allows room for narrative to describe or clarify findings and to **individualize** an assessment, which is documenting information specific to that patient.

INTEGRATED CUED/CHECKLIST FORM

A type of integrated cued/checklist assessment form is a form's integration of assessment data with identification of nursing diagnoses. This type of assessment/nursing diagnoses identification facilitates the progression of steps within the nursing process. It has the advantages of clustering data to facilitate clinical judgment; focusing on data that establish and support nursing diagnoses; ensuring correct, consistent, and acceptable nursing diagnoses labels; and combining an assessment and problem list into one form. This particular assessment form also has the advantage of integrating data collection by different levels of caregivers, while carefully indicating on the form which sections may be completed by registered nurses, licensed practical nurses, or nursing care assistants (see display, Nursing Admission Assessment, Duke University Medical Center).

Use of an Assessment Form

Even if a nurse is using an assessment form checklist, questions should not be asked in a rote manner during an interview. In reviewing body systems, if a nurse asks a patient, "Do you have blurring, double vision, cataracts, or glaucoma?" a patient will probably consider only these problems. But an open-ended question such as, "How are your eyes and your vision?" will keep the interview focused on concerns rather than checklist categories. Then a patient can give more thought before answering.

When a patient's answer is, "No difficulty," a nurse can follow with a brief review of common problems: "No cataracts, nearsightedness, or glaucoma?" When the answer is again "No," go on to the next area. Ideally, the patient should not realize questions are being asked according to a checklist.

When collecting data on an assessment form, the nurse should be aware of information already documented in the clinical record and avoid extensive repetition of questions covering information already obtained from another reliable health source or discipline. The nurse should merely verify the information. Patients can become anxious or angry if they think an interviewer is going to repeat all the questions asked by another caregiver. If verification, and thus repetition is necessary, reassure the patient by explaining that clarification is needed.

A nurse can use spaces provided within the checklist in various ways: with a check (✔) indicating the presence of a symptom, or a notation, such as, "Appetite good." A dash (−) or a "no" in a space would indicate a symptom is not present. An organization's policy and procedure manual will present guidelines on appropriate entries. When there is insufficient room to document information, use the comment area.

A comment section at the end of every checklist gives space to record specific behaviors or symptoms whose presence (or absence) contribute toward diagnoses of patient needs. For example, a patient's appetite is checked as poor. The comment section includes a descriptive statement stating "patient is eating approx 50% of each meal and refusing between meal snacks, stating concern about gaining weight while hospitalized."

A comment section permits further explanations, circumstances, cause and effect relationships, and expanded descriptions of a problem or symptom. Descriptions should be complete. For example, documentation regarding pain should include whether the pain is dull, sharp, or radiating; location; onset; duration; what precipitates it; and what relieves it. Especially when documenting subjective information such as pain, the nurse should include the patient's own words and so indicate by using quotation marks. This method offers the most candid and accurate picture.

Another use of a comment section is to record how the patient is coping with a problem, whether the patient knows the diagnosis of a problem, the patient's understanding of a diagnosis or symptom, and whether advice is being followed.

Special Considerations in Documenting Assessments

Although a variety of information is documented during assessments, sometimes important general information is omitted. Clinical judgment will assist nurses to determine in what depth and detail special considerations should be included on assessments. The following key points apply to most assessments.

(text continues on page 83)

NURSING ADMISSION ASSESSMENT FORM—ADULT INTERMEDIATE CARE

DUKE UNIVERSITY MEDICAL CENTER
Nursing Admission Assessment
ADULT INTERMEDIATE CARE

Check only applicable boxes
Section I
General Admission Information
May be completed by RN, LPN, Nursing Care Assistant

Date: _____ Time arrived on unit: _____ am/pm

Age: _____ Sex: _____ Marital status: _____

Address: _____

_____

Person(s) to contact: **1.** _____ Relationship: _____ phone # _____

2. _____ Relationship: _____ phone # _____

Primary language: _____

Mode of Arrival:	**Accompanied by:**	**Arrived from:**	**Pre-admission tests?** ☐ NA
			(Check of completed)
☐ Ambulatory	☐ Family	☐ Home	
☐ Wheelchair	☐ Friend	☐ Nursing home	☐ Lab ☐ EKG
☐ Stretcher	☐ Ambulance staff	☐ Other hospital	☐ U/A ☐ X-ray
☐ Bed	☐ Self _____	☐ _____	☐ Other _____

Valuables:

	With Patient	Hospital Vault	Sent Home
Hearing aid	☐	☐	☐
Dentures/Upper	☐	☐	☐
Lower	☐	☐	☐
Glasses/Contacts	☐	☐	☐
_____	☐	☐	☐
_____	☐	☐	☐

Oriented to room/nursing unit
☐ Yes   ☐ No (reason) _____

_____

Vital Signs:

B/P _____ R Arm   ☐ Lying   ☐ Standing   ☐ Sitting   How obtained (cuff, arterial line, etc.) _____

_____ L Arm

Heart rate _____   Height _____ (cm/feet, inches) (actual/stated)

Respirations _____   Weight _____ (kg/lbs.) (actual/stated)

Temperature _____   Type of scale _____

Have you been in a hospital/health care facility in the last 15 days? ☐ No ☐ Yes, name of facility: _____

Allergies/Sensitivities (ie, medicine, food, dust, etc.)   ☐ None known

Source	Reaction
_____	_____
_____	_____

Section I completed by _____ Signature/Title _____ Date/Time

(If other than admitting RN)

(continued)

NURSING ADMISSION ASSESSMENT FORM—ADULT
INTERMEDIATE CARE (Continued)

Section II
Functional Health Patterns   Source of information: _____

Nonshaded areas completed by RN or LPN. Shaded areas completed by RN

HEALTH PERCEPTION/HEALTH MANAGEMENT PATTERN

1. What health problems or event caused you to come to the hospital? _____
_____

2. Preexisting conditions/previous surgeries, procedures: _____
_____
_____
_____
_____

3. Have you been exposed to any communicable diseases within the past year?   ☐ No   ☐ Yes (List) _____

4. Females: Is there a possibility you are pregnant?   ☐ No   ☐ Yes

5. Medication taken at home (prescription/over the counter drugs)

	Name	Dose/Frequency/Route	Time	Reason for Taking	Last Dose
1.					
2.					
3.					
4.					
5.					
6.					
7.					
8.					
9.					
10.					

Medications: ☐ Left at home   ☐ Sent home   ☐ _____

6. Do you experience any problems from your medications?   ☐ No   ☐ Yes, _____

What do you do about it? _____

7. Do you experience any problem buying/obtaining your medications/supplies?   ☐ No ☐ Yes

If yes, explain _____

8. Have you ever had a blood transfusion?   ☐ No   ☐ Yes   ☐ Reaction? (type) _____

9. Did you have the following health screenings done within the past year? (check if yes)

☐ breast self-exam   ☐ prostrate check   ☐ vision check
☐ mammogram   date _____   ☐ testicular check   ☐ glaucoma check
☐ pelvic exam/pap smear date _____ ☐ rectal check   ☐ dental exam

> **NURSING DIAGNOSIS:**
> ☐ Noncompliance
> ☐ High Risk for Injury
> ☐ Health-Seeking Behaviors
> (specify) _____
> ☐ Altered Health Maintenance
> ☐ Altered Protection
> ☐ Impaired Adjustment

10. Do you use tobacco?   ☐ No ☐ Yes   Years used _____   Amount per day _____   Form of tobacco _____

11. Do you use alcohol?   ☐ No ☐ Yes   Years used _____   Amount per day _____   Week _____

12. Do you use drugs?   ☐ No ☐ Yes   What drugs? _____   Amount _____   Frequency _____

(continued)

NURSING ADMISSION ASSESSMENT FORM—ADULT
INTERMEDIATE CARE *(Continued)*

NUTRITIONAL—METABOLIC PATTERN

1. Do you follow a special diet? ☐ No ☐ Yes, _____

2. When was the last time you ate? _____

3. Have you been asked to increase/restrict your fluid intake? ☐ No ☐ Yes _____
   Amount _____ /day

4. Appetite ☐ Normal ☐ Increased ☐ Decreased

5. Do you have difficulty with? ☐ No ☐ Choking ☐ Smell ☐ Chewing
   ☐ Swallowing ☐ Tasting ☐ Following diet
   Related to: _____

6. Do you have? ☐ No ☐ Nausea ☐ Vomiting
   ☐ Indigestion ☐ Weight loss/gain _____ lbs.
   ☐ Mouth soreness Time frame _____
   ☐ Persistent fever

7. Skin/Mucosa
   Color: ☐ Pink ☐ _____
   Temperature/Moisture: ☐ Warm ☐ Dry ☐ _____
   Turgor: ☐ Normal ☐ _____
   Edema: ☐ None ☐ Generalized ☐ Localized _____

8. Wounds/Drains/Tubes/Catheters/Dressings: ☐ None _____
   _____
   _____

☐	Fluid Volume Deficit _____
☐	Fluid Volume Excess
☐	Impaired Swallowing
☐	High Risk for Aspiration
☐	Altered Nutrition: Less Than Body Requirements
☐	Altered Nutrition: More Than Body Requirements
☐	Altered Oral Mucus Membrane
☐	High Risk for Altered Body Temperature
☐	Hypothermia
☐	Hyperthermia
**☐	Impaired Skin Integrity
**☐	Impaired Tissue Integrity
☐	High Risk for Infection
☐	_____

ELIMINATION PATTERN

1. Are you having any problems with bowel/bladder elimination? ☐ No
   ☐ Yes, describe _____

2. Abdomen: ☐ Flat ☐ Soft ☐ Nontender ☐ _____

3. Bowel sounds: ☐ Present ☐ Absent

4. Bladder: ☐ Nondistended ☐ Distended
   Comments: _____
   _____

☐	Constipation
☐	Diarrhea
☐	Bowel Incontinence
☐	Altered Patterns of Urinary Elimination
☐	Urinary Retention
☐	Total Incontinence
☐	Stress Incontinence
☐	_____

ACTIVITY EXERCISE PATTERN

1. Do you have enough energy for desired/required activities? ☐ Yes ☐ No

2. Do you need assistance with? ☐ NA
   ☐ Eating/Drinking ☐ Walking ☐ Sitting
   ☐ Toileting ☐ Getting up from bed/chair ☐ Preparing meals
   ☐ Bathing ☐ Stair climbing ☐ Shopping for food/Necessities
   ☐ Dressing ☐ Turning
   Comments: _____

3. Mobility Impairments ☐ None ☐ Unable to assess
   ☐ History of Falling ☐ Tremors/Spasms _____
   ☐ Dizziness ☐ Paralysis _____
   ☐ Unsteadiness/Balance ☐ Decreased Function _____
   ☐ Amputation _____ ☐ Numbness, Tingling, Burning _____
   ☐ Impaired Limb _____
   Gross Motor Movements:

	Normal	Abnormal	Comments: _____
Gain	☐	☐	_____
Posture	☐	☐	_____
ROM	☐	☐	

☐	Fatigue
☐	Activity Intolerance
☐	Self-Care Deficit (specify) _____
☐	Impaired Home Maintenance Management
☐	Impaired Physical Mobility
☐	High Risk for Disuse Syndrome
☐	High Risk for Injury
☐	_____
☐	_____

(continued)

NURSING ADMISSION ASSESSMENT FORM—ADULT
INTERMEDIATE CARE *(Continued)*

4. Do you use any assistive devices at home? ☐ No ☐ Yes

5. Respiratory Pattern: **6.** Cardiovascular Pattern:

☐ Regular ☐ Irregular   Rhythm _____

Breath Sounds: Heart Sounds _____

	R	L
☐ Clear	____	____
☐ Diminished	____	____
☐ Coarse/Rhonchi	____	____
☐ Crackles/Rales	____	____
☐ Wheezing	____	____
☐ Absent	____	____

Neck Veins Flat ☐   Distended ☐

Comments: _____

_____

_____

_____

_____

☐ Ineffective Airway Clearance
☐ Impaired Gas Exchange
☐ Ineffective Breathing Patterns
☐ Cardiac Output, Decreased
☐ Altered _____
Tissue Perfusion

SLEEP REST PATTERN ☐ N.A. for this admission
☐ Deferred

1. Have you had difficulty sleeping prior to admission?

☐ No ☐ If, yes, describe _____

☐ Sleep Pattern Disturbance

COGNITIVE–PERCEPTUAL PATTERN

A. 1. Level of Consciousness: ☐ Alert ☐ Oriented ☐ _____

B. ☐ Deferred

1. What is the highest grade in school you have completed? _____

2. Occupation: _____

3. Do you have problems with your memory? ☐ No ☐ Yes _____

4. Do you have any problems with your vision/hearing/speech?

☐ No ☐ Yes Describe: _____

5. Do you have any problem with your ability to feel pain, temperature? ☐ No ☐ Yes

Describe: _____

6. Have you ever had a seizure? ☐ No ☐ Yes How often? _____

Describe your seizure _____

When was your last seizure? _____

7. Do you have pain? ☐ No ☐ Yes

If yes, (type, duration, location) Describe: _____

_____

How do you get relief from your pain? _____

_____

8. What do you need to learn to be able to care for yourself after discharge? _____

_____

☐ Impaired Verbal Communication
☐ Sensory–Perceptual Alteration (specify) _____
☐ High Risk for Injury

☐ Pain
☐ Chronic Pain

☐ Knowledge Deficit
(specify) _____
_____

SELF-PERCEPTION PATTERN ☐ Deferred

1. What outcome do you expect from this hospitalization? _____

_____

Evidence of anxiety, fear? ☐ No ☐ Yes
If yes, ☐ Mild ☐ Moderate ☐ Severe

☐ Self-Concept Disturbance
☐ Body Image Disturbance
☐ Anxiety
☐ Fear

(continued)

NURSING ADMISSION ASSESSMENT FORM—ADULT
INTERMEDIATE CARE (Continued)

ROLE–RELATIONSHIP PATTERN

□ Altered Family Processes
□ Altered Role Performance
□ Impaired Social Interaction
□ Social Isolation

1. Lives   □ alone   □ with _____

2. Who will assist you with your care after discharge?

_____

3. Resides: □ House   □ Apartment   □ _____
4. Environmental/Safety concerns (stairs, inaccessible bathrooms, etc.)   □ none

   Describe: _____

SEXUALITY–REPRODUCTIVE PATTERN   □ NA for this Admission
                                      □ Deferred

□ Sexual Dysfunction
□ Altered Sexuality Patterns

1. Do you have any questions/concerns about the effects your physical condition/medications

   may have on your sexual activity?   □ No   □ Yes, _____

2. Females: Date of last menstrual period? _____

COPING–STRESS TOLERANCE PATTERN   □ NA for this Admission
                                      □ Deferred

□ Impaired Adjustment
□ Ineffective Individual Coping
□ _____

1. Have you had any recent major life-style changes?   □ No

   □ Yes, describe: _____

2. How do you deal with stressful situations?

_____

_____

_____

VALUE–BELIEF PATTERN

□ Spiritual Distress

1. Religious preference: _____
2. Are there any religious or cultural practices that may be affected by this hospitalization?

   □ No   □ Yes;   Describe: _____

_____

3. Would you like to see a Chaplain?   □ No   □ Yes
4. Advance Directives: MO123 reviewed for completion   □ Yes   □ No
   Has patient discussed Advance Directives with physician?   □ Yes   □ No
   Further actions, if applicable: □ patient given additional information   □ see progress notes

   □ patient referred to: □ social work   □ pastoral services   □ other, _____

Section II Date Collected by _____   **Date:** _____   **Time:** _____
                                 (if other than admitting RN)

Additional Data/Assessments:

_____

_____

_____

_____

_____

_____

_____

_____

_____

_____

(continued)

NURSING ADMISSION ASSESSMENT FORM—ADULT
INTERMEDIATE CARE *(Continued)*

_____
_____
_____
_____
_____
_____

Section III   1. List Nursing Diagnoses/Teaching needs in order of priority.
   2. Document initial plan of care.

Focus: **Nursing Diagnoses**   **Teaching Needs**

   _____   _____

   _____   _____

   _____   _____

Date Assessed by _____   Date: _____   Time: _____
                        (Signature of Registered Nurse)

NA: Not applicable
RN: Registered Nurse
LPN: Licensed Practical Nurse
* Offer smoking cessation material
** Implement Braden Scale

(Courtesy of Duke University Medical Center, Durham, NC.)

Include additional assessment content. Basic demographic and identifying information should be verified from a referral or intake form. In facilities such as hospitals or long-term care facilities, how a patient arrived (by car alone or with family, by ambulance), and orientation to a room are included on assessments. In home care, documenting who is the caregiver, the caregiver's capability, type of care given in the home, and last physician contact are areas of information documented. In all settings, a nurse needs to document a history of present illness and past disabilities, allergies, most recent treatment and medication, and vital signs at admission. Important additional information to include is a family's medical history and their attitude and adjustment toward a patient and the patient's illness and treatment.

Start with the chief complaint. How a nurse asks information of a patient often determines the quality and completeness of assessment data collected. Starting an assessment interview with "How are you feeling?" expresses concern and allows the patient an opportunity to communicate a chief complaint and what is most important to resolve. For a nurse to show concern about a patient's priority problem conveys that a nurse cares and will work toward mutual goals.

Follow a problem. When questioning uncovers a symptom or problem during a nursing history interview, subsequent questions should concentrate on all the characteristics and variables of that problem. Questions should then focus on what the patient is doing, or has tried to do, to cope with that problem. Record the degree of a patient's success when pertinent. For example, a checklist shows, "incontinence ✔ occ." Comments would include: "Cause—medical diagnosis of nerve injury; current approach—attempting a daily 11 am bowel training with 75% success."

Determine reasons. If a patient is doing nothing about a problem or is noncompliant to prescribed therapy, try to find the reason. Questions to ask and document would be: "Have you contacted a physician?" "What did the physician say?" "Do you understand what the physician meant?" "Is there some reason not to do it?" Just asking the patient "Why?" often gets no information when the patient answers, "I don't know." Rather than ask why, it is better to repeat the patient's comment and encourage details.

Learn about past experiences. Also, a nurse should listen for what may later turn out to be useful information. For instance, in home health care nursing, occupational nursing, or another specialty outside the hospital, a nurse can ask the patient what hospital is preferred for inpatient treatment. This method not only gives information to document on a history, it creates an opportunity for a patient to share any earlier good or bad experiences. One home care patient and family member interviewed said that while in a certain hospital, the patient fell and broke a hip during a transfer from bed to chair. In the home the patient was so fearful of another fall the patient did not want to get out of bed. It helped to have the patient share the experience. To name the fear is an important element in planning nursing interventions to change patient behavior.

Involve the caregiver. The nursing history completed in any health care setting should include documentation of the patient's primary caregiver at home. Usually the caregiver is a family member. Nurses can work with that family member, teaching and demonstrating caregiving skills, to enhance a caregiver's capabilities, quality of care, and stamina. This involvement results in benefit to the patient and caregiver and can contribute to preventing readmission to hospital, extended care, or home care services.

Organization of Assessment Data

Although assessment forms vary, they generally include similar content. Content can be clustered differently, however, depending on the framework used to categorize data to be collected.

Traditionally, health care organizations determine their format according to specific needs of patients they service or documentation they wish to capture. Although the most frequently used **nursing model** still organizes data around the medical model that focuses on body systems and parts, some organizations are revising their assessment forms according to holistic models such as Gordon's functional health patterns model or the human response patterns from the North American Nursing Diagnosis Association (NANDA) taxonomy. When applied to an assessment, these classification systems create a logical consistent framework for data to easily flow from assessment to care plan (see display, Categories of Information in Selected Assessment Frameworks).

The nursing admission assessment form on page 74 uses Gordon's functional health patterns to organize the data. A nursing history using a medical or body systems model combines a nursing history and simplified physical examination record into one nursing assessment form (see display, Patient Admission Data Base, Robinson Memorial Hospital).

A brief form, combining both history and physical examination, has the advantage of shortening assessment documentation time, allowing information to be found quickly, and relating history and physical findings together. Some hospitals prefer to separate the history and physical examination forms of the assessment (see

CATEGORIES OF INFORMATION IN SELECTED ASSESSMENT FRAMEWORKS

Body System Model

EENT (ears, eyes, nose, throat)	Urologic
Respiratory	Musculoskeletal
Circulatory	Reproductive
Gastrointestinal	Integumentary
Neurologic	

Gordon's Functional Health Patterns

Health perception—Health management	Self-perception
	Self-concept
Nutritional—Metabolic	Role-relationship
Elimination	Sexuality—Reproductive
Activity—Exercise	Coping–stress tolerance
Sleep—Rest	Value—Belief
Cognitive perceptual	

NANDA's Human Response Pattern

Exchanging	Moving
Communicating	Perceiving
Relating	Knowing
Valuing	Feeling
Choosing	

display, Physical Assessment Data portion of University Hospitals of Cleveland assessment forms, page 88).

An assessment form that uses the NANDA human response patterns would have the assessment data base separated into areas of:

▲ Communicating—a pattern involving the sending of messages

▲ Valuing—a pattern involving the assigning of relative worth

▲ Relating—a pattern involving establishing bonds

▲ Knowing—a pattern involving the meaning associated with information

▲ Feeling—a pattern involving the subjective awareness of information

▲ Moving—a pattern involving activity

(text continues on page 87)

PATIENT ADMISSION DATA BASE FORM

ROBINSON MEMORIAL HOSPITAL

PATIENT ADMISSION DATA BASE

Date _____ Time _____ Ht. _____ Wt. _____

T. _____ P. _____ R. _____ AP, _____ BP: R _____ L _____

Mode of Adm: W/C _____ Walk _____ Cart _____

From: EC _____ Admitting _____ ER _____

Informant: _____

I.D. Band _____ Orient to Unit _____

Valuables _____

_____

Disposition _____

REASON FOR ADMISSION (Chief Concern)

_____

_____

_____

Analysis of Chief Concern if applicable. Date of onset ___

Location/Radiation _____

Quality/Character _____

Environmental Factors (setting) _____

Aggravating/alleviating factors _____

Other symptoms _____

Have you been a pt. in hospital before? _____

ALLERGIES (Indicate Reactions)

Drugs _____ Reactions _____

_____

_____

_____

_____

Foods _____

Other _____

Allergy band on _____

PRESENT MEDICATIONS

Name	Dose	Frequency	Last Dose

Do you have any medications with you? __ yes __ no

List _____

Disposition _____

Do you take any meds not prescribed by a doctor?

____ yes ____ no

Alcohol (drinks/day) _____ Tobacco (#/day) _____

(Number of years) _____ (Number of years) _____

Previous blood transfusion   yes   no

Previous reactions _____

ACTIVITY/EXERCISE

Energy level:

_____ Tires easily _____ Average _____ Very Active

ADL: Independent _____ Assistance _____

Cane _____ Walker _____ W/C _____

Other _____

PAST HEALTH HISTORY

Past Surgeries/Disabilities _____

_____

Past Illnesses: "Have You Ever Had...?"

_____ Heart disease   _____ Bleeding disorder

_____ Hypertension   _____ Hepatitis

_____ Stroke   _____ Cir. problems

_____ Cancer   _____ Emotional

_____ Seizures   _____ Muscle/Joint dis.

_____ Diabetes: Difficult to control

_____ Yes   _____ No

_____ Other _____

NUTRITIONAL/METABOLIC

Diet _____

Coffee/Tea/Soft Drinks (cups/day) _____

Appetite _____ Dysphagia _____

Wt. Loss _____   Amount _____

Wt. Gain _____   Amount _____

Skin Problems/Lesions-Mark Drawing/Appropriate Letter

A-Amputation
B-Burn
Br-Bruises
C-Cath/tubes
D-Deformity
Dc-Decubitus
L-Laceration
R-Rash
S-Scar
Sc-Scratches
St-Stoma
P-Petechiae

(continued)

PATIENT ADMISSION DATA BASE FORM (Continued)

Describe: _____

_____

CARDIOVASCULAR

Any problems? _____ Chest pain _____

Palpitations _____ Pacemaker _____

Other _____

_____

RESPIRATORY

Any problems? _____

Dyspnea _____ With exercise _____

At Rest _____ Cough _____ Sputum _____

Other _____

_____

ELIMINATION

Bowel: Date last BM _____

Any Problems? _____ Stools/Day _____

Nausea _____ Constipation _____

Vomiting _____ Diarrhea _____

Bladder: Time last void _____

No Problem _____ Dysuria _____

Frequency _____ Nocturia _____

Urgency _____ Hematuria _____ Incontinence _____

Ostomies _____

Catheter: _____ Yes _____ No Type _____

Insertion Date: _____

SEXUAL/REPRODUCTIVE

Date of last period _____

Could you be pregnant? _____

Any problems? _____ Menstrual problem _____

Date of menopause _____

Date of last PAP Test? _____

Abnormal discharge _____

Describe _____

BREAST: "DO YOU"

Check your own breasts? _____ Yes _____ No

Patient Teaching _____

Have any lumps, swelling or tenderness _ yes _ no

Have any discharge from the nipples _ yes _ no

If yes, explain _____

PROSTATE PROBLEM _____

COGNITIVE/SENSORY MOTOR

Any problems? _____ Dizzy/fainting _____

Memory loss _____ Numbness/Tingling _____

Memory change _____ Speech _____

Are you having pain? _ yes _ no Describe _____

_____

Ears _____ Throat _____ Vision _____

EMOTIONAL: "Do you have any?"

Mood changes _____ Yes _____ No

Depression? _____ Yes _____ No

Insomnia? _____ Yes _____ No

Sleeping pill _____ Yes _____ No

Recent stresses? _____ Yes _____ No

Explain _____

PROTHESIS

_____ Glasses/Contact lens _____ Artificial limb (R/L)

_____ Hearing aid (R/L) _____ Breast

_____ Artificial eye (R/L) _____ Tracheostomy

_____ Dentures: Upper/Lower _____ Lower bridge

Other _____

PRESSURE ULCER RISK ASSESSMENT

_ Impaired mental status _ Incontinent/Involuntary

_ Limited ROM _ Activity (bed/chair only)

_ Altered nutrition

If one is checked initiate skin car protocol

FALL RISK ASSESSMENT

_____ Impaired mental status _____ Previous fall

_____ Impaired sensory function _____ Impaired mobility

_____ Sedated/Severe pain

If one is checked initiate fall protocol

ROLE RELATIONSHIP/VALUE BELIEF

Occupation _____

Religion _____

Could being here interfere with any religious practice?

_____ yes _____ no

Explain _____

(Dietary restrictions, blood transfusions, medications, etc.)

ANTICIPATED DISCHARGE NEEDS

Do you live alone? _____ yes _____ no

With whom do you live _____

(continued)

PATIENT ADMISSION DATA BASE FORM (Continued)

Have steps to climb	_____ yes	_____ no
Will you need help	_____ yes	_____ no
Need transport home	_____ yes	_____ no
Need financial aid	_____ yes	_____ no
Need medical equip	_____ yes	_____ no

Anticipate need for extended care facility ___ yes ___ no

Will help be needed at home while you are in the hospital?

_____ yes _____ no

Home treatments or services utilized presently? (ie, VNA,

hospice, O_2) Explain _____

Social service needs to be notified

_____ yes _____ no   Date notified _____

Is there anything you or your significant other would like to know regarding your care in the hospital or after discharge?

_____ yes _____ no

Explain _____

TEACHING NEEDS

_____
_____
_____
_____

DISCHARGE/GOAL MUTUALLY SET WITH PATIENT/FAMILY

_____
_____
_____
_____
Signature of Patient/Family

Advanced directive information received,   yes   no

Admitting notified   yes   no

Living Will on chart   yes   no

Durable power of attorney on chart   yes   no

ATTENDING PHYSICIAN OR NURSE CLINICIAN/ RESIDENT NOTIFIED FOR H&P   Time _____

By _____

_____
Signature/Title of Nurse completing   Date

_____
RN Signature   Date

(Courtesy of Robinson Memorial Hospital, Ravenna, OH.)

▲ Perceiving—a pattern involving the reception of information

▲ Exchanging—a pattern involving mutual giving and receiving

▲ Choosing—a pattern involving the selection of alternatives (Guzzetta, Bunton, Prinkey, Sherer, & Seifert, 1989, pp. 15–22)

Although this taxonomy was not designed for assessment application, it is being used as an assessment format structure in many health care organizations.

Specialty Assessment Forms

In addition to general information, some assessments often need to include special information related to ongoing observation or related to specific care settings.

Frequent Assessment

Recent emphasis is being placed on frequent assessments, or sometimes called reassessments, of the patient. In the hospital, assessments can be made frequently depending on the patient's condition. A flow sheet format is most efficient for recording and retrieving

this data for easy and rapid comparison of patient information (see display, Frequent Assessment Form: Neurologic Flow Sheet).

Specialty Area Assessment Forms

Specialty areas like operating rooms, emergency rooms, day surgery, and maternity customize their assessment forms to gather information needed to provide safe and comprehensive care within the time frame a patient is there.

Operating room, emergency room, and day surgery assessments include specific assessment data related to those service areas. These assessments may include:

▲ Reason patient states request for care

▲ Most recent circumstances contributing to presenting problem

▲ Height, weight

▲ Vital signs, including present cardiorespiratory status

▲ Previous surgeries, anesthesia

▲ Treatments for the same condition

▲ Allergies, including allergies/reactions to anesthesia, antibiotics, antibiotic skin cleansers

(text continues on page 90)

PHYSICAL ASSESSMENT DATA FORM

UNIVERSITY HOSPITAL OF CLEVELAND
PHYSICAL ASSESSMENT DATA

GENERAL

Admitted from:
( ) Home   ( ) Clinic/Office: _____
( ) Emergency room   ( ) Extended care facility: _____
                     ( ) Other: _____

Arrived Via: ( ) Walking   ( ) Wheelchair   ( ) Cart
Accompanied by: _____

Explanations ( ) Primary nursing   ( ) Smoking policy
Given: ( ) Use of signal light/intercom   ( ) Meal times
              ( ) Use of bed control   ( ) Visiting hours
              ( ) Location of bathroom   ( ) Telephone service
              ( ) Closet   ( ) TV
              ( ) Bedside and tray tables ( ) Newspapers
              ( ) Urine collection   ( ) Valuables: _____
                                          Given to: _____

NUTRITIONAL METABOLIC

Height _____   Weight _____

Skin: ( ) healthy   ( ) ashen   ( ) mottled   ( ) jaundiced
Color: ( ) pale   ( ) flushed   ( ) cyanotic

Temperature: ( ) warm   ( ) cool
              ( ) hot   ( ) cold/clammy

Turgor: ( ) good
              ( ) poor

Edema: _____
Describe location and degree (1–4+)

Oral Mucous Membranes: ( ) Not applicable

( ) intact   ( ) lesions _____
( ) moist   ( ) dry

Color: ( ) pink   ( ) cyanotic
        ( ) pale   ( ) other _____

_____ _____
SHADE AND LABEL ANY IDENTIFYING MARKS
(scars, bruises, rash, cuts, ulcers, etc)
( ) not applicable

front   back

ELIMINATION   ( ) not applicable
Abdomen: ( ) soft   ( ) firm
          ( ) nontender   ( ) tender: location _____
          ( ) nondistended ( ) distended: girth _____
          ( ) ostomies/tubes: type _____
          care (circle): independent, needs assistance

Bowel Sounds: ( ) present
               ( ) absent
               ( ) other: _____

(continued)

PHYSICAL ASSESSMENT DATA FORM (Continued)

ACTIVITY-EXERCISE

Respiratory effort: ( ) easy ( ) use of accessory muscles: _____

Cough: ( ) no ( ) yes Sputum: ( ) no ( ) yes _____

Breath Sounds: _____
( ) Not applicable

Peripheral pulses: ( ) not applicable
Key: +0 - absent +1 - weak +2 - normal +3 - bounding

	dorsalis pedis	posterior tibial	radial	other: _____
Right				
Left				

Gait: ( ) not ambulatory ( ) steady ( ) unsteady _____

Range of Motion
( ) not applicable

	Full	Limited (describe)
LA		
RA		
LL		
RL		

Muscle Strength (see key)
( ) not applicable

LA	
RA	
LL	
RL	

Muscle Strength Key
+5 - able to move against full resistance
+4 - able to move against gravity and moderate resistance
+3 - able to move against gravity but no resistance
+2 - weak movement, unable to overcome gravity
+1 - flicker of muscle movement
  0 - no movement

Additional data: list and/or describe (eg prostheses, AV fistula/shunt, vascular access device, pacemaker, etc)
_____
_____
_____

COGNITION-PERCEPTION

Orientation: circle one
  0 - not oriented
  ×1 - oriented to person
  ×2 - oriented to person, place
  ×3 - oriented to person, place, time

Level of consciousness: circle one
  5 - conscious
  4 - Lethargy, somnolence, drowsiness
  3 - stupor-aroused by verbal stimuli but responds poorly to pain
  2 - light coma-no response to verbal stimuli but responds to pain
  1 - deep coma-no response to painful stimuli

Clarity of speech: ( ) clear ( ) slurred ( ) aphasic
( ) primary language if not English: _____
Pupils: ( ) not applicable ( ) describe _____
Thought processes: ( ) logical ( ) illogical (confused) ( ) flight of ideas
Behavioral: ( ) not applicable ( ) guarding ( ) grimacing
signs of pain: ( ) other _____

SELF-PERCEPTION/SELF-CONCEPT

Behavior indicates the following:

Mood:	( ) clam	( ) agitated	( ) angry
	( ) anxious	( ) sad	( ) other _____
Affect:	( ) normal	( ) labile	( ) flat
Verbal style:	( ) interactive	( ) quiet	( ) talkative ( ) guarded

(continued)

PHYSICAL ASSESSMENT DATA FORM (Continued)

Additional data (if indicated): _____

_____

_____

_____

_____	_____
Primary Nurse signature/date reviewed	Admitting Nurse signature/date
_____	_____
Primary Nurse—printed name	Admitting Nurse—printed name

(Courtesy of University Hospitals of Cleveland, Cleveland, OH.)

▲ Time and content of last meal
▲ Time and type of medication taken within past 24 hours
▲ Presence of dentures, contact lenses
▲ When and where most recent laboratory work or x-rays taken

For clinical judgments in maternity care, nurses require specific assessment and reassessment information related to maternal health care needs. Assessment information to be collected includes:

▲ Gravida and para (how many pregnancies and how many deliveries)
▲ Prenatal care
▲ Previous ultrasound and prenatal tests
▲ Past difficult and high-risk pregnancies or deliveries
▲ Past type of anesthesia and any untoward reactions
▲ Intended method of feeding infant
▲ Pericare and lochia (reassessment following delivery)
▲ Level of fundus (reassessment following delivery)
▲ Learning needs in infant care
▲ Family planning history and plan for after delivery

Specific Patient Population Assessment Forms

A **patient population** or group of the same type of patients often has similar characteristics, similar problems, and similar needs. For instance, pediatric or child health, psychiatric, and mental health nursing and geriatric units require that additional and specific information be collected and documented during assessment for appropriate, safe, and comprehensive care.

PEDIATRIC ASSESSMENT

Growth and development, feeding and sleep patterns, toilet training, and special toys are just some of the pediatric-specific assessment areas necessary to help a pediatric patient adjust to other caregivers and maintain the current level of functioning (see display, Cleveland Clinic Foundation Pediatrics Admission Nursing Assessment). Knowing this information also allows a nurse to determine any variation that would indicate a problem. For example, if a pediatric patient is toilet trained, a bedwetting episode is an indication of a problem. That problem could have a physical cause because bedwetting could be a sign of urinary urgency, which is a symptom of a urinary tract infection. Or that problem could have a psychological cause because bedwetting could be a symptom of anxiety due to a new environment and separation from parents and home.

Additional assessment information specific to pediatric patients includes:

▲ Type of delivery (for infant assessments)
▲ Growth and development
▲ Type of food, food likes/dislikes, eating methods (fingers or utensils, bottle or cup with lid)
▲ Meal pattern (mealtimes and snacks)
▲ Sleeping pattern, nighttime and naps
▲ Immunization status
▲ Sibling and playmate relationships

PSYCHIATRIC ASSESSMENT

A variety of assessment forms focus on psychiatric problems. A critical documentation flow sheet is the suicide assessment, which is documented each shift. A yes–no checklist format includes a comment area for the following questions. Does the patient:

▲ Verbalize suicidal ideation?
▲ Verbalize suicidal intention? Want to die?
▲ Verbalize suicidal plan? How patient intends to harm self? Have access to means to harm self? Where would this occur?
▲ Verbalize feelings of hopelessness/helplessness? Verbalize should not have been born?
▲ Show sudden changes in mood, behavior, affect, thoughts, activity level, giving belongings away?

An initial suicide assessment also includes determining whether the patient has ever known anyone who

FREQUENT ASSESSMENT FORM

NEUROLOGIC FLOW SHEET

PUPILS: SIZE 1m 2m 3m 4m 5m 6m

	Time															
Level of Consciousness	Alert															
	Oriented X3															
	Confused															
	Arouse to light pain															
	Arouse to deep pain															
	Comatose															
Pattern of Speech	Coherent															
	Incoherent															
	Slurred speech															
	Aphasic															
Motor Response	Facial symmetry															
	Obeys commands															
	Localizes pain															
	Withdraw from pain															
	Flaccid															
Motor Strength 0 to +4 Absent Strong	Right arm															
	Right leg															
	Left arm															
	Left leg															
	Equal grasp															
Pupils (see chart)	PERRLA															
	Right (size)															
	Left (size)															

attempted suicide and whether the patient ever made an actual attempt (J. K. Hogan, Windsor Hospital, Chagrin Falls, Ohio, personal communication, November, 1992).

Additional assessment information specific to psychiatric patients includes:

▲ History of abuse, including drugs
▲ Addictive behavior, including food, drugs, alcohol
▲ Behavior and mannerisms, mood and affect

▲ Attention span, goal-directed activities/plans
▲ Communication characteristics, including eye contact
▲ Communication and behavior with family or significant other
▲ Mental status, orientation to person, place, time
▲ Aggression assessment
▲ Assessment of traumatic events
▲ Reality testing

PEDIATRICS ADMISSION NURSING ASSESSMENT FORM

CLEVELAND CLINIC FOUNDATION
Pediatrics
ADMISSION NURSING ASSESMENT

Date	
Time	

VITAL STAT	Age	Pulse A R	Weight	Height	Nickname
	Temp.	Rhythm	Resp.	B.P.	Person to contact
	Adm. from		Accompanied by		Phone religion
					sibs

Admitting diagnosis
1.

2.

Family's understanding of illness
3.

Past hospitalization and recent illness

Immunizations Up-to-date Yes No	If no, why?	Exposure to communicable disesae

Allergies (food or drug)

Medications

Drugs taken today

Growth and development

A. Sleep pattern   Naps   Lights on   off
    Sleeps through night   Special toys, blanket (describe)

Comments

B. Nutrition
    General appearance

Recent gain/loss _____
Formula: type   warm   cold   amount per feed & frequency

Diet   Bottle   Cup   Foods avoided

Eats by self   High chair

Condition of mouth & teeth

Comments

C. Elimination: Bladder _____ Bowel _____   Day _____ Night _____
    Potty trained: must be asked _____   asks for potty _____
    Names for urine _____   For stool _____
    Frequency of stools _____   Type _____
    Comments _____

(Courtesy of Cleveland Clinic Foundation, Cleveland, OH.)

GERIATRIC ASSESSMENT

In addition to generic information collected in assessments, other assessment data can and should be investigated at assessment or at reassessments when a patient is elderly. These data cue on intermittent or chronic problems common to the geriatric population. Regardless of duration of the problem, these aspects can be pivotal in medical and nursing diagnoses, care planning, intervention, and evaluation. This additional assessment information specific to geriatric patients includes:

▲ Short-term memory, orientation ×3, confusion
▲ Mobility, including balance, gait, and assistive devices
▲ Bowel evacuation pattern, including medication and use of enemas
▲ Nutritional status, meal pattern
▲ Role relationship with adult children
▲ Social activities or social isolation
▲ Death of friends, relatives, and change in social activities
▲ Helplessness, hopelessness, sadness, depression
▲ Attitude toward living, toward dying
▲ Importance of religious activities, ability to attend church
▲ Sensory deficits such as hearing, vision, and speech and the effect on communication
▲ Decrease in economic resources and related anxiety
▲ Change in life-style due to spouse death, economics, illness

HIGH RISK FOR FALLS—ASSESSMENT DATA

In geriatric settings or in acute care settings in which a geriatric patient is admitted, nurses need to assess patients to prevent common injuries of the elderly. Documentation of these aspects of assessment information is important in determining risk for injury. One of the biggest risks and cause of frequent injuries of geriatric patients is falls.

Common problems of the elderly are also risk factors in determination of falls. Still, regardless of a patient's age, the following factors need to be assessed to determine the potential for falls:

▲ Altered mobility
▲ Neurologic impairment
▲ Altered hemodynamic state
▲ Dizziness or other untoward reaction of medication
▲ Confusion
▲ Generalized weakness
▲ Previous falls

Most high risk for falls assessments include a rating scale with a benchmark total, above which the patient is considered to be at risk for falls (see display, Assessment for Risk for Falls).

Abuse Assessment

Unfortunately, abuse is becoming more common in patients of all ages; however, pediatric, geriatric, and spouse abuse are most frequent. Many states have adopted legislation, including reporting laws and protective services laws, to provide procedures and support for victims of abuse. Some states make reporting mandatory for anyone who has reasonable cause to suspect or believe that an individual is a victim of abuse, neglect, or exploitation. Adequate assessment is important. Abuse can be physical abuse, negligence, financial abuse (often called exploitation), and psychological (emotional) abuse. Symptoms to assess and document include:

▲ Undernourishment as evidenced by dehydration symptoms and low body weight
▲ Bruises
▲ Suspiciously shaped burns
▲ Unexplainable or multiple fractures
▲ Unlikely or inconsistent explanations of cause of injury
▲ Evasion, fear, or anxiety during conversation
▲ Patient explanation for injury of "fell down stairs" or "walked into door"

Any one, and especially two or more, of the above situations are indications that abuse may be a factor.

Procedures in documenting and reporting abuse should be reviewed when a nurse suspects its occurrence. Documentation here, as in general assessments, is focused on what is seen. Additionally, focus in abuse assessments includes reaction of the patient to questions concerning the cause of injuries.

ASSESSMENT FOR POTENTIAL/HIGH-RISK PRESSURE ULCER FORMATION

Assessment data to determine the potential or high risk for pressure ulcers, also called pressure sores, include patients with evidence of:

▲ Debilitated physical condition
▲ Limited activity and mobility
▲ Presence of sensory deficits
▲ Inadequate nutrition and fluid intake
▲ Diaphoresis
▲ Incontinence of bowel or bladder
▲ Inadequate circulation
▲ Edema
▲ Inadequate oxygenation

The Skin Risk Assessment Record identifies patients at risk for pressure sore formation. Scoring provides measurable assessment data and background support for

ASSESSMENT FOR RISK FOR FALLS FORM

ASSESSMENT FOR RISK OF FALL POTENTIAL

Name _____ Room # _____ Age _____ Sex _____

Diagnosis _____ Admission Wt. _____

Physician _____

Risk Score _____ Date _____

Parameters	0	1	2	3	Score
Level of consciousness	Alert Wakefulness	Alert but often drowsy	Drowsy Score ×2	Stupor Score ×2	
Mental status	Never confused	Rarely confused	Occasionally confused	Always confused	
Weight	<100 lbs	100–150 lbs	150–200 lbs	>200 lbs	
Vision	Optimum vision with or without corrective lenses	Distinguishes caregivers	Distinguishes between light and dark only	Totally blind	
Hearing	Full hearing both ears	Deaf or hearing impaired one ear only	Hearing impaired both ears	Deaf both ears	
Physical status	Use of all extremities; fully mobile	Impaired use of extremities uses walker or cane	Limited use of extremities; chairfast Score ×2	Immobile rarely out of bed Score ×2	
Verbal	Able to make needs known	Some difficulty communicating needs	Always has difficulty communicating needs	Unable to make needs known	
History of falls	No falls within last 30 days	1 fall within last 30 days	2 falls within last 30 days Score ×2	3 falls within last 30 days Score ×2	

Note: Residents with scores above (12) should be considered at risk for potential falls.

(Courtesy of Lakeside Plantation, Naples, FL.)

a nurse to establish likelihood of a high-risk situation for a patient (see display, Skin Risk Assessment Form).

KEY POINTS

▲ A nursing assessment is documented to collect information for analysis in clinical decision-making, which in turn supports a nursing diagnosis, leaning toward establishing a plan of care.

▲ The framework used to collect assessment data in a particular health care organization influences the type of format used for nursing assessment. Common frameworks include body systems, Gordon's functional health patterns, or the NANDA human response patterns.

▲ A nursing history includes physical, psychosocial, environmental, functional, and learning needs and health care management information regarding a patient.

▲ A nursing assessment consists of a nursing history component and a physical examination component. The physical examination may be extensive or brief, focusing on just one or two health needs or problems.

▲ The advantages of cued or flow sheet assessments are that assessments are standardized and data entry is fast. Comment areas allow for individualizing and clarifying checked entries.

▲ Periodic reassessments, or ongoing daily or by-shift assessments, are important in determining patient status, progress, and continuing needs.

SKIN RISK ASSESSMENT FORM

SKIN RISK ASSESSMENT RECORD
ASSESS ON ADMISSION AND QUARTERLY

Identify any patient at risk to develop skin conditions assessing the eight clinical condition parameters and assigning a score. Patient with a score of 8 or above should be considered at risk to develop skin conditions. Initiate prevention protocol.

Directions: Choose the number for each parameter that applies to the patient's status. Total the eight numbers to determine the patient's risk potential.

Dates & Year				
Scores				

Clinical Condition Parameters

General Physical Condition (health problem)
Good (minor) 0
Fair (major but stable) 1
Poor (chronic/serious not stable) 2

Level of Consciousness (to commands)
Alert (responds readily) 0
Lethargic (slow to respond) 1
Confused 2
Semicomatose (responds only to verbal or painful stimuli) 3
Comatose (no response to stimuli) 4

Activity
Ambulate without assistance 0
Ambulate with assistance 1
Chairfast 2
Bedfast 3

Mobility (extremities)
Full active range 0
Limited movement with assistance 1
Moves only with assistance 2
Immobile 3

Incontinence (bowel and/or bladder)
None 0
Occasional (<2 per 24 h) 1
Usually Incontinent (urine & stool, incl. catheter) 2
Double Incontinence (urine & stool) 3

Nutrition (for age and size)
Good (eats/drinks adequately 3/4 of meal) 0
Fair (eats/drinks less than 3/4 of meal) N/G, G, TUBE OR TPN 1
Poor (unable/refuses to eat/drink—less than 1/2) 2

Skin/Tissue Status
Good (well nourished/skin intact) 0
Fair (poorly nourished/skin intact) 1
Poor (skin not intact) 2

Predisposing Disease (diabetes, COPD, anemia, etc.)
Absent 0
1 disease present 1
2 diseases present 2
3 or more diseases present 3

Suggested Preventive Protocol

		Total				

8–10 Monitor skin closely.
Mild Turn & reposition q2h

11–15 Special mattress; Pressure-relieving devices; elbow heel protectors, if
Mod. indicated. Dietary intervention

16–22 Monitor skin daily. Lab work if indicated.
Severe Treatments as ordered.

Signature & Title

Resident
Name _____ Room # _____   I.D. Number _____

(Courtesy of Lakeside Plantation, Naples, FL.)

▲ Specialty areas have customized assessments for patients' special assessment needs on those units (eg, emergency department patients). Assessments have also been customized for specific patient populations (eg, pediatric patients). Additionally, assessments can be focused on patients' functional abilities to prevent injuries (eg, assessment for high risk for falls in geriatric patients).

REFERENCES

American Nurses Association. (1991). *Standards of clinical nursing practice*. Washington, DC: Author.

Guzzetta, C. E., Bunton, S. D., Prinkey, L. A., Sherer, A. P., & Seifert, P. C. (1989). *Clinical assessment tools for use with nursing diagnoses* (pp. 15–22). St Louis: C. V. Mosby.

Long v. Johnson, 381 N.E.2d 93 (Ind. 1978). In Fiesta, J. (1983). *The law and liability: A guide for nurses* (p. 61). New York: John Wiley & Sons.

Newhall v. Central Vermont Hospital, 349 A.2d 890 (Vt. 1975). In Fiesta, J. (1983). *The law and liability: A guide for nurses* (p. 65). New York: John Wiley & Sons.

BIBLIOGRAPHY

Bellack, J. P., & Edlund, B. J. (1992). *Nursing assessment and diagnosis*. Boston: Jones and Bartlett Publishers.

Camp, D. L., & O'Sullivan, P. S. (1987). Comparison of medical surgical and oncology patients' descriptions of pain and nurses' documentation of pain assessments. *Journal of Advanced Nursing*, 87 (12), 593–598.

Eggland, E. T. (1977). How to take a meaningful history. *Nursing '77*, 7(7), 22–30

Thompson, J. M., & Bowers, A. C. (1988). *Health assessment: An illustrated pocket guide* (2nd ed.). St. Louis: C. V. Mosby.

FILL IN

1. The process of writing collected pertinent data regarding actual and potential problems or needs of a patient is _____ .

2. An initial assessment is completed when a _____ _____ .

3. Clustering information assists in _____ .

4. Determining _____ is one outcome of an initial assessment.

5. Two components of a nursing assessment are _____ and _____ .

6. _____ data is information that a patient tells a nurse.

7. _____ data is information that can be measured, seen, heard, touched, or smelled by a nurse.

8. A disadvantage of an open-ended format is that _____ .

9. When documenting a nursing assessment, priority should be on a patient's _____ , needs, and complaints.

10. Periodic _____ are important in determining patient status and continuing needs.

MATCHING DEFINITIONS

Match the phrase in Column B that matches its definition in Column A.

1. _____ current problem
2. _____ possible complication
3. _____ abbreviated form to collect data
4. _____ free form narrative
5. _____ check mark form

a. reassessment form
b. cued format
c. actual problem
d. open-ended form
e. potential problem

MATCHING TYPES OF DATA

Match the term in column B that describes the type of data in column A

1. _____ teary-eyed
2. _____ pain is bad
3. _____ ate good
4. _____ wheezes
5. _____ feel alright
6. _____ pacing
7. _____ cold to touch
8. _____ making progress
9. _____ urine negative
10. _____ had a bowel movement

a. subjective
b. objective
c. neither

MULTIPLE CHOICE

1. _____ Assessment data may sometimes be collected on
   a) progress notes
   b) reassessment form
   c) standardized assessment flow sheets
   d) all of the above

2. _____ To assess discharge needs for patient care, it is important to gather information on a
   a) patient's culture
   b) family relationships
   c) psychosocial status
   d) all of the above

3. _____ Nursing assessments are used for
   a) eligibility for care and reimbursement
   b) therapists to learn patient needs
   c) determining on which nursing unit the patient should be admitted
   d) all of the above

4. _____ Sources of information for assessments can be the patient or
   a) family or previous caregivers
   b) medical chart or the patient's physician
   c) a and b
   d) friends who visit

5. _____ A nursing assessment can also be called
   a) the analysis sheet
   b) an admission form or data base
   c) an intake
   d) a Kardex

CHALLENGE FOR CRITICAL THINKING

1. In clinical decision-making at assessment time, information is collected and verified than clustered and analyzed to establish nursing diagnoses. Why is a physical examination important following a nursing history?

2. Discuss why a general assessment designed for adults would not be appropriate when assessing a pediatric patient.

3. What is the relationship between an assessment and the development of a teaching plan?

4. Discuss the factors that are important to consider when assessing a geriatric patient's risk of falling.

5. Identify environmental factors that are detrimental to obtaining data in an assessment interview. Role play with another student by interviewing the student about his or her last class. Conduct the interview in a distracting environment, then again in a quiet environment.

LEARNING TO DOCUMENT

1. Divide into groups of four. *Role play by rotating a nurse and patient and two observers. Do not use personal or real patient information in this activity;* instead create fictitious patient situations. Use the patient admission data base form on page 85 to document data collected. The two observers should take notes during the interview, then at the end of the interview, offer constructive advice on how to improve the process of assessment documentation.

2. Mrs. Myra Minka in room 101 is a 50-year-old multiple sclerosis (MS) patient in poor health. She is mentally alert but is unable to get out of bed and needs maximum help to change positions in bed. She weighs 100 lbs, is eating 75% of her meals; she refuses to drink very much because she doesn't like to use the bedpan. She is continent of bowel and bladder, but the nurse and Dr. J.M. Nagle are concerned about the reddened area on her coccyx and both heels. Is Mrs. M. at risk for decubitus ulcer? Fill out the Skin Risk Assessment Form on page 100, to substantiate or refute the potential status for ulcers.

3. Mr. Charles Cody was just admitted to the hospital (12 noon) with the diagnosis of a stroke. He was confused and slurred his speech; he could not move any extremities. His pupils reacted to light, right pupil was 3m and left 5m. At subsequent hourly intervals his condition remained the same, then he became alert and oriented X3 4 hours later. At that time, he is coherent and obeys commands but cannot move his right arm and right leg. At 4:00 Mr. C. could move his left leg and left arm at +2 strength. Mr. C has a very strong grip with the left hand only. At 4:00 both pupils are equal and reactive to light and accommodation, and both measure 3m. Fill out the Neurologic Flow Sheet on page 101 to indicate this assessment for 4 days.

SKIN RISK ASSESSMENT FORM

SKIN RISK ASSESSMENT RECORD
ASSESS ON ADMISSION AND QUARTERLY

Identify any patient at risk to develop skin conditions assessing the eight clinical condition parameters and assigning a score. Patient with a score of 8 or above should be considered at risk to develop skin conditions. Initiate prevention protocol.

Directions: Choose the number for each parameter that applies to the patient's status. Total the eight numbers to determine the patient's risk potential.

Clinical Condition Parameters	Dates & Year			
	Scores			
General Physical Condition (health problem)				
Good (minor) 0				
Fair (major but stable) 1				
Poor (chronic/serious not stable) 2				
Level of Consciousness (to commands)				
Alert (responds readily) 0				
Lethargic (slow to respond) 1				
Confused 2				
Semicomatose (responds only to verbal or painful stimuli) 3				
Comatose (no response to stimuli) 4				
Activity				
Ambulate without assistance 0				
Ambulate with assistance 1				
Chairfast 2				
Bedfast 3				
Mobility (extremities)				
Full active range 0				
Limited movement with assistance 1				
Moves only with assistance 2				
Immobile 3				
Incontinence (bowel and/or bladder)				
None 0				
Occasional (<2 per 24 h) 1				
Usually Incontinent (urine & stool, incl. catheter) 2				
Double Incontinence (urine & stool) 3				
Nutrition (for age and size)				
Good (eats/drinks adequately 3/4 of meal) 0				
Fair (eats/drinks less than 3/4 of meal) N/G, G, TUBE OR TPN 1				
Poor (unable/refuses to eat/drink—less than 1/2) 2				
Skin/Tissue Status				
Good (well nourished/skin intact) 0				
Fair (poorly nourished/skin intact) 1				
Poor (skin not intact) 2				
Predisposing Disease (diabetes, COPD, anemia, etc.)				
Absent 0				
1 disease present 1				
2 diseases present 2				
3 or more diseases present 3				

Suggested Preventive Protocol	Total			

Suggested Preventive Protocol

8–10 Mild	Monitor skin closely. Turn & reposition q2h
11–15 Mod.	Special mattress; Pressure-relieving devices; elbow heel protectors, if indicated. Dietary intervention
16–22 Severe	Monitor skin daily. Lab work if indicated. Treatments as ordered.

Resident
Name _____ Room # _____   I.D. Number _____

(Courtesy of Lakeside Plantation, Naples, FL.)

FREQUENT ASSESSMENT FORM

NEUROLOGIC FLOW SHEET

PUPILS: SIZE   1m   2m   3m   4m   5m   6m

	Time														
Level of Consciousness	Alert														
	Oriented X3														
	Confused														
	Arouse to light pain														
	Arouse to deep pain														
	Comatose														
Pattern of Speech	Coherent														
	Incoherent														
	Slurred speech														
	Aphasic														
Motor Response	Facial symmetry														
	Obeys commands														
	Localizes pain														
	Withdraw from pain														
	Flaccid														
Motor Strength 0 to +4 Absent Strong	Right arm														
	Right leg														
	Left arm														
	Left leg														
	Equal grasp														
Pupils (see chart)	PERRLA														
	Right (size)														
	Left (size)														

Documenting Nursing Diagnoses and Care Plans

LEARNING OBJECTIVES

After studying this chapter, the learner should be able to:

▲   Explain the formulation of nursing diagnoses as the second step in documentation of the nursing process.

▲   Identify components of the nursing diagnosis.

▲   Formulate the documented care plan as the third step in documentation of the nursing process.

▲   Identify components of a nursing care plan.

▲   Define key terms as applied to nursing diagnoses and care plans.

▲   Compare traditional and standardized models of nursing care plans and special considerations in developing the care plan.

▲   Explain how to individualize standardized care plans.

▲   List the advantages and disadvantages of standardized care plans and nursing guidelines.

KEY TERMS

Clinical decision-making	Expected outcomes	Nursing diagnosis	Signs and symptoms
Defining characteristics	NANDA	Nursing interventions	Taxonomy
Etiology	Nursing care plan	Related factors	

After assessment data are collected, validated, clustered into patterns, and analyzed, a nurse uses clinical decision-making based on nursing knowledge and theory to proceed to the next step of the nursing process. This next step is to identify health problems and strengths of the patient. When a health problem can be resolved with independent nursing interventions, the nurse labels it as a nursing diagnosis. A **nursing diagnosis** is a clinical judgment about individual, family, or community responses to actual or potential health problems. Nursing diagnoses provide the basis for selection of nursing interventions for which the nurse is accountable (North American Nursing Diagnosis Association, 1992).

The nurse then establishes a plan of care to achieve **expected outcomes**, which are measurable, patient-focused goals of care. **Nursing interventions** eliminate or minimize health problems, enhance wellness strengths and behaviors, and assist the patient to achieve the expected outcomes. The American Nurses Association (ANA) defines nursing as "the diagnosis and treatment of human responses" (ANA, 1980). In the ANA *Standards of Clinical Practice*, the second standard proposes that validated nursing diagnoses are derived from the assessment data and documented in a clinical decision-making process that establishes a plan of care to achieve expected outcomes (ANA, 1991).

A **nursing care plan** or **plan of care** is a comprehensive outline of proposed interventions to achieve established expected outcomes within a definite time frame. The nursing care plan must include the following components:

▲ Nursing diagnoses
▲ Expected outcomes (goals)
▲ Nursing interventions

Importance of Documenting Nursing Diagnoses and Care Planning

The nursing diagnosis and care planning steps are dynamically important because the **clinical decision-making**, knowledgeable and intuitive judgment of the nurse, is most autonomous at this point of the nursing process. Here, a clinical judgment is important because the nurse is making decisions regarding the:

▲ Actual nursing diagnoses of the patient
▲ High risk-nursing diagnoses of the patient
▲ Health care priority of patient problems
▲ Interventions effective for the patient's health care needs related to the diagnosis

▲ Interventions effective for the patient's individual needs

Because the nursing diagnosis and plan of care establish the direction for care, clinical decisions made in the process of planning are crucial in the care, progress, and ultimate outcome of the patient. When the nurse establishes nursing diagnoses, each nursing diagnosis directs the development of expected outcomes on the care plan. In turn, expected outcomes direct the action and focus of independent (nurse-initiated) nursing interventions.

The Purpose of a Nursing Care Plan

In today's documentation framework, care plans are a key component of better documentation because they contribute to:

▲ Goal direction and coordination of care
▲ Continuity of care
▲ Communication
▲ Reflection of nursing care standards
▲ Appropriateness of care for reimbursement
▲ Related and future use
  • A basis for the potential of costing out nursing care
  • A component for nursing management functions such as staffing, patient acuity determinations, and patient assignments

Goal Direction and Coordination of Care

A written care plan gives direction to patient care. All nursing and interdisciplinary caregivers can see expected outcomes and can see planned interventions to reach expected outcomes within a time frame.

A care plan establishes priorities for care. When a number of caregivers are focused on the same high-priority expected outcomes, goals will be accomplished at a faster rate because interventions are reinforced toward the achievement of outcomes. The efforts of caregivers who are guided in the same direction are more effective than efforts of caregivers who do not communicate goals and purpose.

Continuity of Care

A patient often has many nurses and therapists providing care through the course of hospitalization, even if the patient remains on one nursing unit. By routinely reviewing the care plan and revising the plan when the condition of the patient changes, continuity of care is facilitated.

Some patients see groups of caregivers change because of transfers to different departments within a facility or because more than one health care organization is involved in care. Because of the direction the care plan gives to caregivers in different departments, continuity of care is provided as the patient is transferred between hospital patient care units. Similarly, expected outcomes and progress toward outcomes is documented and shared with caregivers in other settings; continuity is maintained and coordinated interventions toward expected outcomes continue even when the patient is discharged.

Communication

A care plan provides a means of communication between the nurse and other health professionals. The care plan communicates the content and intent of the plans for care of the patient. Further, care plan revisions quickly show progress the patient is making in accomplishing expected outcomes.

A care plan is also a communication tool between caregivers and the patient. Using the care plan as a base, the patient is more likely to stay involved in care planning. Motivation is enhanced by viewing progress in achieving outcomes. Viewing progress is possible when outcomes are expressed in solid, measurable terms and directed toward mutually established goals.

Reflection of Nursing Care Standards

A nursing care plan provides nurses an opportunity to document patient needs and planned interventions that reflect accepted standards of nursing care (see display, American Nurses Association Standards of Care). The ANA and nursing specialty groups define standards of professional care. Regulatory (Health Care Financing Agency [HCFA]) and accrediting organizations (Joint Commission on Accreditation of Healthcare Organizations [JCAHO], National League for Nursing [NLN]) and other health care organizations establish guidelines of what needs should be addressed, and sometimes include related aspects that should be documented. For example, the standards of JCAHO require nurses to document discharge planning from the time of admission. This documentation can be completed on the care plan or on an attached discharge plan form. Further, JCAHO delineates what aspects of the discharge plan should be included in documentation. For example, the discharge plan must contain identified patient problems and whether expected outcomes were met. If not met, progress toward reaching outcomes is documented. Progress is based on expected outcomes and planned interventions documented in the care plan and is derived from progress documented in the clinical notes.

Appropriateness of Care for Reimbursement

Because a care plan shows problems and reasons for care, it supports the need for care and level of care that qualifies for reimbursement. For example, Medicare-reimbursed care requires skilled nursing be provided for primary and secondary diagnoses. These diagnoses reflect a patient's acute condition. For Medicare-reimbursed care, documentation including the care plan, must justify the medical diagnoses represented by a diagnosis-related group (DRG) code, which in turn establishes patient length of stay (LOS). The DRG and LOS establish the reimbursement rate the government will pay for a patient's care. (See case management in Chapter 9 for information on DRGs and documentation.) Sometimes a complication causes a patient to need a longer

---

 ### AMERICAN NURSES ASSOCIATION STANDARDS OF CARE

Standard I. Assessment

The nurse collects client health data.

Standard II. Diagnosis

The nurse analyzes the assessment data in determining diagnoses.

Standard III. Outcome Identification

The nurse identifies expected outcomes individualized to the client.

Standard IV. Planning

The nurse develops a plan of care that prescribes the interventions to attain expected outcomes.

Standard V. Implementation

The nurse implements the interventions identified in the plan of care.

Standard VI. Evaluation

The nurse evaluates the client's progress toward attainment of outcomes.

Reprinted with permission, American Nurses Association. (1991) *Standards of Clinical Practice.* Washington, DC: Author.

stay or an additional type of care. The care needs to be included in a revised care plan and substantiated in progress notes.

Rates of reimbursement by insurance companies and other third-party payers also depend on care plans to show that skilled care is being provided. Reimbursed skilled care is that which by law can only be provided by a licensed nurse. Examples of skilled care are injections, catheterizations, and other invasive procedures. Before reimbursement is made, most insurance companies specifically require that a need for skilled care be shown on the care plan and proof of skilled care be documented on clinical notes. Further, some insurance companies will review progress notes to see if specific planned interventions on the care plan were performed.

Use of Nursing Care Plans

Nursing care plans are used as a primary source of information during nursing care rounds, interdisciplinary team conferences, change of shift reports, and discharge planning. This use is discussed in Chapter 10.

Care plans can also be used to determine patient acuity or to establish costs for nursing care. This can be accomplished by assigning specific numeric values to each intervention on a care plan. Numeric values can be determined according to skill, duration, and frequency of that intervention. Added totals of numeric values establish how much care a patient needs. If a total numeric value for a patient is 12 and a range for moderate level of care is 10 to 15, that patient is in a middle patient acuity level classification.

With an acuity system attached to care plan interventions, cost of nursing care and staffing can be determined. When a time duration is multiplied by nursing salaries, a cost value can be placed on nursing care provided. For example, if it takes a nurse 10 minutes to perform a wound care treatment and the nurse's salary is $24/hour, the labor cost for that portion of nursing care is $4. Duration and frequency of care can be computed for full-time equivalents of care, and staffing for the next shift (by discipline) can be determined. For example, if 24 patients on a unit have skilled nursing needs that total 1 hour for each patient during the evening shift, four licensed nurses would be needed for staffing.

Characteristics of a Successful Care Plan

Nursing care plans are a permanent and important part of the chart. They must be individualized, complete, concise, accurate, and realistic.

The Care Plan Is Individualized and Patient Focused

After formulating the nursing diagnosis, the next step in the nursing process is to plan care for the patient. "The patient" is a significant phrase because the care plan must be individualized or customized to the patient, both in describing needs and expected outcomes and establishing interventions to respond to those specific needs and expected outcomes. Nursing care plans must be developed with input from the patient and significant others when appropriate, and modifications to standardized care plans must be documented to support individualization of care.

The Care Plan Is Realistic

In planning patient care, the goals and interventions must be realistic for the nursing practice setting. If the patient is depressed and wants to go outside, an intervention to have an aide take the patient outside every day for an hour is certainly realistic in a long-term care setting, but not usually possible in an acute care setting.

When planning patient care, the nurse must consider health care facilities, community resources, and costs. In looking at costs, weigh the probability of achieving the desired outcome, the efforts involved in reaching the desired outcome, and the potential meaning to the patient to accomplish (or fail to accomplish) the desired outcome. For example, a young man named Joe was badly injured in an automobile accident. A cervical spine injury required extensive physical therapy for rehabilitation, with little or no guarantee that any progress could be made. Options were home care with in-home physical therapy, outpatient physical therapy with gait training rails and other stationary equipment, or inpatient care in a rehabilitation facility. Joe was anxious to rehabilitate but feared that little progress would be made. Concerns about cost were addressed by trying to value cost in each setting in relation to relative chance for success in the setting. Finally, he received in-home continuous care with outpatient physical therapy and made progress in rehabilitation. Nurses can help patients look at costs by referring to community resources, offering care provider alternatives, and planning affordable and accessible care.

The Care Plan Includes Strengths and Barriers in Achieving Goals

When planning patient care, the nurse should consider the patient's age and developmental level, recognize the patient's strengths and weaknesses, and allow for changeable and unchangeable barriers to interventions and patient learning. An unchangeable barrier could be a limited intelligence level or communication or language ability. A changeable barrier could be available resources or support of family and caregivers. When the patient participates in setting goals and agrees to the stated interventions, the nurse and patient overcome some of these barriers and motivate the patient to learn and start to assume self-care.

The Care Plan Lists Measurable, Achievable, Mutually Agreeable Expected Outcomes

A walk in the hall does not measure an outcome; walk 100 yards without shortness of breath (SOB) is measurable. Describing an expected outcome for the tenth day when the average LOS for a diagnosis is 7 days is not achievable. For example, if 7 days is the average LOS in the hospital for a patient who had coronary artery bypass surgery, a nurse does not include in the care plan that on the tenth day, or by discharge, the patient will be ambulating 500 yards in the hall four times a day. First, a good deal more time may be required before the patient is able to do that; second, the patient is not likely to be in the facility on the tenth day and therefore expected outcomes could be measured as a false negative. (See Chapter 6 for discussion of expected outcomes.) Similarly, in planning for care, propose adequate, feasible actions for the patient, taking into consideration present life-style, culture, patient objectives and goals, and current physical and emotional status in response to illness and treatment. When focusing on the patient, considering all these facets, the patient is more likely to truly feel involved in and then agree to the plan of care.

The Care Plan Reflects Priorities of Care

The nurse can establish priorities for care by listing nursing diagnoses in priority of importance. To find the most important, look at the primary diagnosis or the reason for admission or the patient's chief complaint. That is the starting point. The highest priority nursing diagnoses will be the most urgent needs. Determine which is the most serious in terms of patient condition or even threat to life. The next priority would be any related diagnoses. For example, if a postoperative patient has a primary medical diagnosis of breast cancer, based on the patient's data, the most important nursing diagnosis second day postoperatively may be Ineffective Airway Clearance R/T (as explained in more detail later, R/T means related to) poor cough/deep breathing effort. A second nursing diagnosis in priority listing could be Body Image Disturbance R/T missing body part (mastectomy). Lower priority nursing diagnoses are those that may or may not refer to the patient's primary or secondary illness or

symptoms and are not life threatening. One may be Altered Nutrition: Less than Body Requirements R/T lack of interest in food.

One example of an outline for setting priorities describes the nursing diagnoses related to physiologic needs first, then nursing diagnoses related to psychosocial needs. Because most patients need to feel physically free of pain and discomfort before psychosocial needs can be addressed, one priority progression of categories of needs may be physical, psychological, emotional, social, and spiritual needs. Remember that spiritual needs are not necessarily any less important than other needs, but most patients focus on and react to daily functioning needs first, then turn toward spiritual needs. In some situations, however, spiritual needs may be a priority for the patient and family. Generally, by prioritizing the patient's physical problems or diagnoses first, the patient is physically comfortable to be able to work through other problems of psychological, emotional, social, and spiritual diagnoses.

Within each of these categories (physical, psychological, emotional, social, and spiritual), nursing diagnoses can be listed in this priority: life-threatening health response problems, the patient's own priorities, followed by other concerns.

EXAMPLE: A patient with congestive heart failure

(*Life-threatening health response problem*):
Decreased Cardiac Output R/T decreased myocardial contractility, altered cardiac rhythm, and fluid volume overload

(*Patient priority*):
Activity Intolerance R/T decreased cardiac output and impaired gas exchange

(*Other concern*):
Ineffective Family Coping R/T disruption of patient's homemaking role during rehabilitation

Nursing diagnoses concerning knowledge deficit (teaching/patient education) can be listed on the care plan within each category of physical or psychosocial needs. Or the nursing diagnosis of Knowledge Deficit can be separated onto a teaching plan as an addendum to the care plan. Either way, it is helpful to have all learning needs grouped together for better patient education planning. The last nursing diagnosis to be listed in this example, then, can be Knowledge Deficit, which requires patient teaching. The nursing diagnosis could read Knowledge Deficit R/T disease process and treatment, or more individualized for this patient Knowledge Deficit R/T chronic congestive heart failure and care management. When a patient has difficulty in medication administration the knowledge deficit can be more specific to read Knowledge Deficit R/T congestive heart failure and medication regimen.

Special Considerations When Writing a Care Plan

How Much Detail Is Necessary?

A consideration in writing care plans is the amount of detail necessary for clarification. The rule of thumb is to follow hospital policy, procedures, and recognized standards or protocols. For example, a complex wound care procedure can be documented in detail for fast reference and for accuracy in treatment when procedures change as the wound status changes.

What Are Normal Ranges?

The nurse should also consider the normal limits in outcome goal specifications. Most patient care problems can be compared to standards or identifiable norms or patient-specific norms. The care plan can identify these normal parameters. For example, if the patient's own normal limits fall outside the average normal range, then instead of "vital signs WNL" document "vital signs within physician-designated parameter" or "vital signs within patient's normal range."

Should the Care Plan Include Patient Requests?

Patient and family personal requests or preferences should be noted on the care plan. Few things are more frustrating for a patient than to have to repeat preferences and requests to a caregiver on every shift for more than a couple of days. Moreover, if a nurse does not acknowledge and attempt to comply with patient or family requests, an unnecessary barrier arises in the nurse–patient relationship. This can potentially affect the patient's motivation, involvement in plan of care, and compliance. If a nurse mutually develops goals with a patient and family, particular requests of the patient can be easily integrated into the care plan.

Who Writes the Care Plan? When? Who's Involved?

When documenting the plan of care the nurse should adhere to some traditional principles. The registered nurse who writes the assessment should write the initial care plan, taking information from the assessment and writing the care plan as soon as possible within 48 hours after the assessment. Patient and family involvement in development of the care plan and approval of revisions

of the care plan should be documented on the care plan. Involvement of interdisciplinary health care members in planning care should be indicated on an interdisciplinary care plan or indicated on the nursing care plan to refer to the separate disciplinary care plan. Finally, the care plan should be written so that it can accurately be understood by all levels of nursing personnel and interdisciplinary caregivers, whomever shall be reading the care plan.

When Should the Care Plan Be Revised?

A care plan is efficient and useful only when it is kept accurate and updated. A nurse makes revisions if the nursing diagnosis is no longer accurate as the patient progresses or regresses in the illness or in response to the illness and treatment. Revisions need to be made if the nursing interventions were carried out and the patient failed to meet or make any progress toward achieving expected outcomes. If this occurs, the nurse investigates the need to reorder priorities or revise outcome goals or interventions. Important questions are:

▲ Have the nursing needs of the patient been met?
▲ Has the patient's condition improved, deteriorated, or remained the same?
▲ Have the interventions been carried out as designated in the care plan, and if not, has it been due to a content problem, a communication problem, a nursing problem, or a patient problem?

Remember, any nurse-initiated intervention can be added, deleted, or revised because it is a nursing order, not a medical order.

The Current Care Plan Controversy

Care planning has changed significantly over the past couple of decades. Before the introduction of principles in care plan development and use of standardized care plans, nurses became frustrated with the time-consuming function of documenting planned care. With the nursing shortage and the increase of paperwork requirements, nurses were faced with a care planning task that took even more time away from bedside care. Today, frustrations still exist.

In addition, depending on how the nursing care plan is written, some nurses feel that the documentation of the care plan is cumbersome. Although some accrediting organizations and documentation authors seek to eliminate care plans, the purpose and function of care plans remain important to nursing care.

In 1991, JCAHO eliminated any reference to a requirement for a separate care plan. However, in the 1992 JCAHO *Accreditation Manual for Hospitals*, the requirement for clinical record data includes patient assessments, nursing diagnoses and/or patient needs, nursing interventions, and patient outcomes (Standard NC.1.3.5). All of these are components of a care plan. Rather than strictly eliminating care plans, the JCAHO still requires evidence of planned care. It can however, be in any format—PIE, SOAP, narrative critical path, or guidelines method (see Chapter 9 for these formats).

Care Plan Types

Traditional Care Plan

Traditional narrative care plans allow health care organizations to revise forms easily and establish guidelines in documentation without form changes. Additionally, an open format (lined form for writing free narrative) allows a nurse to individualize outcomes and interventions, choosing interventions and tips from nursing textbooks, procedure manuals, or standardized care plan books.

Standardized Care Plan

In comparison, a standardized or generic care plan saves time because a nurse does not need to refer to experiential memory, professional nursing texts, or procedure manuals to gather content. Using a standard care plan, the nurse is assured of the inclusion of important outcome goals and interventions. Standard care plans also decrease redundancy for nurses who need to write the same generic intervention and outcomes for patients with the same diagnoses. They are efficient and helpful for new graduates or nurses inexperienced in caring for particular patients. They are also a major contribution to quality because the quality assurance program can incorporate standards into the nursing care plan (see display, Standardized Nursing Care Plan).

Standardized care plans have the disadvantage of depersonalization or lack of individualization. This can be remedied by allowing space for individualized revisions and additional text. Another disadvantage of standardized care plans is the combining of different (diagnoses) standard care plans and individualized additions to the care plan. It results in care plans stapled together of which some accrediting and auditing organizations disapprove.

A remedy to that problem is computerized documentation. Phrases can be chosen to create one individualized care plan from standardized phrases and individualized input. Or a care plan can be written from a checklist format, which some computer software programs have done. Computerization facilitates the individualization of standardized care plans by the ability to easily add, delete, or revise text without crossed out or unused sections of text in the final care plan.

Avoiding Pitfalls in Documenting Nursing Care Plans

A successful care plan begins with an adequate and complete assessment. A major reason for difficulty in documenting nursing care plans is inaccurate or incomplete data to complete the problem-solving process. Clinical problem-solving depends on a logical progression of nursing documentation. The assessment may be inadequate or out of date and that causes a failure in planning nursing care. If assessment data are inadequate because the patient or family member cannot provide an adequate history, document that the nurse has an insufficient data base. The nurse should attempt to get information from other health provider sources or other family members or caregivers. If the assessment is adequate but the nurse obtains more information that is incomplete or unclear, or if significant information learned after assessment is not added to documentation, then the care plan will not provide direction for the quality care desired.

Including the patient and family in care planning contributes to assessment data that considers the patient's life-style, culture, and beliefs. Ignoring the patient or family in care planning results in choosing interventions that are inappropriate or incompatible with daily activities and preferences. If patient and family preferences are not considered, important aspects of the care plan will fail.

A successful care plan is specific. If a plan is not specific enough, a care plan will be inadequate. Communication will then include assumption, and measurable criteria will not be appropriate for good outcome evaluation. If an intervention involves observation, the care plan should state how frequently to observe. If a procedure can be performed in various ways, and yet should be done in a consist manner, the care plan should describe how to do it.

A successful care plan is legible. A common and long-standing problem of documentation is illegibility. If even one caregiver cannot read the care plan because of illegible handwriting, the care of that patient, even if for only one shift, is affected. Multiply that by many shifts, and communication and thus effectiveness of the documented plan are affected.

Writing a Nursing Diagnosis

A nursing diagnosis is different from a medical diagnosis. A nursing diagnosis focuses on a patient response to a health problem that can be altered or prevented by nursing interventions. A medical diagnosis is a statement of illness with a focus on curing pathology that determines medical orders or protocols. Although some medical and even nursing professionals object to the term

STANDARDIZED NURSING CARE PLAN

NAPLES COMMUNITY HOSPITAL
Naples, FL

IMPAIRED GAS EXCHANGE

Date and Initials	Patients Care Problems	Patient Expected Outcome	Target Date	Date and Initials	Specific Nursing Interventions	C/RV/RS Status
	_____ Actual _____ Potential	Patient will:			[ ] Ensure adequate alveolar ventilations	
	IMPAIRED GAS EXCHANGE, related to:	[ ] Verbalize that breathing is more comfortable			[ ] Provide frequent stimulation	
	[ ] Reduction of functional lung tissue	[ ] Prevent/reduce risk or presence of infection by _____			[ ] Teach pursed-lip breathing to prolong, expiratory phase and slow rate	
	[ ] Reduced lung elasticity				[ ] Avoid use of respiratory depressants	
	[ ] Altered chest wall movement/structure	[ ] Demonstrate improved vital signs and diagnostic studies such as _____			[ ] Postural drainage, vibration, percussion q _____	
	[ ] Hypoventilation	_____			[ ] Avoid unnecessary activity/provide assistance with ADL	
	[ ] Bronchospasm				[ ] Bath	
	[ ] Medications	[ ] Modify ADL to decrease oxygen consumption			[ ] Feeding	
	[ ] Infection				[ ] Transfer activity	
	[ ] Allergy	[ ] State three activities that may control or prevent progression of hypoxemia and/or hypercapnia			[ ] Hydrate _____ cc/shift	
	[ ] Smoking				[ ] Small, frequent meals (soft, minimize milk/cheese products) supplements q _____	
	[ ] Inflammation	[ ] Slow, steady inspiration and hold for 3 seconds			[ ] Teach energy conservation techniques	
	[ ] Altered level of consciousness	[ ] Uses relaxation techniques			[ ] Exhale on standing, lifting, pulling, bending	
	[ ] Other _____	[ ] Coordinates breathing pattern with functional activities			[ ] Administer O_2 with any exercise (as ordered)	
	_____	[ ] Identify two measures to avoid infection			[ ] Determine degree of hypoxemia during ambulation or transfer activities	
	_____	[ ] Avoid crowds			[ ] Administer and instruct on the appropriate use of bronchodilators (oral/inhaled), antibiotics, diuretics, oxygen	
		[ ] Reduce contact with individuals with colds				

Initials _____ Signature _____

_____ _____

Patient care problem initiated by _____ (Signature) _____ RN _____ (Date)

Patient care problem resolved by _____ (Signature) _____ RN _____ (Date)

NCH Front   Revised: 6/92
Courtesy of Naples Community Hospital, Naples, FL.

diagnosis, appropriately used and documented nursing diagnoses are effective and desirable within professional nursing practice.

For ease and consistency in identifying a patient problem by a label, standardized nursing diagnoses are increasingly used by nurses. A growing number of health care organizations establish in their policies and procedures or list of standardized nursing diagnoses that are approved for use in their nursing documentation system. The most widely used list of standardized nursing diagnoses is that of the North American Nursing Diagnosis Association (NANDA), who has been endorsed by ANA as the official organization to develop a taxonomy of nursing diagnoses. NANDA's purpose is to identify, develop, and classify nursing diagnoses (see display, Nursing Diagnoses, North American Nursing Diagnosis Association, April 1992). When standardized language is used, communication is clear and consistent regarding needs and problems of a patient.

To establish relationships and patterns, nursing diagnoses have been grouped into classes and subclasses within a classification system. This classification structure is called a **taxonomy**. By looking at a taxonomy, the nurse learns more about the nature and facets of nursing diagnoses and can determine how to find a nursing diagnosis within a taxonomy.

Types of Nursing Diagnoses

According to NANDA (1992), an actual nursing diagnosis describes a human response to a health problem that a nurse is licensed to treat. It is supported by defining characteristics (manifestations/**signs and symptoms**) that cluster in patterns of related cues or inferences. **Related factors** (**etiologies**) are factors that contribute to the development or maintenance of an actual diagnosis.

A high-risk nursing diagnosis describes a human response to a health condition or life process that may develop in a vulnerable individual. A high-risk diagnosis is supported by *risk factors* that contribute to increased vulnerability (NANDA, 1992).

In recognition of the importance of identifying patient strengths, NANDA has added wellness nursing diagnoses to the list. These diagnoses describe a human response that has the potential for enhancement (NANDA, 1992), for example, Family Coping: Potential for Growth.

Components of a Nursing Diagnosis

An actual diagnosis consists of a three-part statement: the problem (human response), the related factor, and the defining characteristics (see display, Components of a Nursing Diagnosis). The first part of human response describes the problem, for example, Fluid Volume Excess.

The second part is the related factors or etiology. For this example the second part of the diagnosis is written as follows:

R/T excess fluid intake

As you can see, the related factor is most often abbreviated to read R/T (related to), for example, Colonic Constipation, R/T *immobility*. Having a different related factor, such as Colonic Constipation, R/T *chronic use of medication and enemas* creates a different patient condition that calls for different nursing interventions. The related factors, then, are critical in communicating accurate patient condition and are important when individualizing nursing interventions.

The third component, often not included on the written care plan, is the signs and symptoms, called **defining characteristics**. This is the assessment information that led the nurse to the nursing diagnosis decision because the characteristics are essential clues for assigning the diagnosis.

as evidenced by 3+ lower extremity periph edema

shortness of breath

A high-risk diagnosis consists of a two-part statement: the problem (human response) and the risk factors that contribute to increased vulnerability. For example, High Risk for Infection (problem) related to immunosuppression (risk factor).

The diagnosis in the care plan is usually written without signs and symptoms, so a complete nursing diagnosis would read:

Fluid Volume Excess R/T excess fluid intake

However, if a health care organization chooses to list defining characteristics in the care plans, the defining characteristics can be listed below the diagnosis and related factors. For example,

Fluid Volume Excess R/T excess fluid and sodium intake

Defining characteristics:

- ▲ edema
- ▲ effusion
- ▲ anasarca
- ▲ weight gain
- ▲ shortness of breath
- ▲ abnormal breath sounds
- ▲ orthopnea
- ▲ S_3 heart sound
- ▲ pulmonary congestion
- ▲ blood pressure and central venous pressure changes
- ▲ decreased hemoglobin and hematocrit

NURSING DIAGNOSES, NORTH AMERICAN NURSING DIAGNOSIS ASSOCIATION

Activity Intolerance
Activity Intolerance, High Risk for
Adjustment, Impaired
Airway Clearance, Ineffective
Anxiety
Aspiration, High Risk for
Body Image Disturbance
Body Temperature, High Risk for Altered
Breastfeeding, Effective
Breastfeeding, Ineffective
Breastfeeding, Interrupted
Breathing Pattern, Ineffective
Cardiac Output, Decreased
Caregiver Role Strain
Caregiver Role Strain, High Risk for
Communication, Impaired Verbal
Constipation
Constipation, Colonic
Constipation, Perceived
Coping, Defensive
Coping, Ineffective Individual
Decisional Conflict (Specify)
Denial, Ineffective
Diarrhea
Disuse Syndrome, High Risk for
Diversional Activity Deficit
Dysreflexia
Family Coping: Compromised, Ineffective
Family Coping: Disabling, Ineffective
Family Coping: Potential for Growth
Family Processes, Altered
Fatigue
Fear
Fluid Volume Deficit
Fluid Volume Deficit, High Risk for
Fluid Volume Excess
Gas Exchange, Impaired
Grieving, Anticipatory
Grieving, Dysfunctional
Growth and Development, Altered
Health Maintenance, Altered
Health-Seeking Behaviors (Specify)
Home Maintenance Management, Impaired
Hopelessness
Hyperthermia
Hypothermia
Incontinence, Bowel
Incontinence, Functional
Incontinence, Reflex
Incontinence, Stress
Incontinence, Total
Incontinence, Urge
Infant Feeding Pattern, Ineffective
Infection, High Risk for
Injury, High Risk for
Knowledge Deficit (Specify)
Noncompliance (Specify)

Nutrition, Altered: Less than Body Requirements
Nutrition, Altered: More than Body Requirements
Nutrition, Altered: Potential for More than Body Requirements
Oral Mucous Membrane, Altered
Pain
Pain, Chronic
Parental Role Conflict
Parenting, Altered
Parenting, High Risk for Altered
Peripheral Neurovascular Dysfunction, High Risk for
Personal Identity Disturbance
Physical Mobility, Impaired
Poisoning, High Risk for
Post-Trauma Response
Powerlessness
Protection, Altered
Rape Trauma Syndrome
Rape Trauma Syndrome: Compound Reaction
Rape Trauma Syndrome: Silent Reaction
Relocation Stress Syndrome
Role Performance, Altered
Self-Care Deficit
    Bathing/Hygiene
    Dressing/Grooming
    Feeding
    Toileting
Self-Esteem, Chronic Low
Self-Esteem, Situational Low
Self-Esteem Disturbance
Self-Mutilation, High Risk for
Sensory-Perceptual Alterations (Specify) (visual, auditory, kinesthetic, gustatory, tactile, olfactory)
Sexual Dysfunction
Sexuality Patterns, Altered
Skin Integrity, High Risk for Impaired
Skin Integrity, Impaired
Sleep Pattern Disturbance
Social Interaction, Impaired
Social Isolation
Spiritual Distress
Suffocation, High Risk for
Swallowing, Impaired
Therapeutic Regimen, Ineffective Management of
Thermoregulation, Ineffective
Thought Processes, Altered
Tissue Integrity, Impaired
Tissue Perfusion, Altered (Specify Type) (renal, cerebral, cardiopulmonary, gastrointestinal, peripheral)
Trauma, High Risk for
Unilateral Neglect
Urinary Elimination, Altered
Urinary Retention
Ventilation, Inability to Sustain Spontaneous
Ventilatory Weaning Response, Dysfunctional
Violence, High Risk for: Self-Directed or Directed at Others

▲ COMPONENTS OF A NURSING DIAGNOSIS

ACTUAL HEALTH PROBLEM
(Human Response)

"related to"

RELATED FACTORS
(Etiology)

"as evidenced by"

DEFINING CHARACTERISTICS
(Signs and Symptoms)

KEY POINTS

▲ The components of the nursing diagnosis include the patient's actual or potential health problems, related factors (etiology), and signs and symptoms (defining characteristics).

▲ In documentation of the nursing care, the care plan is developed from ongoing, measurable assessment data. The care plan includes the nursing diagnoses, expected outcomes, and nursing interventions.

▲ The care plan should be outcome directed with interventions that are clear and specific and designed to contribute to the achievement of expected outcomes.

▲ The expected outcomes are the basis to evaluate the progress the patient is or is not making toward the achievement of established outcomes.

▲ The nursing care planning portion of the nursing process is an important key within the dynamic continuum. The documented care plan is a guideline for direction or any change in direction of care. Nursing diagnosis and care planning are procedurally important because the decision-making judgment of the nurse sets the direction for patient care within the nursing process. Because the nursing diagnosis and planning of care establish the direction and provision of nursing care, they are crucial to patient progress and the ultimate patient outcome.

▲ Standardized care plans or guidelines assist the nurse in documenting complete and comprehen-

sive care plans, which positively affect quality assurance and reimbursement issues. The individualization of these care plans, however, is an important responsibility of nurses caring for patients.

REFERENCES

American Nurses Association. (1991). *Standards of clinical nursing practice*. Washington, DC: Author.

American Nurses Association. (1980). *Nursing: A social policy statement*. Washington, DC: Author.

North American Nursing Diagnosis Association (1992). *NANDA nursing diagnoses: Definitions and classification*. St. Louis: Author.

North American Nursing Diagnosis Association. (1989). *Taxonomy I, revised 1989, with official diagnostic categories* (pp. 2, 5, 6–8). St. Louis: Author.

Tribulski, J. A. (1988). Nursing diagnosis: Waste of time or valued tool? *RN, 51(12)*, 30–40.

Yura, H. (1987). *The nursing process* (5th ed.). Norwalk, CT: Appleton & Lange.

Yura, H., & Walsh, M. (1988). *The nursing process* (p. 141). Norwalk, CT: Appleton & Lange.

BIBLIOGRAPHY

Brider, P. (1991). Who killed the nursing care plan? *American Journal of Nursing, 91(5)*, 34–39.

Dennison, P. D., & Keeling, A. W. (1989). Clinical support for eliminating the nursing diagnosis of knowledge deficit. *Image: Journal of Nursing Scholarship, 21*(3), 142.

Eggland, E. T. (1990). Osteoarthritis. In Dolan, M. *Community and home health care plans* (p. 185). Springhouse, PA: Springhouse Corp.

Holloway, N. M. (1988). *Medical surgical care plans* (p. 273, 388). Springhouse, PA: Springhouse Corp.

Krenz, M., Karlik, B., & Kiniry, S. (1989). A nursing diagnosis based model: Guiding nursing practice. *Journal of Nursing Administration, 19*(5), 32–36.

Leddy, S., & Pepper, J. M. (1985). *Conceptual bases of professional nursing* (pp. 216–217, 225). Philadelphia: J. B. Lippincott.

Lunney, M. (1982). Nursing diagnosis: Refining the system. *American Journal of Nursing, 82(3)*, 456–459.

McCloskey, J. C., & Bulechek, G. M. (1992). *Nursing interventions classification (NIC)*. St. Louis: Mosby–Year Book.

McCourt, A. E. (1987). Implementation of nursing diagnoses through integration with quality assurance. *Nursing Clinics of North America, 22*(4), 903.

PRACTICE SESSION

FILL IN

1. A comprehensive, biopsychosocial outline of proposed interventions to achieve established expected outcomes with a definite time frame is referred to as a _____ .

2. The second step of documentation of the nursing process is the documentation of _____ .

3. A problem expressed as a definite alteration in health is _____ .

4. After determining a nursing diagnosis, the next step in the nursing process is _____ .

5. A nursing care plan includes _____ , _____ , and _____ .

6. Actions taken by a nurse to assist a patient to reach stated expected outcomes are _____ .

7. Nursing diagnoses direct the development of _____ , which influences the development of _____ .

8. The nurse can establish priorities for care by _____ .

9. A nursing diagnosis is different from a _____ .

10. Nurses are responsible to _____ standardized care plans.

MATCHING

Match the term in Column B with its definition in Column A.

1. _____ type of classification system
2. _____ human response to health need
3. _____ scheme classifying nursing diagnostic labels
4. _____ second component of nursing diagnoses
5. _____ third component of nursing diagnoses

a. related factor or etiology
b. taxonomy
c. nursing diagnosis
d. NANDA
e. signs and symptoms or defining characteristics

IDENTIFYING NURSING DIAGNOSES

Identify whether these (NANDA) nursing diagnoses labels are accurately written. If not, rephrase so that it is correct.

1. _____ altered urinary elimination
2. _____ colitis

3. _____ immobility

4. _____ decreased endurance

5. _____ impaired appetite

6. _____ ineffective breathing pattern

7. _____ self-esteem disturbance

8. _____ potential for infection

9. _____ decubitus ulcer or pressure sore

10. _____ confusion

MULTIPLE CHOICE

1. _____ Care plans contribute toward
   a) goal direction
   b) coordination of care
   c) continuity of care
   d) all of the above

2. _____ Some standards that influence how care planning is developed are from organizations such as
   a) ANA
   b) JCAHO
   c) NLN
   d) all of the above

3. _____ Care plans are not just for meeting documentation requirements, they are also used for
   a) change-of-shift reports
   b) team conferences
   c) discharge planning
   d) all of the above

4. _____ The R/T in a nursing diagnosis means
   a) rationale toward
   b) related to
   c) reason/theory
   d) reverse/toward

5. _____ A nursing diagnosis is composed of three parts, including
   a) health problem, etiology, signs and symptoms
   b) patient need, reason/theory, signs to watch for
   c) nursing diagnosis, medical diagnosis, disease complications
   d) none of the above

CHALLENGE FOR CRITICAL THINKING

1. Define nursing diagnosis, including components.

2. Why is it important to list nursing diagnoses in priority of importance when developing an initial nursing care plan or nursing problem list? How would you determine priority?

3. Reimbursement for health care is a national concern. How does a care plan influence reimbursement?

4. How does a nurse individualize a care plan?

5. Discuss the pros and cons of documenting separate care plans.

LEARNING TO DOCUMENT

1. A 44-year-old woman underwent a right-sided mastectomy 2 days ago. The doctor has told the patient and family that chemotherapy will be necessary because of cancer metastases to the lung. In appropriate terms what probable nursing diagnoses can you identify for this patient and family? List at least three diagnoses in priority.

2. A 50-year-old man was admitted to the hospital following an acute asthma attack that was precipitated by an upper respiratory viral infection and smoking. List in appropriate terms possible expected outcomes for this patient.

3. A 65-year-old woman has had a mild myocardial infarct (heart attack). She was told not to exert herself for the next 6 weeks. She complained of "never being well again" and unable to keep a clean, neat house as she is accustomed. How should care plan interventions be documented for these two problems?

4. Choose one of the three patients above and develop a nursing care plan, using the care plan column format in the Standardized Nursing Care Plan.

6

Documenting Nursing Interventions and Outcomes

LEARNING OBJECTIVES

After studying this chapter, the learner should be able to:

▲   Define structure components of a narrative clinical progress note to reflect clinical judgment and the nursing process.

▲   Identify two types of nursing interventions.

▲   List types of nursing activities to document in clinical progress notes.

▲   Explain the relationship of expected outcomes to progress note patient outcomes.

▲   Describe three ways in which patient outcomes are currently documented to meet new outcome documentation requirements.

KEY TERMS

Expected outcomes
Nursing activities
Nurse-initiated treatments

Nursing interventions
Outcome criteria
Patient outcomes

Physician-initiated treatment
Target date

Eggland ET, Heinemann DS. NURSING DOCUMENTATION:
CHARTING, RECORDING, AND REPORTING.
© 1994 J.B. Lippincott Company.

In the fourth step of documenting the nursing process, the nurse implements the care plan by performing the nursing interventions described on the care plan. **Nursing interventions** are composed of a series of nursing activities or actions. After the nurse performs these nursing activities, the nurse documents on the clinical progress notes that these activities were completed. Clinical progress notes documented by nurses caring for a patient are also called nurses notes.

Nursing interventions that the nurse performs include actions that assist the patient in reaching expected outcomes. Some nursing interventions decrease or eliminate the patient problems identified in the nursing diagnosis. Nursing interventions also include actions that contribute to enhancing patient capabilities. In the *Nursing Interventions Classification* (*NIC*) of McCloskey and Bulechek (1992), nursing interventions include nurse-initiated treatments and physician-initiated treatments. These authors also describe nursing interventions as composed of a series of concrete **nursing activities** or actions, which together carry out a nursing intervention. For example, a nursing intervention "assess tissue perfusion" includes the activities of monitoring the blood pressure and pulse every hour, monitoring intake and output every 8 hours, monitoring the level of consciousness every 4 hours, and auscultating the lungs every 4 hours.

Abbreviations used in clinical progress notes, as in other documentation forms, must be accepted abbreviations approved by the health care organization in which the nurse is working. Using only approved abbreviations eliminates confusion as to what an abbreviation means. Eliminating confusion prevents errors in clinical judgment and patient care.

A nurse documents on the clinical progress note the nursing interventions, which are composed of:

▲ Nursing actions initiated by medical order
▲ Nursing actions initiated by nursing order
▲ Nursing actions resulting from medical and nursing collaborative care

Nursing actions initiated by medical order, also called **physician-initiated treatments**, are usually medical treatments or medication administrations the nurse performs as directed by a medical order. Nursing actions initiated by nursing order, also called **nurse-initiated treatments**, include a wide variety of nursing interventions. These interventions include ongoing assessment or monitoring, teaching, counseling, treatment administration, and referrals. Documentation of these interventions is also done on the clinical progress note. Nursing actions, which are the result of nursing and medical collaborative care, are assessment oriented.

Patient outcomes that are documented in clinical progress notes reflect evaluation of nursing care and are a description of the patient's actual status after nursing interventions for an identified nursing diagnosis. For example, a patient has a nursing diagnosis of Pain. A planned intervention is pain management. Nurse activities for pain management include changing the position of the patient, instructing the patient in relaxation techniques, and administering medication for pain relief. The documented outcome for that pain management intervention would be whether or how much the intervention alleviated the pain. The patient outcome could be documented "patient states pain decreased to +3 pain level," 30 minutes after nursing interventions.

Documentation of interventions and outcomes provides an important link between the steps of assessing and planning for care and evaluating whether care has been effective. The record shows the sequence of clinical judgment implementation and the active cycle of the nursing process.

Clinical progress notes include clinical data, nursing interventions, and patient outcomes. Clinical data are collected by ongoing assessment of the patient. Nursing actions or interventions are developed in response to identified needs and are performed according to the care plan. Outcomes reflect the result of care. Because clinical notes include data, interventions, and outcomes, notes reflect steps of the nursing process and data to support clinical judgments. Finally, clinical progress notes should represent a record of the implementation of planned care.

Documentation of nursing interventions and outcomes contributes to:

▲ Evaluating patient goal attainment as a result of nursing care
▲ Determining current progress toward expected outcomes
▲ Ensuring opportunity for communication among caregivers, by a central record of data regarding ongoing care
▲ Determining if care implemented meets established standards
▲ Determining care provided, for reimbursement purposes
▲ Determining care provided, for legal protection
▲ Contributing available data for nursing research, thus enhancing nursing theory and knowledge

Documenting Nursing Interventions

Traditional questions in documenting nursing interventions have included the question of how much or how little information needs to be documented. A second question of nurses is how nursing interventions from the nursing care plan can be repeated on clinical progress notes.

What to Document

The outline of what to document for a particular patient is listed on the individualized care plan. The nursing diagnoses provide the topic of a clinical note, and expected outcomes and nursing actions provide the specific detail as they compare to a patient's present health status. Current and updated versions of the care plan provide the outline, as new patient needs are assessed and expected outcomes and proposed interventions develop. A nursing diagnosis (or diagnoses) is the focus or topic of a note. The nursing orders or (proposed) nursing interventions should be the basis of documenting actual interventions implemented. The expected outcome on the care plan should be the guideline for documenting the response of the patient to the nursing intervention or the progress the patient is making toward the expected patient outcome.

"If it wasn't documented, it wasn't done" is an accepted axiom in nursing documentation. Nursing action documentation then covers all aspects of providing patient care and includes the following interventions:

▲ Autonomous or nurse-initiated treatment/interventions
- Observing, assessing, and monitoring the patient's condition
- Providing comfort measures, in pain, positioning, and so forth
- Monitoring and assisting in problems related to physiologic functions of hydration, nutrition, respiration, and elimination
- Assisting in activities of daily living or giving direction and supervision in that assistance
- Teaching and counseling
- Instructing and performing actions to prevent infection, injury, or complications of the disease process
- Providing emotional support
- Providing a therapeutic milieu
- Referring to appropriate resources and, when appropriate, instructing the patient in how to gain access to and use resources

▲ Physician-initiated treatment/interventions
- Administering therapeutic interventions by written or verbal medical orders

▲ Collaborative or care management interventions
- Consulting with physicians or other disciplines in collaborative or multidisciplinary care. Nursing actions include collaborative monitoring, care planning, and intervening to prevent complications or treat health care problems that exist or are high risk due to pathology or treatment. Collaborative interventions involve nurses with physicians; physical, speech, respiratory and occupational therapists; dietitians, and medical social service personnel.

All nursing actions should be documented when performed. If these nursing actions are not performed but were prescribed in care planning, a nurse should document the reason they were not completed. Reasons may include patient refusal, NPO (nothing by mouth) due to diagnostic tests or surgery, or patient not available for scheduled treatment. In addition to the above nursing actions, other actions or other vital information important for inclusion in nursing notes will have been documented in the patient's individualized care plan.

How to Write a Clinical Progress Note

A clinical progress note always begins with documenting the time and date it is being written. This information is important in terms of patient assessment, patient progress, and validation of time of treatment interventions. Timed documentation affects the level of quality care and provides legal protection.

The outline of a nursing clinical progress note should reflect the nursing process:

1. Nursing diagnosis
2. What was assessed
3. Clinical data
4. Interventions
5. Patient outcome or response
6. Any further plans (may also be included)

The nursing diagnosis is the topic of the note or a topic of a paragraph in the note. What was assessed can be a brief statement that indicates what skilled nursing assessment was performed on which body part or system. Recall that skilled nursing is nursing activity that requires, by law, a licensed registered nurse (or a licensed practical nurse under the supervision of a registered nurse) to perform. This part of the clinical progress note is optional, but it is helpful in establishing skilled care for reimbursement that requires skilled interventions. Clinical data are the symptoms, measurements, and pertinent information from the patient, which are directly related to the specific nursing diagnosis addressed. Interventions should be listed in the order of what was assessed, what was implemented, or what was taught to the patient or caregiver. The patient response or outcome is the patient's subjective response to the intervention and the measurable, objective outcome of patient status as it compares to the expected outcome on the care plan. The following is an example of a clinical progress note:

12/22/92 4:30 pm

Nursing diagnosis: Ineffective Airway Clearance R/T tenacious sputum and poor cough effort. *Assessed*: VS, SOB, breath sounds, cardiopulmonary status. *Clinical data*: Pt c/o "chest tight and can't breathe." BP160/100, P110, R30. Exhibits stridor and nasal flaring. Respiratory wheeze evident with auscultation, left lower lobe. Pt coughed up 10 mL thick, tenacious, yellow mucus.

Interventions: Administered bronchodilator medications as ordered. Instructed pt in coughing and deep breathing. *Outcome*: Pt demonstrated effective controlled coughing and deep breathing and responded to bronchodilator medications with relief. States "no difficulty breathing now." BP130/90, P82, R22.

There is an important point to make in the difference between a structured narrative note (an example above) and traditional narrative notes without subject topics. Adding structure by topics related to the nursing process creates organization and interrelation among the data, which reflects critical thinking, professional judgment, and decision-making. This method results in quickly seeing progress toward patient care goals and quality patient care. In narrative notes, structure is possible and desirable to facilitate documentation of clinical judgment and retrieval of information for multidisciplinary communication.

How to Write Interventions on the Clinical Progress Note

Newly practicing nurses sometimes ask how to take the interventions from the care plan and document them on the clinical progress notes. Simply copying proposed interventions from the care plan, putting them into past tense, and documenting them onto clinical progress notes is not appropriate because it shows no active participation in clinical judgment. Although the documented nursing interventions must be consistent with the established plan of care, and may repeat some of the same terminology, clinical progress notes must include more information. Interventions documented on clinical notes must be supported by substantiating data, should show some relation toward achievement of expected outcomes, and should result in a documented patient response or outcome. If documented nursing actions indicate an expected outcome is not being achieved, then the corresponding nursing intervention in care

planning would be one factor to be evaluated and possibly revised.

Frequently Used Clinical Progress Note Formats

The format of clinical notes is determined by the policy of the health care organization. The following are examples of SOAPIER, (*S*ubjective, *O*bjective, *A*ssessment, *P*lan, *I*ntervention, *E*valuation, *R*evision), traditional narrative, and PIE (*P*roblem, *I*ntervention, *E*valuation) progress notes, which are commonly used. Focus notes of *D*ata, *A*ction, *R*esults (DAR) are presented in Chapter 9, Comparing Charting Methods, along with detailed explanations of SOAPIER and PIE charting.

SOAPIER

The acronym SOAPIER stands for subjective, objective, assessment, plan, intervention, evaluation, and revision. Essentially this information includes the categories of clinical data, intervention, and patient outcome. In this multidisciplinary problem-oriented medical record, the problem is written as a medical problem by all caregivers, including nurses.

Problem #3. Acute glomerulonephritis

S: Pt claims burning on urination, frequency, urgency, and nocturia. Pt states she "cries because of pain" while voiding and is uncomfortable using a bedpan.

O: Pt voided ×6 from 11 pm to 7 am. Observed pt crying while sitting on bedpan. Urine test: positive for α-hemolytic streptococci. Taking Pyridiate 200 mg PO qid since yesterday (first dose 8 am).

A: Altered Urinary Elimination pattern and Pain R/T urinary tract infection. Urinary culture of 8/19/92 positive.

P: Maintain medication regimen, protein-restricted diet, and bed rest per MD. Force fluids. Maintain accurate I&O. Observe for symptoms of hypertension, renal failure, and depression.

I: Encouraged patient to drink 12 oz water q2h. Assisted patient onto bedpan. Called MD to report continued pain and requested order for increased activity of OOB to bedside commode.

E: Patient still experiencing pain 3 hours after Pyridiate administration. Current medication has not relieved symptoms.

The evaluation (*E*) shows that the patient has made limited progress toward an expected outcome of absence of pain. A revision (*R*) could be added to modify the nursing intervention so that progress is made toward the expected outcome. An example could be to increase fluids to 1000 mL/day and encourage patient to drink cranberry juice.

The SOAPIER note includes a patient's primary symptoms, secondary problems, complaints, response to treatment, and progress or lack of it. In SOAPIER or in any format, subsequent clinical notes should include documentation of pain status or any unresolved patient need, until relieved.

TRADITIONAL NARRATIVE

Clinical progress notes are still frequently written in a traditional narrative form. For locating data quickly, it is helpful to document nursing topics addressed throughout the note, such as UTI management, incontinence, hydration, and potential complications in the following note.

Date: 9/22/92

Time: 6:30 am

UTI management: Pt c/o urgency and dysuria. Sleeping since 10:30 pm. 12:00 am c/o of dull pain in L flank area. Pyridium 200 mg PO administered per order. *Incontinence*: Incontinent of urine. Bed linen changed ×4. I&O maintained with notation of times incontinent. *Hydration*: Offered fruit juices, soda, and water; encouraged increase in fluids. Taking fluids poorly—intake 30 mL from 11 pm to 6:30 am despite instruction and rationale for greater intake/hydration. *Potential complications*: No c/o of headache or potential hypertensive symptoms.

The order of a narrative note should be the same as a structure note (SOAPIER, PIE): patient need or problem, nursing actions, and patient response or outcome when possible. Each problem or nursing diagnosis should be addressed in this manner.

PIE

A problem, action, and response is easier to retrieve in a structured format such as PIE:

P: Altered Urinary Elimination related to Foley catheter obstruction. Foley catheter not draining due to large amount of white sediment in urine.

I: Attempted to irrigate Foley with 200 mL of Soln G but unable to instill any irrigant. Catheter removed with balloon deflated and intact. New #18 Foley catheter with 10-mL balloon inserted. Balloon inflated with 8 mL sterile NS.

E: Catheter draining well—100 mL in first 30 min, 9 am to 9:30 am.

Nursing note information should be documented by date and time of occurrence and signed by the documenting nurse. If a nurse documents about many nursing diagnoses in one note, diagnoses should be listed in the same priority as in the care plan. Within each topic of a nursing diagnosis, aspects of physical health, daily function, and overall well-being should be included.

Flow Sheets for Monitoring Patient Status and Documenting Interventions

Revising clinical note forms into a checklist or flow sheet format is becoming increasingly popular because of the flow sheet speed of entry, ease in retrieving information, and ease in making fast comparisons for monitoring data. In documenting interventions, flow sheet forms can be focused on assessment information, interventions, or a combination of both assessment and interventions encountered during a defined time of nursing care. Forms can be customized for particular disease entities or special patient populations (eg, type of patient). Today, in an increasing number of hospitals, flow sheets are customized for particular departments, such as medical/surgical areas and especially intensive care areas. Four-page foldout "daily records" or "care flow sheets" bring together many types of documentation categories: vital signs, procedures, diagnostics, therapeutics, patient activity, hygiene interventions, dressing changes, teaching checklists, assessments, and treatments (see displays, Robinson Memorial Hospital Daily Observation Record and Robinson Memorial Hospital Treatment Flow Sheet).

Assessment and treatment patient care notes are also used to record routine, frequent care observations, such as nutrition (assisted feeding, NPO, tube feeding) and treatments (wound care, suctioning, moist packs, traction). These items are checked off with a nurse's initials when completed. If necessary, treatments or response can be further described in nursing narrative notes on the back of the form. For example, a dressing change would be checked off with initials on the flow sheet when it was performed. A narrative on the back of the form would describe the characteristics and appearance of the wound, wound care treatment, and the type of dressing applied. Topics needing further description in narrative notes are usually marked with an asterisk to remind nurses that descriptive narrative charting is needed. A portion of a flow sheet form could look like this:

	Date 7-3	3-11	11-7
* Wound Care			
Dressing change	✔		

A printed asterisk (*) or written check mark (✔) indicates: Additional documentation (necessary) in narrative notes.

(text continues on page 122)

DAILY OBSERVATION FORM

ROBINSON MEMORIAL HOSPITAL
Patient Progress Notes
DAILY OBSERVATION RECORD

Date:

								LEGEND	PULSE GRADING
B E H A V I O R / **L. O. C.**	Time:							P-Person	O-Absent
	Alert:							PL-Place	1+-Easily occuled
	Oriented	P PL T C	P PL T C	P PL T C	P PL T C	P PL T C		T-Time	2+-Occluded with
	Disoriented							C-Circumstance	mild pressure
	Lethargic							+-Present	3+-Normal
	Unresponsive							--Absent	4+-Bounding
	Cooperative							R-Right	D-Doppler
	Uncooperative							L-Left	
	Anxious								**Patient Teaching**
	Eye Contact	Yes No	Yes No	Yes No	Yes No	Yes No			

S K I N	Temp: Warm						
	Hot						
	Cool						
	Cold						
	Moisture: Dry						
	Moist						
	Diaphoretic						
	Turgor: Elastic						
	Non-Elastic						
	Color:						
	Integrity: Intact						
	Impaired						

C A R D I O V A S C U L A R	Heart Sounds: Regular							
	Irregular							
	Apical Radial Deficit	+ −	+ −	+ −	+ −	+ −		**Team Leader**
	JVD @ 45	+ −	+ −	+ −	+ −	+ −		**Responsible**
	Pulses	R L	R L	R L	R L	R L		7-3
	Temporal							
	Carotid							
	Brachial							3-11
	Radial							
	Femoral							
	Post. tibial							11-7
	Dorsalis pedis							
	Calf tenderness:							
	on palpatation							**OR**
	on dorsiflexion							
	Edema:	R L	R L	R L	R L	R L		7^A-7^P
	Facial							
	ABD							
	Sacral							7^P-7^A
	Arms							
	Hands							
	Legs							
	Ankles							**Other**
	Pedal							

Signatures

Courtesy of Robinson Memorial Hospital, Ravenna, Ohio

TREATMENT FLOW SHEET

DATE _____   **TREATMENT FLOW SHEET**

	7ᴬ	8ᴬ	9ᴬ	10ᴬ	11ᴬ	12ᴾ	1ᴾ	2ᴾ	3ᴾ	4ᴾ	5ᴾ	6ᴾ	7ᴾ	8ᴾ	9ᴾ	10ᴾ	11ᴾ	12ᴬ	1ᴬ	2ᴬ	3ᴬ	4ᴬ	5ᴬ	6ᴬ
Nursing Rounds																								
Activity: BR (1), BSC (2), Chair (3), Ambulate c Assist (4), Self Ambulate (5)																								
Bath: Self (1), Assist (2), Complete (3), Shower (4)																								
Back Care																								
Oral Care																								
Pericare/Foley Care																								
Turn and Reposition R-Right, S-Side, L-Left, B-Back																								
Bed in Prevention Mode																								
Restraints: Soft (1), Vest (2), Wrists (3), Ankles (4), Leathers (5), Remove q8O-check skin condition-then reapply (6), (R) Right, (L) Left																								
Side Rails: (▲▲), (▲▼), (▼▼)																								
Call Light in Reach																								
Antiembolism Hose: Knee High (1), Thigh High (2), ICS (3)																								
Urine Color: Straw (1), Amber (2), Pink (3), Red (4), Orange (5), Tea (6), Clear (7), Cloudy (8), Sediment (9), Foley (10), Suprapubic (11), External Cath (12), Incontinent (13)																								
Oxygen																								
Cough/Deep Breathe (1), Incentive Spirometry (2)																								
Suctioning																								
	7ᴬ	8ᴬ	9ᴬ	10ᴬ	11ᴬ	12ᴾ	1ᴾ	2ᴾ	3ᴾ	4ᴾ	5ᴾ	6ᴾ	7ᴾ	8ᴾ	9ᴾ	10ᴾ	11ᴾ	12ᴬ	1ᴬ	2ᴬ	3ᴬ	4ᴬ	5ᴬ	6ᴬ

Initials	Signature		Initials	Signature		Initials	Signature

Courtesy of Robinson Memorial Hospital, Ravenna, Ohio

Documenting Medication Administration

Intervention flow sheets, like the medication administration record (MAR), give the opportunity to document repetitious procedures for fast verification of completed interventions.

An example of an intervention flow sheet is the MAR, which comes in various forms, sizes, and functions. Each form should have the following information regarding ordered medications: name, dose, frequency, administration route, administration site, side effects, order date, discontinue date, the medical orders update, the documentation of medication given, and the documentation of any medication withheld or refused.

The route of administration is also important to document, especially for patients with multiple intravenous access devices such as central venous catheters and peripheral intravenous lines. Documentation of intramuscular (IM) injections is important too, for example, "11/30/92 2:00 am Demerol 100 mg IM administered in left hip." Subcutaneous injection sites for heparin and insulin administration should also clearly reflect the rotation of sites. Clear detail in medication administration documentation has a benefit of legal protection for the nurse and health care organization.

Nursing documentation should include the patient's knowledge of the medication and knowledge of administration including route and injection site rotation; any patient teaching regarding the medication; the patient's willingness to take the medication; the effectiveness of the medication (eg, alleviate pain or nausea); the patient's response to the medication (eg, any side effects or untoward reactions); and the patient's feelings about taking the medication (eg, apprehensive about taking medication due to c/o "difficulty in swallowing such a large pill").

Medication should be charted when it is given, not before. If the patient takes his or her own medication, write "patient self-medicated"; this often occurs in home care. Chart accurately the time medication is given; always date and sign each medication entry. The medication column is used to list the drug name, the route of administration, the dosage, frequency, and times to administer the medication (see display, Medication Charting Sheet).

Routine medications are usually listed at the top and PRN medications listed at the bottom of the form. Each day is divided into three columns; each column represents an entire shift and should be used only for that shift

(designated shift time is noted on the back of the form with the narrative notes).

Enter the time the medication was administered in the appropriate column, for example, 10 am. If the medication is withheld, enter the time the medication was to be administered and circle it. Document on the back (in narrative form) the reason the medication was withheld.

Example: (10 am)

The nurse's note should read:

NPO from 7 am for upper GI series. Valium 5 mg not given 10 am per Dr. Peak order.

The bottom of the page is used for signatures. The nurse signs with full name and title under all times he or she administered medication or observed the patient self-administering medication.

As in other areas of documentation, if a nurse makes an error, the procedure is to draw a line through the error; write "error," "void," or "mistake in entry"; and sign with initials. If the correction is not legible, a nurse should rewrite the note, but all original forms with errors must be attached.

On some medication forms, medication times are listed then crossed off and initialed after they are given.

EE   AJ   AJ

Valium 5 mg po qid   10 am   2 pm   6 pm   10 pm

Documenting Expected Outcomes

Requiring health care organizations to document outcomes is one of many attempts by accreditation groups to halt rising health care costs by investigating direction and effectiveness of health care services. Documenting outcomes enhances quality of care by focusing on actual patient outcomes and revising care planning to achieve expected outcomes. From a nursing perspective, documenting outcomes shows patient progress in achieving nurse–patient mutually agreeable goals documented on the care plan. A nurse can also document reasons why an outcome is not met, or only partially met, and document plans to remedy lack of progress in achieving goals. A multidisciplinary care plan reflects expected outcomes

MEDICATION CHARTING SHEET

HEALTHCARE PERSONNEL
Medication CHARTING Sheet

Give meds according to the Current Medication Status Sheet (D6-a).
Please note this is a CHARTING sheet only.

Patient Name _John Thomas_   Social Security # _123-45-6789_

Week Ending: _9-11-92_   Address   _123 Windchime Lane_

Medications	Dates:	9-5 SATURDAY			9-6 SUNDAY			9-7 MONDAY			9-8 TUESDAY			9-9 WEDNESDAY			9-10 THURSDAY			9-11 FRIDAY		
List Dose, Route, Frequency	Hour Due ↓	DAY	EVE	NITE	DAY	EVE	NITE	DAY	EVE	NITE	DAY	EVE	NITE	DAY	EVE	NITE	DAY	EVE	NITE	DAY	EVE	NITE
po qd Digoxin 0.25 mg	10A	10A			10A			NPO (10A) Over														
po q 6 h Keflex 250 mg	8 / 2	8A / 2P	8P	2A	8A / 2P	8P	2A	8A / 2P														

Patient Self-Administed:

Please write time med. given in appropriate box. If not given, state med., time, and reason with your signature on reverse side of form.

Employee Signature Each Shift:
Jacqueline Shore RN
Sandy Beach LPN
Cathy Driftwood CNA
Jacqueline Shore RN
Sandy Beach LPN
Cathy Driftwood CNA
Jacqueline Shore RN

mutually agreed on by a patient and interdisciplinary caregivers.

Expected outcomes should be individualized. For example, a care plan expected nursing diagnosis could read Knowledge Deficit R/T disease process and treatment, or more individualized for this patient, Knowledge Deficit R/T chronic congestive heart failure (CHF) and care management. When a patient has difficulty in medication administration, the knowledge deficit can be more specific, reading Knowledge Deficit R/T CHF and medication regimen.

Expected Outcomes and Outcome Criteria

In traditional care plan documentation, goals were nursing goals that were the objectives of nursing care. For example, the nursing goal for the diagnosis Impaired Skin Integrity R/T surgical incision was to promote wound healing and prevent infection. In contemporary documentation, however, emphasis is on the patient outcome, and goals are patient focused and are labelled expected outcomes. This **expected outcome** is a statement of the desired conditions or status of the patient as a result of nursing interventions performed. It reflects either an enhanced capability, such as being able to ambulate progressive distances, or it reflects a diminished response, such as experiencing less pain. It involves the physical condition of the patient, the learning of the patient, or the emotional response or feelings of the patient. This expected outcome is important in establishing progress or lack of progress of the patient in decreasing or eliminating a problem, need, or dysfunctional area. This expected outcome is also used in the evaluation phase of the nursing process, comparing the expected outcome to the patient outcome. Because outcomes are used to evaluate patient progress, the expected outcome and patient outcome must be patient oriented and measurable.

Regulatory and standard-setting organizations emphasize outcome-directed, problem-solving care. Documenting expected outcomes now has become more common and more helpful in care planning and is often required. Expected outcomes give visible direction to interventions, communicate and clarify that direction to the interdisciplinary health care team, serve as a tool to evaluate care, and promote patient/family involvement in setting the objectives of care. This involvement motivates the patient and family toward treatment compliance and subsequent positive health-related behaviors.

Patient-oriented expected outcomes provide criteria for measuring patient readiness for discharge. Having the patient and family involved in setting goals and outcomes keeps them aware of patient progress toward discharge. Outcomes, when achieved, are also a starting point for plans necessary for a smooth transition to the next level of care and subsequent care planning in that setting. For example, a patient who is diabetic may not be discharged until the patient or family member can learn to give insulin injections. Or the patient can be discharged to a home health agency who will administer injections until a caregiver assumes administration of insulin. At the same time, a home health agency nurse will continue to teach the family about diabetes and its treatment regimen.

Outcome criteria are specific, measurable, realistic statements of goal attainment. They present information that will guide the evaluation phase of the nursing process. Outcome criteria answer the questions, who, what actions, under what circumstances, how well and when (Alfaro, 1990). For the stroke patient whose goal is ambulation with a quad cane, the outcome criteria would be: The patient (who) ambulates (what action) with a quad cane (under what circumstances) 30 feet (how well) before shift change (when) (Craven & Hirnle, 1992). Outcome criteria clarify the expected outcome—what is expected as a result of nursing care.

The nurse usually documents one expected outcome for each nursing diagnosis. If more than one expected outcome is necessary, they should be listed in priority, beginning with the most urgent outcome and ending with the least urgent. If they are sequential outcomes, list them in the expected chronological order.

Nursing leaders are attempting to standardize expected outcomes, as standardization of nursing diagnoses and nursing interventions has been accomplished. Below are some examples of standardized expected outcomes that address patient condition, pain, learning, function, treatment, preventive measures, and referrals (see display, Examples of Standardized Outcomes).

Characteristics of Expected Outcomes

Expected outcomes should be based on assessment and nursing diagnosis information, initially determined within 24 hours of admission to a hospital, updated as patient needs change or as the care plan is revised, and measurable. Expected outcomes should be appropriate and realistic, attainable by the patient, and compatible with the physician's medical regimen. Patients or significant others should be involved in the development of expected outcomes for motivation and for advice regarding what is realistic and attainable based on the patient's education, attitude, culture, behavior pattern, and life-style. By using input from family and caregivers, a nurse can determine barriers and strengths a patient has to meeting standardized expected outcomes. The nurse then individualizes expected outcomes to meet the patient's particular needs or unchangeable circumstances.

▲ **EXAMPLES OF STANDARDIZED OUTCOMES**

▲ __(C/P)__ status will stabilize as evidenced by _____ .
▲ Nutrition/hydration will be restored to acceptable level by _____ .
▲ Patient or caregiver will achieve independence in ADL within limits of disease process (or postoperatively).

Or, patient will

▲ Express partial or complete relief from pain following palliative measures within _____ .
▲ Regain acceptable level of joint mobility and muscle strength to transfer, ambulate, or use assistive devices safely.
▲ Verbalize understanding of disease process by stating _____ .
▲ Explain and demonstrate treatment regimen.
▲ Identify signs and symptoms of complications to be reported to the RN/MD.
▲ List __(cardiac)__ risk factors and any necessary changes in life-style.
▲ Verbalize preventive measures for __(infection control)__ .
▲ Verbalize understanding/demonstrate willingness to comply to follow-up care/referral to appropriate resources.
▲ Prepare for a peaceful, dignified death.

Components of Expected Outcomes

Components of an expected outcome statement include:

▲ Desired patient behavior or physical improvement derived from the nursing diagnosis (described in general measurable terms with all circumstantial conditions defined)
▲ Signs and symptoms or conditions that verify the attainment of the expected outcome. When signs and symptoms are added, they are linked to the improvement statement with "as evidenced by."
▲ Time frame in which the patient's final desired improvement will be accomplished

For example:

Pt will maintain adequate mobility as evidenced by progressive activity and absence of complicating factors within (*1 week*).

The expected outcome statement used in care plans should reflect the highest level of realistic, attainable function or need fulfillment possible for an individual patient. It is the end result of care; it measures the condition or behavioral change; it does not measure the process of nursing intervention to affect the change.

The subject of the expected outcome should be written when someone other than the patient is the subject of the expected outcome, for example when Mrs. D, the patient's wife, will be learning to administer insulin injections. In that case the shortest expected outcome could read "Mrs. D will verbalize medication and rationale for administration and demonstrate appropriate insulin injection technique, before pt discharge."

Expected Outcome Revision

A patient outcome is the actual result of nursing intervention; it can fall short of complete achievement of an expected outcome. A deviation from an expected outcome occurs when the expected outcome (as measured by the patient outcome) is not met, is partially met, or is not met appropriately. Consider Mr. D, a diabetic patient learning insulin self-injection. The expected outcomes read, "(Patient will) verbalize rationale of insulin injection; appropriately demonstrate insulin self-administration within 3 days." On the third day if Mr. D can verbalize medication and rationale for administration and demonstrate unassisted insulin self-administration, the goals are met. If instead he can inject himself every morning but forgets to rotate administration sites, the goal is partially met. If he inappropriately insists on visiting an outpatient clinic every morning to have his insulin administered to him, the goal is not met. When a deviation to a desired outcome occurs, goals and interventions must be reassessed and reasons determined as to why the desired outcome is not achieved. Expected outcomes on the care plan are then changed, planned interventions may be changed, or both may be changed. An expected outcome could be changed to "Mr. D will verbalize medication and rationale for administration and demonstrate appropriate insulin injection technique before discharge." Interventions could be changed to include a different learning media such as a video instead of reading material and could include referral to a diabetic support group or a home health nurse.

Resolution and Target Dates for Expected Outcomes

Two decades ago, care plans consisted of two columns. One was the need or problem and the other was approach or actions. After the addition of goals, now referred to as expected outcomes, time frames were added to the goal. Resolution dates were the first innovation added, then target dates.

RESOLUTION DATES

The *resolution date* is when the problem or nursing diagnosis is no longer active so interventions for that problem or diagnosis have been discontinued. With the advent of problem-oriented medical records, a resolution date was noted to differentiate between an active problem and a discontinued or resolved problem. Today that resolution date is still used where old problems or nursing diagnoses are retained on the care plan. Resolution dates inform nurses that a problem is resolved, and the patient no longer needs related interventions.

TARGET DATES

The **target date** is the expected date or the expected period of time it will take to meet the stated expected outcome. Target dates are written on the care plan to designate when goals or outcome results are expected. In concise, contemporary care plans a target date is included in an expected outcome following the American Nurses Association (ANA) standards, which call for a time measurement for outcomes (see display, ANA Standard for Outcome Identification).

> The specification of the date will reflect the best judgment of the nurse considering the time needed to reverse the alteration, the condition of the client, the availability of support systems (family, friends, neighbors, etc.), the impact of the alteration for the client, and the type and duration of interventions required....
> A significant level of logical thinking and critical judgment by the nurse is needed to realistically designate the expected goal and the date for the realization of that goal. (Yura, 1988)

In writing a time frame in the care plan, the most definite reference would be to write the date. Adding the day would prevent errors when writing the date, and it

▲ ANA STANDARD FOR OUTCOME IDENTIFICATION

ANA Standard III. Outcome identification includes a measurement criterion that states that "outcomes include a time estimate for attainment." (ANA, 1991, p. 10).

Target dates can be written in many different ways:

▲ By actual day, "Monday," or
▲ By actual date, "1/21," or
▲ By combination of both "Monday, 1/21," or
▲ By a time frame, "within 3 days," or
▲ By a relative date, "by HD2" (hospital day 2) or "POD3" (postoperative day 3)

would be a more accurate, faster reference communicating when someone is reading the actual target date. Reading hospital day 2 (HD2) or postoperative day 3 (POD3) necessitates looking up the admission or surgery day if the date is not written on that form. In a standardized care plan in which HD2 or POD3 is preprinted, writing the date beside it is helpful for fast reference.

WHEN TARGET DATES ARE NOT MET

The difficulty with target dates is the concreteness of the estimated length of time for expected achievement of the expected outcome. If the outcome is not achieved by a certain time, it appears that nursing care was inadequate, which may not be the case. Estimating target dates must be done judiciously, then documentation regarding meeting or not meeting the target date should be specific. Documentation should include reasons or extenuating circumstances that impeded achievement of expected outcomes within the allotted time frame. Such extenuating circumstances could be a disabling complication (such as infection or fever), disorientation, or a personal or family crisis.

Sometimes expected outcomes need to be revised, whether or not the nursing diagnosis is revised. An example of a reason for goal revision is if the original goal is not realistic or achievable for the patient after reassessment finds new barriers to accomplishing the stated goals. Expected outcomes, along with the rest of the care plan, should be reviewed and updated as needed according to the health care organization's policy. Some acute care organizations review the care plan every 24 hours, and certified home health care agencies review the plan of treatment every 30 days.

Interventions can continue beyond target dates, until the resolution date shows that the problem or need has been met. A nurse should change the time frame in a care plan when a target date is not met and needs revision. The nurse then documents in clinical notes the reason for not meeting the date and the continuation or updated plans to meet the next target date. If the time frame or target dates are written on a separate column on a care plan, do not repeat the time frame or target dates in the expected outcome as well.

Documenting Patient Outcomes

Some organizations use progress notes or weekly outcome summary notes to document actual patient outcomes. In this way they use patient outcome information to focus on resolution or revision of unmet expected outcomes. Other organizations use flow sheets and document patient outcomes only at the end of care on a discharge summary.

At present, health care organizations are using three methods to meet this outcome documentation requirement. They usually use only one of the systems below.

Weekly Narrative Outcome Summary Note

Some organizations require a patient's primary nurse or case manager to write a narrative summary of outcomes on a weekly basis, usually on Friday. In this summary note a nurse identifies patient problems, expected outcomes, and progress being made in achieving those expected outcomes. This summary is based on information observed in caring for a patient and on information documented on daily progress notes. These notes should represent a logical progression of nursing actions to resolve patient problems and identified needs.

> *Problem*: Impaired Skin Integrity R/T abdominal incision. *Expected outcome criteria*: Pt and caregiver will demonstrate wound care and dressing change using aseptic technique. *Patient outcome*: Pt and wife instructed in wound care cleansing with H_2O_2 and DSD. Pt cleansed wound appropriately, but contaminated 4×4 when opening package. Pt has difficulty due to arthritic stiffness in hands. RN reinforced principles of aseptic technique and demonstrated DSD application again. Wife willing to do wound care and was able to demonstrate skill appropriately.

Nursing Plan Outcome Record

Interim Health Care, a home health agency located in Cleveland, Ohio developed a concise outcome record form that was computerized by MedPad, Inc. of Atlanta, Georgia. This outcome record duplicates a patient's documented care plan inclusive of identified patient problems (written as nursing diagnoses) and goals related to identified problems. Lines to the right of each identified problem and goal allow for entry of date completed and progress notes on each patient outcome. Interventions are included on the form, so that process outcomes can be dated or rationale for interventions not implemented can be stated. This is helpful when there is a need for monitoring due to noncompliance or untoward reaction of a patient to an intervention. This form is completed by a nursing case manager at the time of recertification every 60 days and at discharge of the patient from service.

The form is in the following format:

	Pt Outcome	Resolv Date
Problem: Impaired Skin Integrity R/T abdominal incision.	_____	_____
Interventions: (care plan nursing actions are listed here . . .)		
Expected outcome criteria: Pt and caregiver will demonstrate wound care and dressing change using aseptic technique.	_____	_____
Problem: High Risk for Infection R/T abdominal incision.	_____	_____
(care plan nursing actions are listed here . . .)		
Expected outcome criteria: Pt will list S/S of infection and whom to call.	_____	_____

Criteria-Based Outcome Record

Some organizations are experimenting with criteria-based outcome forms in which long-term and short-term goals are in a flow sheet format, and dates with comments can be entered at set intervals of time. As stated in Chapter 5, goals (expected outcomes) are those documented on a care plan. Outcome criteria are specific, measurable, realistic care steps leading to achievement statements of goal attainment and are documented instead of, or in addition to, expected outcome criteria. The following outcome example is for an identified problem of pain related to postoperative incision.

Patient Outcome	Goal Date	Date Accom	Comment
Long-term			
Verbalizes pain mgmt strategies			
Short-term			
Verbalizes factors that initiate or aggravate pain symptoms			
Identifies appropriate interventions to decrease or alleviate pain			
Describes level and characteristics of pain			
Reports pain above established level			
Long-term			
Uses pain management techniques			
Short-term			
Demonstrates pillow-splinting technique			
Maintaining q4h medication regimen			
Demonstrates change of position to relieve pain			

KEY POINTS

▲ Narrative clinical progress notes reflect clinical judgment and the nursing process. These can be separated into categories of clinical data, intervention, and patient response or outcome.

▲ Nurses perform two main types of nursing interventions that must be documented in the clinical progress note: nurse-initiated treatments and physician-initiated treatments. Nurse—physician and multidisciplinary collaborative actions are also documented.

▲ Nursing actions documented in clinical progress notes include observing, assessing, monitoring, providing care and support, referring, consulting, administering, teaching, and counseling.

▲ Outcome criteria include desired patient behavior or physical improvement expressed in observable, measurable patient activities or characteristics of patient status. Criteria also include specific circumstances or conditions under which behavior will occur within a designated time frame.

▲ Outcomes are currently documented to meet new outcome documentation requirements. In some organizations, outcomes are documented in the weekly narrative outcome summary note, nursing plan outcome record, or criteria-based outcome record.

▲ A nurse compares patient outcomes to the expected outcomes on a patient's care plan and documents what progress the patient has made.

REFERENCES

Alfaro, R. (1990). *Applying nursing diagnosis and nursing process, 2/e* (p. 100). Philadelphia: J. B. Lippincott.

American Nurses Association (1991). *Standards of clinical nursing practice* (p. 9). Washington, DC: Author.

Craven, R., & Hirnle, C. (1992). *Nursing fundamentals: Human health and function*. Philadelphia: J. B. Lippincott.

McCloskey, J. C., & Bulechek, G. M. (1992). *Nursing interventions classification (NIC)*. St. Louis: Mosby–Year Book.

Yura, H. & Walsh, M. (1988). *The nursing process* (p. 141). Norwalk, CT: Appleton & Lange.

BIBLIOGRAPHY

American Nurses Association and Arthritis Health Professions Association. (1983). *Outcome standards for rheumatology nursing practice*. Washington, DC: American Nurses Association.

Calley, I. S., & Siler, P. V. (1987). Nursing process: A framework for documentation. *Emphasis Nursing, 22*(2), 84–91.

Camilleri, R. (1987). Nurses' note: Six ways to write right. *Image: Journal of Nursing Scholarship, 19*(4), 210–212.

Carpenito, L. J. (1989). *Nursing diagnosis: Application to clinical practice* (3rd ed.). Philadelphia: J. B. Lippincott.

Eggland, E. T. (1988). Charting: How and why to chart your care daily—and fully. *Nursing '88, 18*(11), 81.

▰ PRACTICE SESSION ▰

FILL IN

1. Nursing interventions arise out of a _____ .

2. Nursing interventions are documented on _____
   _____ .

3. Nursing interventions are of three types:
   _____ and
   _____ and
   _____ .

4. Actual patient status results following intervention for an identified nursing diagnosis is
   termed a _____ .

5. A nursing clinical progress note should reflect _____
   _____ , _____ ,
   _____ , _____ , and
   _____ .

6. Regardless of format, nursing documentation should include _____ , _____ ,
   and _____ .

7. A mental checklist for writing descriptions on clinical progress notes includes: _____ ,
   _____ , _____ , _____ , _____ , and _____ .

8. The expected date or period of time it will take to meet an expected outcome is a _____ .

9. Components of expected outcomes include _____ .

10. An example of an intervention flow sheet is a _____ , which charts medication
    that was administered.

MULTIPLE CHOICE

1. _____ Documentation of implemented interventions and outcomes provides an important link
   between the steps of
   a) planning of care and evaluation of care
   b) nursing history and evaluation of patient condition
   c) nursing diagnosis and care planning
   d) patient teaching and patient return demonstrations

2. _____ The most commonly used structured nursing notes are
   a) SOAP or SOAPIER
   b) PIE
   c) DAR
   d) all of the above

3. _____ Contributions of accurately documented implemented nursing interventions include
   a) monitoring goal direction of care
   b) coordinating and communicating among caregivers

    c) determining if care meets established standards

    d) all of the above

4. _____ Reasons why planned nursing interventions are not implemented nor documented include

    a) patient refuses treatment

    b) NPO due to diagnostic tests or surgery

    c) patient not available for scheduled treatment

    d) all of the above

5. _____ Advantages of standardized intervention flow sheets include

    a) easier filing

    b) more space for narrative descriptions

    c) facilitates comparison of data

    d) all of the above

MATCHING

Match the type of order in Column B with nursing action listed in Column A.

1. _____ Tylenol #3 q4h, PRN   **a.** nursing order

2. _____ Cipro 500 mg bid   **b.** medical order

3. _____ refer to social worker   **c.** collaborative action

4. _____ check pedal edema q4h

5. _____ emotional support

6. _____ ROM q4h

7. _____ chest x-ray

8. _____ teach diabetic diet

9. _____ back rub qhs

10. _____ NPO

11. _____ putting side rails up

12. _____ ambulate in hall ×3

13. _____ throat culture

14. _____ refer to physical therapy

15. _____ assess bowel sounds

CHALLENGE FOR CRITICAL THINKING

1. Why might expected outcome criteria need revision? Cite two examples.

2. Discuss the advantages and disadvantages of customized flow sheets in terms of documentation.

3. Explain the relationship between expected outcomes and patient outcomes.

4. Compare and contrast three different ways that a health care organization documents outcomes. Discuss advantages and disadvantages of each.

5. Define nursing interventions and describe why some can be categorized as nursing orders.

LEARNING TO DOCUMENT

1. List the components of SOAPIE notes, PIE notes, and DAR notes. Compare the components to see how they are similar. Fill in the table below.

COMPARING CLINICAL PROGRESS NOTES

Note Components	SOAPIE	PIE	DAR
Data			
Problem			
Intervention			
Evaluation			

2. Pretend you are caring for a 50-year-old man; salesperson for a large advertising firm; he is married; has two teenagers; has admitted to alcohol abuse; and is experiencing blackouts. You enter the room and determine that he is oriented to person and place but not to time and circumstance. He keeps his eyes closed as he tells you he's too tired to bathe this morning. He looks very pale and he is perspiring. When you take check his R (radial) pulse (65), his skin is cool and moist. On auscultation you find his heart sounds are regular (70) but his hands, ankles, and feet are slightly swollen. With this information, use the Daily Observation Record on page 134 to document your day's observation at 8:00 am.

3. Pretend you are caring for a 45-year-old woman, recently divorced after 25 years of marriage. She has a high school education and has not been gainfully employed since marriage. The patient took an overdose of sleeping pills. Orders allow her to ambulate to the bathroom with assistance. She gave most of her own bath but you provided pericare, Foley catheter care, gave her a back rub, and helped her put on her knee-high TED stockings. The Foley was patent, and you emptied the bag of 500 mL of cloudy amber urine. You taught her how to cough and deep breathe, then put the nasal cannula back on so she could receive oxygen at 2 L/min. When you left for lunch you put both side rails up and attached the call light at the side of the bed. With this information, use the Treatment Flow Sheet on page 135 to document your actions at 8:00 am.

DAILY OBSERVATION FORM

ROBINSON MEMORIAL HOSPITAL
Patient Progress Notes
DAILY OBSERVATION RECORD

Date:

								LEGEND	PULSE GRADING
B E H A V I O R / **L. O. C.**	Time:							P-Person	O-Absent
	Alert:							PL-Place	1+-Easily occuled
	Oriented	P PL T C	P PL T C	P PL T C	P PL T C	P PL T C		T-Time	2+-Occluded with
	Disoriented							C-Circumstance	mild pressure
	Lethargic							+-Present	3+-Normal
	Unresponsive							--Absent	4+-Bounding
	Cooperative							R-Right	D-Doppler
	Uncooperative							L-Left	
	Anxious								**Patient Teaching**
	Eye Contact	Yes No	Yes No	Yes No	Yes No	Yes No			
S K I N	Temp: Warm								
	Hot								
	Cool								
	Cold								
	Moisture: Dry								
	Moist								
	Diaphoretic								
	Turgor: Elastic								
	Non-Elastic								
	Color:								
	Integrity: Intact								
	Impaired								
C A R D I O V A S C U L A R	Heart Sounds: Regular								
	Irregular								
	Apical Radial Deficit	+ −	+ −	+ −	+ −	+ −		**Team Leader**	
	JVD @ 45	+ −	+ −	+ −	+ −	+ −		**Responsible**	
	Pulses	R L	R L	R L	R L	R L		7-3	
	Temporal								
	Carotid								
	Brachial							3-11	
	Radial								
	Femoral								
	Post. tibial							11-7	
	Dorsalis pedis								
	Calf tenderness:								
	on palpatation							**OR**	
	on dorsiflexion								
	Edema:	R L	R L	R L	R L	R L		7ᴬ-7ᴾ	
	Facial								
	ABD								
	Sacral							7ᴾ-7ᴬ	
	Arms								
	Hands								
	Legs								
	Ankles							**Other**	
	Pedal								
Signatures									

Courtesy of Robinson Memorial Hospital, Ravenna, Ohio

TREATMENT FLOW SHEET

DATE _____   **TREATMENT FLOW SHEET**

	7ᴬ	8ᴬ	9ᴬ	10ᴬ	11ᴬ	12ᴾ	1ᴾ	2ᴾ	3ᴾ	4ᴾ	5ᴾ	6ᴾ	7ᴾ	8ᴾ	9ᴾ	10ᴾ	11ᴾ	12ᴬ	1ᴬ	2ᴬ	3ᴬ	4ᴬ	5ᴬ	6ᴬ
Nursing Rounds																								
Activity: BR (1), BSC (2), Chair (3), Ambulate c Assist (4), Self Ambulate (5)																								
Bath: Self (1), Assist (2), Complete (3), Shower (4)																								
Back Care																								
Oral Care																								
Pericare/Foley Care																								
Turn and Reposition R-Right, S-Side, L-Left, B-Back																								
Bed in Prevention Mode																								
Restraints: Soft (1), Vest (2), Wrists (3), Ankles (4), Leathers (5), Remove q8O-check skin condition-then reapply (6), (R) Right, (L) Left																								
Side Rails: (▲▲), (▲▼), (▼▼)																								
Call Light in Reach																								
Antiembolism Hose: Knee High (1), Thigh High (2), ICS (3)																								
Urine Color: Straw (1), Amber (2), Pink (3), Red (4), Orange (5), Tea (6), Clear (7), Cloudy (8), Sediment (9), Foley (10), Suprapubic (11), External Cath (12), Incontinent (13)																								
Oxygen																								
Cough/Deep Breathe (1), Incentive Spirometry (2)																								
Suctioning																								
	7ᴬ	8ᴬ	9ᴬ	10ᴬ	11ᴬ	12ᴾ	1ᴾ	2ᴾ	3ᴾ	4ᴾ	5ᴾ	6ᴾ	7ᴾ	8ᴾ	9ᴾ	10ᴾ	11ᴾ	12ᴬ	1ᴬ	2ᴬ	3ᴬ	4ᴬ	5ᴬ	6ᴬ

Initials	Signature	Initials	Signature	Initials	Signature

Courtesy of Robinson Memorial Hospital, Ravenna, Ohio

CHAPTER 7

Legal and Ethical Considerations in Documentation

LEARNING OBJECTIVES

After studying this chapter, the learner should be able to:

▲ Describe four critical elements of a negligence or malpractice case.

▲ Explain how legal problems occur due to omitted or altered content or incorrect documentation mechanics.

▲ Demonstrate documentation guidelines and procedures for errors.

▲ List nine characteristics of documentation content that result in legal risk.

▲ List seven characteristics of documentation mechanics that result in legal risk.

▲ Describe key concepts of six potentially liable events.

▲ Identify three types of advance directives.

▲ Explain the similarities and differences between law and ethics.

▲ State the four principles of ethics and discuss how two relate to legal issues.

KEY TERMS

Autonomy	Competency	Foreseeability	Negligence
Beneficence	Damage	Justice	Omission
Breach of duty	Defendant	Legal duty owed a patient	Plaintiff
Causation	Electroencephalogram	Litigation	Proximate cause
Comatose	Fidelity	Malpractice	Surrogate
Commission			

Eggland ET, Heinemann DS. NURSING DOCUMENTATION:
CHARTING, RECORDING, AND REPORTING.
© 1994 J.B. Lippincott Company.

The nursing record is a legal document. If a lawsuit is filed against a physician, hospital, or nurse, the medical record will be brought into court. A nurse involved in care will be asked to testify as a **defendant** (the person being sued) or a witness, and lawyers will question the nurse about the content in the patient record. The content will be considered more accurate than the nurse's recollection of the patient and events surrounding care. The content of the medical record and how the content is documented can be critical in the outcome of a trial.

Guidelines for Documenting Nursing Care

Some basic charting guidelines govern documentation regardless of the types of chart formats used. Legal cases have been won or lost because of charting problems. For example, if errors are not correctly marked, attorneys question a nurse's intention and competency in documenting and therefore in providing care. Also, "if an alteration was dishonest or appears to be dishonest, it could result in a charge of fraud or misrepresentation" (Fiesta, 1983). Good charting has the following characteristics:

- ▲ Conciseness
- ▲ Accuracy
- ▲ Completeness
- ▲ Legibility
- ▲ Timeliness
- ▲ Logical organization

Nurses should follow some basic guidelines when documenting care.

Identifying the Correct Patient's Clinical Record

The patient's clinical record (chart) and all forms within the record should have the patient's identifying information stamped or written on each page. This includes but is not limited to name, address, Social Security number, Medicare number (if appropriate), primary physician, and admission date. Before making any entry on a chart, a nurse should check that it is the correct chart before documenting information. Caution is needed when caring for patients with the same last name. A nurse should not identify charts by room number only; this is a common mistake.

In writing entries, some organizations have a policy to write a patient's name instead of "patient" or the abbreviation "Pt." For example, a nurse writes "Mrs.

Green c/o lower back pain. . . . " instead of "Pt c/o lower back pain. . . . " This specific identification prevents any confusion regarding a patient's identification.

Making Entries

Entries should be started with the complete date including month, day, and year. The month should be stated first, not the day. This is essential for uniformity, fast date identification, and reduced errors. Time of the entry should be noted when charting periodically during a shift. The time of significant incidents should be charted when they occur.

Correcting Errors in Documentation

Mistake in entry/wrong chart. The chart is considered a legal document. What should a nurse do if documenting information in the wrong chart? Some nurses would prefer to throw away notes with errors, rewrite, and have colleagues rewrite copied notes on the new form. The appropriate way, however, is to mark the mistaken "wrong patient entry" and write the date and nurse initials. Incorrect information should be crossed out so the original information is still legible. The original note sheet is retained as part of the chart, even if original notes are rewritten. An important reminder is erasures, white-out, and paste-overs are not permitted in the chart (see display, Correcting Errors in Documentation, sample A). Correct information should be entered near this mistake notation; but if there is inadequate room to write, note where the correct information can be found.

Marking errors. While charting in the correct chart, if a nurse writes something in error, it must be marked as an error. The procedure is to draw a thin line through the entire error, write "error," sign initials, and write in the correct information. Instead of "error" some organizations use the word(s) "Mistake in entry" or "Void" to avoid the indication an error occurred in rendering care (see display, Correcting Errors in Documentation, sample B). Correct information should be entered near a mistake notation. If there is inadequate room to write, a nurse writes a note where the correct information can be found (see display, Correcting Errors in Documentation, sample C). When documenting errors, the procedure is to date and sign initials, being sure that a full signature is on the same form to easily identify a nurse's initials (see display, Correcting Errors in Documentation, sample D).

An important point to remember is that a nurse should

▲ CORRECTING ERRORS IN DOCUMENTATION

A. WRONG PATIENT ENTRY

Wrong patient entry 5-2-90 TD

5-2-90 Lower leg wound 3 cm x 5 cm c̄ 2 cm red raised border tender and warm to touch.

5-2-90 3:00 pm Mrs. Jones c/o dull, constant pain in Ⓛ lower leg. Mottled from knee to ankle.
Bilat pedal pulses strong. Dr. Moon called. T. Dew RN

B. MARKING ERRORS

*Error 5/20 EE see ***

5-20-90 Ⓛ lower leg wound 3 cm x 5 cm c̄ 2 cm red raised border — tender & warm to touch. ~~Foul smelling,~~
thin white drainage. *No odor present from wound (see following note re: flatus). Erma Edward, RN

C. ENTERING CORRECT INFORMATION

Error 5-4-90. See correct info 5-4 note. EE

5-3-90 Dr. Stone visited. ~~Soaks d/c.~~ Dry, sterile dssg d/c. Wound to be under U/V light tid.
Pt instructed re: wound care, for disch. 5-4-90. E. Eggland, RN

5-4-90 9 am Pt to be disch at 11 am. Warm, moist soaks to continue x 20 min 3 x day, and no dssg on wound.
U/V light tx d/c. Pt able to give rationale for soaks & do return demo. No further questions/concerns per pt.
See disch instruc sheet. Copy given to pt. E. Eggland, RN

D. LABELING ERRORS AND INCLUDING SIGNATURES

Treatments	5/1/90		
Warm, moist soaks to wound x 20 min tid	10 am TD 2 pm TD 6 pm JR		
Dry sterile dssg to wound	Error ~~8 am~~ EE 10:30 am EE		

RN Signatures: Erma Edward, RN
Terry Dew, RN
Joan Ross, RN

never mark anyone else's documentation as an error or in any way alter documented notes of another caregiver.

Introducing a New Subject

Regardless of the format used, if a space exists between text or at the end of text, a line should be drawn from the end of the text to the end of the right margin on the line, so that no one can add documentation to another nurse's note. A traditional narrative note is the easiest format to show this principle:

4-7-90

7:15 am. Diabetes mellitus. Urine fractional for sugar and acetone negative. Oral hypoglycemic medication given. Instructed patient in 1500 ADA diet; literature given to patient; RN will review information with patient again this afternoon, and answer further questions. Patient able to define diabetes, purpose, dose, and side effects of hypoglycemic agent, dietary regimen, and symptoms of hypoglycemia and hyperglycemia. See teaching sheet.

8:00 Postop cholecystectomy care. Dressing dry and intact. No c/o of pain nor discomfort. Patient ambulating in hallway without difficulty. Ellen Eggland, RN, MN

Signing Notes

Nursing notes must be signed at the end of the entry and subsequent entries if an additional note is later added during the same shift time. Immediately after the name a nurse should write nursing title (RN, LPN), educational degree, or certification. Using full first and last name is preferable, but a first initial and last name is acceptable if organizational policy allows and no other staff person has the same initial and last name. For clarification of confusing identification, a middle initial can be added or first name written out. On certain forms, such as flow sheets, policy may permit entry of only first and last initials. Somewhere on that same form, however, should be a designated space where the full name can be written for easy identification of initials.

If a nurse writes on the last line of a page and needs to enter more information on the next page or reverse side of a page, an acceptable procedure is to write "continued on next page" and sign a full signature. On the next page a nurse writes the date and note "5-31-90 note continued." A nurse signs a full signature again at the end of the entry as usual.

Adding a Nursing Note Addendum

Nursing notes are written on every line but never in between lines. No empty space should be left between entries because someone could insert a note, even in

error. Sign every entry. If a nurse adds a postscript after signing a first entry, the nurse signs again at the end of the postscript. For example:

2:45 pm. Mr. Black c/o dull chronic pain in L foot. Foot warm, pedal pulse satisfactory. VS: BP130/90, P90, R22. Demerol 75 mg IM given per Dr. Bleu telephone order. Ellen Eggland, RN, MN. 3:20 pm. Pt states "Pain is gone." Ellen Eggland, RN, MN

If a day or so later, a nurse recalls omitting some important information regarding an earlier shift, the nurse uses the next available space. Note that day's date and time of entry, and start with the heading, "Addendum to nurse's note of (month, date, time)." A nurse writes an addendum entry then signs as usual. This method has become an acceptable way of documenting complete patient care that was omitted during a previous shift.

Charting When Orders Are Not Implemented

Charting is required for each nursing intervention, whether it be an observation, treatment, nursing procedure, or medication administration. Occasionally an order or planned intervention is omitted because of patient condition, absence, or treatment refusal. When an order or care plan intervention is omitted, a nurse documents what was omitted or refused and why. Use a patient's own words if noncompliance is involved. Also note nursing actions in response to this omission, including who was notified (see display, Guidelines for Daily Charting). Further information on documenting patient noncompliance and refusal of treatment is discussed later.

Determining Charting Frequency

Frequency of charting is determined by:

▲ A health care organization's policy, which will state how often nursing observations and interventions are to be charted on particular units
▲ Nursing guidelines or multidisciplinary protocols, which will state a required frequency of documentation, based on the nursing diagnosis or nursing management problem addressed in the guideline/protocol
▲ Acuity level of the patient, wherein a nurse makes a clinical judgment as to how often a patient should be observed and assessment and intervention documented
▲ Frequency of nursing interventions as noted on the care plan

---

▲ | **GUIDELINES FOR DAILY CHARTING**

DO

- ▲ Read the nursing notes before caring for a patient and before charting care.
- ▲ Use concise phrases. In narratives, begin each phrase with a capital letter and start each new topic on a separate line.
- ▲ Document nursing action taken following indication of a need for action (for example, a leaking Foley catheter).
- ▲ Sign each entry, postscript, and addendum.
- ▲ Be definite. Avoid "apparently," "appears to be." Substantiate with facts.
- ▲ Have the patient's name and identifying number on every sheet.
- ▲ Describe reported symptoms accurately. Use the patient's words in describing them when these words are helpful.
- ▲ Write neatly and legibly in the ink color prescribed.
- ▲ Use accepted hospital abbreviations whenever possible.
- ▲ Put entries in order of consecutive shifts and days. Write the complete date/time of each entry.
- ▲ Chart changes in patient condition, to whom it was reported (or attempts to report), and time of contact (and attempts).

DON'T

- ▲ Begin charting before checking the name on the patient's chart.
- ▲ Pull a chart by room number only. DO use the patient's name, age, sex, and diagnosis.
- ▲ Skip lines between entries or leave space before signing.
- ▲ Chart procedures in advance.
- ▲ Wait until the end of the shift to chart or rely on memory.
- ▲ Use notebook paper or pencil. Always use the appropriate nurses note form of the hospital, and always use ink.
- ▲ Throw away nurses notes that have errors on them. Mark the error. Include the sheet as part of the chart.
- ▲ Use medical terms unless you are sure of their exact meaning.
- ▲ Erase.
- ▲ Backdate, tamper with, or add to notes previously written. Use an addendum if necessary.
- ▲ Repeat in your narrative what you have written on forms in other parts of the chart, unless further explanations are needed.

(Reprinted/adapted with permission from *Nursing '88*, November. Copyright 1988. Springhouse Corporation, 1111 Bethlehem Pike, Springhouse, PA 19477-0908. All rights reserved.)

- ▲ Time designated in expected outcome, often written as "by third postop day," "before discharge," "within 30 minutes"
- ▲ Frequency guidelines of a published charting system, such as PIE whose authors suggest documenting every shift (8 hours)
- ▲ Designated times for entries on some flow sheets or standardized forms

Shift charting. For stable long-term care patients, some health care organizations traditionally accept shift charting. The example below will show contemporary shift charting, which includes specific times of observations and interventions.

4-8-90

7 am–3 pm. FRACTURE, LEFT LOWER TIBIA. 8 am and 2 pm—Lower L leg cast clean and dry. No weight bearing maintained with 3-point crutch ambulation. No complaint of pain. PERIPHERAL CIRCULATION. No tingling or loss of sensation in L toes. Able to move all toes. No edema. Pedal pulse strong and regular. Foot pink and warm. 12 noon—Ambulating in hall without difficulty and no complaint of pain. NUTRITION. Intake of food and fluids adequate for stage of disease: ate complete

meals at breakfast and lunch, and fluid intake approx. 40 oz water. PSYCHOSOCIAL. 2 pm—Cheerful, talkative. Visiting other patients. E. Eggland RN MN

Proponents state that an advantage of shift charting is the saving in time in documentation to present a summary within a single time frame. In an overworked, understaffed unit, however, more detailed charting for legal protection seems to outweigh the benefit of time saved. A disadvantage of shift charting is the question of frequency of intermittent observations of the patient. It is evident that the narrative was written at the end of the shift; thus, questions regarding accuracy of memory can be made because specific times are not documented at time of occurrence. In terms of content, a disadvantage is that notes can tend to be vague, without structure and without quick identification and location of problems. The above adaptation of capitalizing subject content can help alleviate that problem.

Topic-a-day charting. Some long-term care settings advocate the topic-a-day method of charting. One day all shift personnel will document with a focus on nutritional needs and food and fluid intake of the patient; the next day, charting may be focused on ambulation and exercise; the next day on psychosocial status and needs. An advantage is that each focus is investigated at different times in a 24-hour day by more than one nurse. Depending on the topic, however, a nurse on the 11 pm to 7 am shift may not have an opportunity to observe and report on a subject for the day. A topic each shift resolves that problem.

Topic-a-shift charting. The same format above broken down into more frequent topic changes brought about more frequent observation of different systems observed. More than one topic observed per shift resulted in more complete and frequent topic investigations as well. For example, the 7 to 3 shift might include in charting the patient's appetite, self-help, personal hygiene, and mental status. The 3 to 11 shift would concentrate on ambulation, communication, and visitors. Finally, the 11 to 7 shift would note sleep, skin condition, and vital signs.

Time entry narrative. These notes are the most frequently used narrative notes. This type of note takes more time to document than the above methods, but it is the most accurate and timely presentation of patient occurrences. The timeliness of some procedures is important for legal protection of the nurse providing care. For example:

> 9:00 am. BP124/78, T99.8°F, P88, R18. IV infusing well in R antecubital fossa. Abdominal operative area has been prepped. Pt states he has been NPO since midnight. Preop checklist completed.

Think about what would happen if, after the nurse leaves the unit, the IV infiltrates? . . . Surgery is postponed till evening? . . . The patient has an emesis during anesthesia? Because of this timed note, morning preoperative nursing activities show that the patient's status was appropriate for scheduled surgery.

Types of Litigation

Lawsuits involving physicians, nurses, and health care organizations generally involve cases of medical malpractice, personal injury, disability, worker's compensation claims, and insurance claims.

The most common types of **litigation** are negligence and malpractice. **Negligence** involves two aspects: omissions and commissions. An **omission** is the failure to provide care. A **commission** involves one performance of care at a level that falls below the standard of care. **Malpractice** involves three aspects: professional misconduct, the improper or unreasonable performance of professional skill, or a deviation from a professional standard of care.

For negligence and malpractice, judges consider four elements in deciding the merits of a case. They are:

▲ **Legal duty owed a patient**
  • What a patient can expect from caregivers based on the standards of care
▲ **Breach of duty**
  • A deviation from the standards of care that involves omissions and commissions
▲ **Proximate cause**, which includes:
  • **Foreseeability**—As a result of professional training it is possible to foresee what could happen to a patient because of nursing action or lack of action
  • **Causation**—Breach of duty caused an injury
▲ **Damage**—Injury (C. Schaffer, Cleveland, personal interview, July 9, 1992)

Breach of duty, proximate cause, and damage are three transgressions that can be supported or refuted by what nurses have documented in a patient's record. Nursing documentation should present what actually occurred with a patient:

1. The patient's condition before an injury
2. What led up to the injury or crisis
3. How the injury actually occurred
4. The circumstances surrounding the injury
5. The results or outcome of the incident
6. The patient's response at the time of injury and within the next 48 hours

If this information is documented, then the record can show if nurses provided all the care that should have been provided in the situation or if they did not (breach of duty); if nurses could have expected or inadvertently caused an injury (proximate cause); and if true injury resulted from what the nurses did or did not do (damage). With appropriate documentation, nurses can protect themselves from potential legal problems.

Potential Legal Problems in Documentation

We have addressed basic knowledge of content to include in nursing documentation and charting techniques to avoid inappropriate entries. Now we will expand the basics to show how potential legal issues and actual legal problems occur because of omitted or altered content and improper mechanics of documentation. This information is important for all nurses, because "omissions and alterations (in the patient chart) . . . are the most frequent problems with charting from the malpractice defense standpoint" (Creighton, 1986).

The following information will present guidelines to prevent omissions and inappropriate alterations in the record. These precautions will minimize risk and maximize protection for nurses and health care organizations in a malpractice or negligence case.

All nurses should document with a view toward the possibility that the patient record may be submitted to a court of law as a central source of information regarding patient condition and nursing care. This attitude is important in liability prevention and claims defense.

What a nurse documents in a record is a major factor in determining liability; the record may protect caregivers or may increase the risk of losing a court case. For this discussion, legal risk means the degree of probable protection of a nurse and health care organization in a law suit. High or low risk is determined by the *content*—pertinent aspects of care—and *mechanics*—charting techniques.

Appropriate content and correctly marked changes would be more likely in a record if a nurse documents in accordance with a health care organization's policies and procedures, professional nursing standards of care, and the nursing process framework. In a court of law, judges and juries will try to determine if a nurse performed in a reasonable and prudent manner and in accordance with standards of care. They will use the following sources to determine standards of care:

▲ Governmental regulations
▲ Professional experts (expert witnesses)
▲ Accrediting and professional organizations
▲ The health care organization's policies and procedures (Johnson, 1988)

Documentation Content That Increases Legal Risk

Certain characteristics of documentation *content* create a legal risk (see display, Documentation Content That Increases Legal Risks).

LEGAL RISK 1: CONTENT IS NOT IN ACCORDANCE WITH PROFESSIONAL OR HEALTH CARE ORGANIZATION STANDARDS

Hospital standards determine what information should be collected and documented, how frequently it should be documented, what types of symptoms to document, and conditions under which to follow orders.

Types of data to collect. Data that organizations want to document are included in standards of care policies or on standardized forms. Standards and forms detailing information to be documented should be filled out completely, with nonapplicable data blanks marked N/A or crossed out. Information on the standard form but not available at the time of interview should be noted,

DOCUMENTATION CONTENT THAT INCREASES LEGAL RISK

▲ The content is not in accordance with professional or health care organization standards.
▲ The content does not reflect patient needs.
▲ The content does not include description(s) of situations that are out of the ordinary.
▲ The content overgeneralizes patient assessment or nursing interventions.
▲ The content is not timely or is chronologically disorganized.
▲ The content is incomplete or inconsistent.
▲ The content does not include appropriate medical orders.
▲ The content implies a potential or actual risk situation.
▲ The content implies attitudinal bias.

with a plan to obtain data. Plans can include getting information from relatives or rescheduling an interview at a time when the patient is better able to communicate and is willing to be examined more completely.

Frequency of data collection. If a hospital standard or policy and procedure states the required frequency of data collection, documentation should show that frequency by documented timely entries.

In *Washington Hospital Center v. Martin* (1982) an 83-year-old woman fell from a hospital bed and fractured her left hip. The patient was confused and weak and had previously slipped out of restraints in other attempts to get out of bed. The nursing policy stated that patients in restraints should be checked every half hour. Nursing notes showed entries more than an hour apart and did not mention whether side rails were up or down. The verdict was in favor of the patient.

Symptoms to document and responsibility for communication. Hospital standards of care indicating desirable assessment documentation and reporting of symptoms have been significant in determining outcomes of negligence and malpractice cases. If a standard nursing practice indicates that certain symptoms should be observed, documentation should reflect that. For example, for a patient in a cast, documentation should reflect extremity skin color, temperature, and pulse. In addition, symptoms should be communicated and documented until the problem is resolved.

In *Darling v. Charleston Community Memorial Hospital* (1965), nurses documented pain, odor, and pale skin color of a casted leg. When the primary physician took no action on the information, the nurses continued to document symptoms but did not report the problem to anyone else. The leg was amputated and the patient successfully sued.

The responsibility of documentation does not end with writing symptoms. The nurses should have reported the lack of physician action to the nursing supervisor. Nurses should have documented the physician's comments on a personal record at home to remember information before they testified in court.

LEGAL RISK 2: CONTENT DOES NOT REFLECT PATIENT NEEDS

According to the nursing process and nursing standards, documentation of care should be linked to identified patient problems. The documentation of a nursing assessment should be measurable, the care planning goal directed, the interventions clear and specific, and the evaluation an indication of the patient's progress toward the achievement of the goal(s). At assessment and throughout care if a nurse fails to document important patient needs, a nurse could be found negligent. Needs must be addressed in nursing notes, patient teaching when appropriate, and in discharge summaries.

> A hospital in New Jersey was sued by the family of a maternity patient who died 3 hours after an uncomplicated delivery. An expert witness testified that vital signs were poorly monitored, nurses' notes poorly kept, and the nursing diagnosis should have led nurses to conclude hemorrhage was possible. (*Maslonka v. Hermann et al*, 1980)

During the critical postdelivery period, nurses should have routinely measured and documented vital signs and vaginal bleeding. Any obstetric delivery, by its nature, has the nursing diagnosis High Risk for Fluid Volume Deficit. Nurses should have focused their interventions and documentation on this problem.

LEGAL RISK 3: CONTENT DOES NOT INCLUDE A DESCRIPTION OF SITUATIONS THAT ARE OUT OF THE ORDINARY

The following unusual events need to be charted according to agency guidelines for the protection of the nurse and facility:

▲ Unusual, unexpected changes in condition or patient situation
▲ Abnormal test results with report of results to physician
▲ Inability to take appropriate action with a potential

or actual problem because a physician cannot be contacted
▲ Direct or indirect threats from patient or family toward nurse or health care organization, including threats of bodily harm to oneself or another or threats of reports to supervising agencies or threats of legal action

When the patient presents risk to self or others, that information should be documented. Consider the following examples that affect care:

▲ The patient is abusing drugs or alcohol.
▲ The patient is taking medication not authorized by the physician.
▲ The patient is using medical equipment inappropriately at home.
▲ The medical equipment is not functioning adequately, or the patient or family is tampering with equipment in the hospital or home.
▲ The patient has refused treatment or medical advice.
▲ The patient has refused continuation of treatment and medical or nursing supervision.

In these situations, the patient's exact words and exact times of occurrence should be documented. The condition of the patient before and after the situation should be described. Nursing interventions and counseling performed should be included. Finally, patient outcomes should be noted. An important part of this documentation is to show the patient's mental status at the time of any refusal of treatment. Important information to document is the patient's behavior indicating competence and resulting dangers posed to self or others due to refusal of care.

LEGAL RISK 4: CONTENT OVERGENERALIZES PATIENT ASSESSMENT OR NURSING INTERVENTIONS

Documenting a global view of the patient's condition and nursing assessment will not be specific enough to protect from liability in incidents. For example, notes documented before a fall stating "patient ambulating without assistance" is not descriptive of the patient's condition. Instead, detailed documentation should support that before the fall, the patient showed no symptoms that would make him at risk for an injury. Documented support for the nurse should have read: "Pt ambulating in hall approx 50 ft and states no pain nor dizziness nor SOB."

LEGAL RISK 5: CONTENT IS NOT TIMELY OR IS CHRONOLOGICALLY DISORGANIZED

If there is an inappropriate period of time between care and actual documentation, the risk of liability increases. Medical and nursing decisions for continued therapy and care can be made on outdated information if assessment, planning, intervention, or outcome documentation updates are not included in the chart in a timely manner.

If not entered in a timely manner, documentation can result in an unnatural order of events or interrupted chronological entries. Subsequent caregivers may provide care based on inaccurately assuming the last entry of care was the current condition of the patient or the most recent treatment provided. If entries are not in chronological order, disorganized documentation encourages attorneys to suggest that care was questionable in timeliness and therefore in appropriateness.

Positive, frequent, and accurate charting have been a determinant in several legal cases.

> In *Engle v. Clarke* (1961), a patient underwent surgery for an epigastric hernia. At 3 pm he was nauseated and was given Dramamine. At 4 pm the patient was restless, pale, and perspiring profusely so the nurse called the physician, who said he would visit. The nurse documented that glucose was ordered and administered, and blood pressure was 120/80. She charted detailed patient assessment entries and interventions at 5 pm and again at 6 pm.

Although the patient died, the clinical record showed that the nurse had accurately assessed and charted hourly observations and had taken appropriate actions. A similar situation and court outcome was found in the case of *Sheppard v. Kimbrough* (1984).

LEGAL RISK 6: CONTENT IS INCOMPLETE OR INCONSISTENT

Standards of documentation require that information be complete. *Omitted information* can lead to increased liability.

> In *St. Paul Fire and Marine Insurance Co. v. Prothro* (1979), a patient who was recuperating from a total hip replacement was injured during a Hubbard tank treatment. The incision was bumped and reopened. An orderly stopped the bleeding and a nurse dressed the wound. The nurse did not document the incident. The wound became infected, the prosthesis had to be removed, and the patient was left with a permanent limp. The patient prevailed because the absence of the information on the chart was detrimental to providing appropriate medical care.

Inconsistent information can lead to increased liability.

> In *Rogers v. Kasdan* (1981), a woman was admitted to the emergency department following an accident. She died 7 days later of brain damage. The court ruled against the hospital because there were discrepancies among various records, intake and output was not totaled correctly, and some records were illegible and incomplete.

Missing documentation in a patient chart is a red flag for lawyers. Opposing lawyers will suggest that gaps in documentation signify gaps and omissions in care. They also may suggest that missing documentation indicates tampering with the clinical record in an attempt to cover up documentation or caregiving errors. The law looks carefully at motive. Even in a legal case that ruled in favor of a doctor and hospital, the court of appeals sent the case back to a trial court to rule whether the hospital's loss of records was caused by negligence or impropriety (*Battocchi v. Washington Hospital Center*, 1990).

LEGAL RISK 7: CONTENT DOES NOT INCLUDE APPROPRIATE MEDICAL ORDERS

Nurses perform certain interventions that require signed medical orders. If medical orders are illegible, ambiguous, not documented, or outside of standards, the nurse has an obligation to question and document appropriate action to clarify orders. The nurse should be respectfully assertive in questioning a physician before orders for treatment are performed. The nurse should contact a nursing supervisor to determine policy and procedure in handling an unclear situation and should keep personal notes on file at home in anticipation of disciplinary action or negligence proceedings.

LEGAL RISK 8: CONTENT IMPLIES A POTENTIAL OR ACTUAL RISK SITUATION

Documenting a risk situation and blaming the health care organization or other caregivers for a patient problem or unexpected outcome only creates evidence for a patient's attorney. Evidence that indicates an organization may be negligent includes the following type of documentation: a "shortage of nurses this shift" resulted in infrequent observations of a patient who fell; a physical therapy "staffing problem resulted in a home care patient visit delay" of 2 weeks, which resulted in decreased range of motion; a "physician didn't have time to answer questions" before a patient signed a treatment authorization. Additional examples of statements that raise questions and concerns include: "the night shift did not perform their duties according to a physician's orders"; or a "home health aide is working outside of the job description."

Instead, nurses should document objective observations regarding patient condition and report any other types of concerns to the head nurse or nursing supervisor.

LEGAL RISK 9: CONTENT IMPLIES ATTITUDINAL BIAS

Any disparaging remarks, accusations, arguments, or name calling within documentation can contribute to a potential defamation of character suit or libel. In addition, if a nurse describes a person with labels such as demanding, obnoxious, dishonest, drunk, lazy, or incompetent, a patient's attorney can stress that such attitudes promoted incomplete or inappropriate care by the nurse. The attorney may also infer that such inappropriate documentation is poor-quality documentation, which directly suggests inadequacy of care. Instead of categorizing patients and documenting slanderous labels, nurses should objectively describe symptoms, behavior, and interactions observed.

Documentation Mechanics That Increase Legal Risks

Beside "what" content a nurse documents, "how" a nurse documents can create legal risks. Documentation mechanics, that is, charting techniques or how a nurse charts information, can also be legally risky if charting is not correctly executed.

Certain common characteristics of documentation *mechanics* pose a legal risk (see display, Documentation Mechanics That Increase Legal Risk).

LINES BETWEEN ENTRIES

If a chart has empty lines between entries, there is a potential for information to be added later by other nurses or caregivers. The nurse's signature below entries makes the nurse accountable for all information written above her name. Nurse managers should never allow one nurse to add notes to another's entry, nor allow one nurse to chart for another nurse. In a court of law, charting for another would be considered hearsay rather than known fact or reliable information. As importantly, it is the responsibility of every nurse to know that charting for another nurse is not a generally appropriate documentation practice. However, a nurse may chart and

DOCUMENTATION MECHANICS THAT INCREASE LEGAL RISK

▲ Lines between entries
▲ Countersigning documentation
▲ Tampering
▲ Different handwriting or obliterations
▲ Illegibility
▲ Dates and time of entries omitted or inconsistently documented
▲ Improper nurse signature or unidentifiable initials

cosign for the care students or auxiliary personnel have given under the supervision of the nurse.

COUNTERSIGNING DOCUMENTATION

Countersigning means a second nurse signs documentation that another nurse has already signed. The policy for countersigning orders is addressed by each health care organization. Countersigning progress notes for supervised staff suggests the countersigning nurse administered the care or observed the ancillary nurse or student administer the care. Legally it means only that the document was read by the countersigning nurse. However, the countersigning nurse accepts responsibility for the intervention and can be sued along with the colleague or ancillary person if a problem arises regarding the action. A good rule to follow is to avoid countersigning unless absolutely necessary by organization policy. If necessary, countersign only in the situation where a nurse has been been actively involved in care and feels comfortable in assuming accountability for it. Nurses should not assume that an adequate defense is "I didn't read the documentation thoroughly." A nurse's signature on any document signifies that the nurse read and verified that documentation.

TAMPERING

Entering data on previously documented forms, entering inaccurate information, rewriting, and dating the record inaccurately can all be considered tampering. If tampering or altering the patient record appears to be dishonest, the nurse can be charged with misrepresentation and fraud. Writing an addendum a day or two after care on the next available space is different from squeezing in writing between spaces to make it appear the information was written at the time of the documentation. Similarly, if a nurse changes a date or adds information to documented observations on a previous documentation entry, the nurse can be accused of fraud and potentially covering up negligence. Leaving no spaces between entries eliminates the potential for late entry of data or tampering with data.

DIFFERENT HANDWRITING OR OBLITERATIONS

Different handwriting within a documentation entry or on a form suggests a second person entered data without signing the entry. This type of documentation is inappropriate. Only one nurse should fill out a form or complete a section of a form, and entries should be clearly marked by the nurse's signature.

Using correction fluid has become a common method of correcting errors in day-to-day communications, but white-out should never be used in professional documentation. Obliterations that do not permit a reader to see the text under the obliteration are suspicious and raise questions about the reason for the obliteration.

Different handwriting, white-out, and obliterations suggest an after-the-fact addition or change to substantiate a position within a potential or actual lawsuit. Erasures of any kind are suspect because what was actually obliterated cannot be proved. Any additions or editing to benefit a defendant could be considered fraud.

> In *Pisel v. Stamford Hospital et al* (1980) a 23-year-old woman with schizophrenia was admitted to a psychiatric unit's quiet room with furniture removed for safety. During the hospitalization, nurses failed to transcribe an order for antipsychotic medication, and the patient was found semiconscious with her neck lodged between the side rails and mattress of the bed that was supposed to have been removed from the room. The director of nursing, against hospital policy, ordered the original patient record removed and a "revised" record rewritten. A $3.6 million verdict was upheld because the substitution of the record indicated the hospital's consciousness of negligence.
>
> In another case (*Quintal v. Laurel Grove Hospital*, 1965), a jury returned a verdict of $4 million against a hospital and physicians. After the lawsuit was filed, the physician altered a vital sign in the preoperative record to show the temperature of a 6-year-old boy was below normal before the child went into minor surgery. The boy, in fact, had a fever, suffered cardiac arrest, and sustained severe brain damage.

ILLEGIBILITY

Poor handwriting, poor spelling, or writing on lines instead of between lines makes documentation difficult to read. Illegibility can result in errors in communication. Also, medication errors can occur from illegible handwriting, often creating a life-threatening situation.

Lawyers will take the opportunity to interpret negatively any questionable legible documentation. Lawyers will purport that illegibility caused errors in communication and errors in care and that illegibility may have been an attempt to obliterate actual conditions or situations. Lawyers will also suggest that the poor quality of documentation is a reflection of the quality of care, which is questionable.

DATES AND TIME OF ENTRIES OMITTED OR INCONSISTENTLY DOCUMENTED

Correct dates and times should be entered for physician visits, verbal orders, phone calls, visitors, and other significant events. Times documented in nursing notes should be consistent with other documents discussing the same issue or incident. Case law supports the contention if there are errors in charting, all documentation in the clinical record could be erroneous (*Hiatt v. Grace*, 1974).

Physicians document when they visit the patient. The dates and times of physician visits on medical progress notes should be consistent with dates and times on daily nursing flow sheets that include a section for this entry. A physician visit log (see display, Physician Visit Log), when located on standardized nursing note flow sheets, helps keep accurate notation of physician visit dates and time. By noting a physician visit on nursing documentation, the nurse can benefit by using that information as a cue to check for new medical orders. As a cue, the notation of the visit can also be a reminder to talk with the patient about the information the physician shared. It gives the nurse the opportunity to determine the patient's comprehension and response to the information the physician may have shared or medical intervention the physician may have performed.

▲ PHYSICIAN VISIT LOG	
Date/Time	**Physician Visit**

IMPROPER SIGNATURE OR UNIDENTIFIABLE INITIALS

A nurse's professional signature is an indication of professionalism and accountability. Improper signatures question the ability and consciousness of a nurse in documentation technique and therefore quality of care. Illegible signatures or initials can bring all staff nurses under scrutiny in a lawsuit investigation because the nurse who made an error may not be identifiable by documentation signature.

As standardized forms become crowded with information, nurse initials are being increasingly used in flow sheets to save space. To solve signature identification problems, most standardized forms have a signature box to have an instant reference to initials to identify the documenter of information (see display, Initials Identification Box).

When a signature box is not printed on a form using initials, most governmental regulations or hospital policies require full signature on an accompanying signature list filed within the patient record.

Law and Ethics in Documentation

We are living in an age in which emphasis and knowledge of legal rights are common. Rights can be defined as "that which a person is entitled to have or to do or to receive from another . . . " (Creighton, 1986). As patient advocates, nurses attempt to ensure the rights of patients while they receive care in a health care organization. Law and ethics are two forces that help people ensure rights, minimize potential harm, and guide human behavior. Laws are mandatory guidelines people must follow, under obligation of fines or incarceration. Ethics are guidelines based on how we wish people would act, under obligation of consciousness. The "force" of the law and the "persuasion" of ethics are intertwined in legal issues of reporting and recording.

Four principles of ethics intertwine with documentation issues, including:

1. Autonomy
2. Beneficence
3. Justice
4. Fidelity

Autonomy is the respect we have for others as human beings, which allows them the right to make judgments and choose actions. The principle of autonomy underlies legal issues of informed consent, advance directives, refusal of treatment, privacy, and confidentiality in access to records.

Beneficence is the duty to do good to others, to help them, and to further their interests, while refraining from harming others (nonmaleficence). This principle underlies discontinuing service and abandonment.

Justice refers to justified distribution of benefits and risks/burdens in a community and can underlie principles of access, distribution, and appropriateness of care.

Fidelity is faithfulness, which includes truthfulness, trust, and keeping promises. This principle is the basis of respect in the nurse–patient relationship.

Legal Issues Related to Autonomy and Beneficence

Autonomy and beneficence are guidelines of behavior that have roots in the law where patient care is involved. Because nurses have respect for a patient's choices and because nurses seek to prevent harm for the patient, they are accountable for the following critical issues involving protection of the patient:

▲ Informed consent

▲	INITIALS IDENTIFICATION BOX	
	Initials and Signature of Nursing Personnel	
EE	Ellen Eggland	

▲ Advance directives
  • Surrogate health care decision-makers
  • Living will
▲ Refusal of treatment
▲ Privacy, access to records
▲ Abandonment

INFORMED CONSENT

All patients have the right to decide what treatment or action can be taken in regard to their own body. Regardless of whether the treatment is desirable for health or for life, the patient or someone designated by the patient must consent to allow that treatment or action to be performed. The consent must meet state statutory law requirements for informed consent. For example, in Ohio the patient must have the ability to understand (capacity determined by age, clear mental state), and the physician must:

▲ Explain the treatment in nonmedical, understandable terms
▲ Explain and discuss the risks associated with the procedure
▲ Explain the risks for the particular patient, including probability of success of the treatment

Sufficient information must be given so that the patient can make a knowledgeable decision in light of other alternatives. Physicians violate their duty if they withhold or minimize risks to persuade the patient to undergo treatment. Finally, all patient's questions should be answered to the patient's satisfaction.

From an ethical view, the four elements of informed consent are disclosure, voluntary choice, patient comprehension, and patient competency. Added to those elements are two variables: the right to a second opinion and the right to stop treatment at any time. Competency is a difficult measurement. **Competency**, sometimes called capacity to make decisions, is defined by the President's Commission for the Study of Ethical Problems in Medicine as requiring:

▲ Possession of a set of values and goals
▲ The ability to communicate and to understand information
▲ The ability to reason and to deliberate about one's choice (President's Commission, 1982)

Although physicians are responsible for obtaining informed consent, nurses should check that consent has been obtained before treatments begin. Nurses can witness patient or family signatures, but in so doing they must be assured that the consent is voluntary, informed, and not given while under the influence of narcotics or other mind-altering drugs.

The explanation of the procedure should include the benefits and risks, alternative treatments, probable success of the various treatments or procedures, and what to expect if the procedure is not performed. Nursing notes can attest to the knowledge the patient has and learns, based on what the patient can verbalize. But nursing notes should not attest to the patient's "understanding" of what the physician explained because understanding is difficult to measure. The nurse, if present during the explanation, can document the patient is able to repeat what the physician said and can appropriately explain what it means.

Consent is given only for the extent of action documented on the informed consent. For example, if a woman consents to a lumpectomy, then a mastectomy cannot be performed during the same surgery if a consent is not written beforehand. To proceed with an action or treatment without consent could generate charges of assault (actual or threat of touch without permission or attempt with force to inflict physical injury) or battery (actual assault with force).

A nurse and a hospital can be held liable along with a physician if there had not been adequate disclosure or other elements of informed consent had not been met. A nurse can detect a problem regarding a patient's consent, when the patient:

▲ Does not seem to understand the procedure or risks
▲ Signed the consent more than a month previously
▲ Had an unauthorized person sign the consent
▲ Did not sign the consent

In any of these events, the staff nurse should quickly bring the situation to the attention of the physician and the nurse manager. If the physician proceeds without appropriate consent, nursing administration should be notified and the nurse should make personal notations outside of the medical record for protection should the situation be brought to court. Also, if a patient reverses a decision and decides against treatment, the nurse is obligated to inform the physician to prevent the unwanted treatment.

ADVANCE DIRECTIVES

Advance directives are signed documents to be followed if a patient becomes unresponsive or incompetent. The documents specify what treatment(s) the patient would choose to accept or refuse if able to do so. One type of advance directive (living will) lists and explains patient wishes. Two other types (durable power of attorney for health care and health care surrogate for health care decisions) designate persons to make decisions for the patient based on what the patient's expressed wishes were or would be.

The federal Patient Self-Determination Act of 1991

mandates all health care organizations receiving Medicare or Medicaid to:

▲ Maintain policies and procedures that provide written information to patients concerning their rights under state law to make decisions regarding their care. Rights include the right to accept or refuse medical treatment and the right to formulate advance directives. (Advance directives are in the form of living wills or durable powers of attorney for health care decisions, and some states like Florida, have a third method called designate surrogates for health care decisions.)
▲ Ensure that advance directive information is provided to patients
▲ Document in the patient record whether or not an advance directive has been executed
▲ Ensure compliance to the patient's advance directive, consistent with state law, and not discriminate or condition the provision of care, based on the presence or absence of an advance directive
▲ Provide education on advance directives to patients and to staff

If a patient is unsure about advance directives, the nurse should encourage the patient and family to contact their physician, lawyer, or clergyman for information and counsel.

The presence or absence of an advance directive must be documented in the patient record. The nurse should document the existence and location of the advance directive and whether a copy was given to the physician. A copy should be requested for the patient's file at the health care organization. Verification should be made that the advance directive complies with the state law where the organization is located. This is particularly important for documents executed in another state.

The health care organization cannot discriminate or establish any condition of care, based on the presence or absence of an advance directive. Nursing documentation should not include any entries that might contradict this requirement.

Organizations should include in their policy and procedures that the organization will not assist a patient in euthanasia, whether or not due to a terminal condition. Nursing documentation should not include entries that may even remotely suggest assistance in dying.

Nursing documentation should reflect the following patients' rights. The patient has the right to:

▲ Accept or reject prescribed medical treatment, in accordance with the law
▲ Formulate an advance directive in the form of a living will or durable power of attorney for health care or designation of a health care surrogate
▲ Receive care whether or not the patient chooses to formulate an advance directive

▲ Change the intent of the advance directive at any time
▲ Transfer to another health care provider if the health care organization cannot follow the advance directive because it is in conflict with organizational policy or caregivers' conscience

Depending on the health care organization, nurses have the responsibility to facilitate informed decision-making regarding advance directives and to ensure that advance directives are current, reflecting any change in patient intent. The competency level of the patient should be addressed in documentation at least every 30 days. Although some families believe a patient should initial and date the original document periodically to indicate continuing conviction regarding the directives, some lawyers suggest otherwise. Legal thought is that the living will remains valid whether or not it is initialed on a continuing basis. In addition, initialing the will imposes an obligation on the patient (to initial the will every 30 days) that the law does not.

Surrogate health care decision-makers. In 1990, the Florida legislature revised the durable power of attorney statute to allow a patient to give a designated person (**surrogate**) authority to make a patient's health care decisions. The legislature also passed the Health Care Surrogate Act, which created a statutory framework for appointment of a health care surrogate decision-maker. There are minor differences between the durable power of attorney and health care surrogate in terms of requirements and responsibilities. Both represent the designated decision-maker for the patient who can no longer make decisions regarding care. The durable power of attorney or the health care surrogate can provide informed consent for an incompetent patient except for abortion, sterilization, electroshock therapy, or experimental treatments. The durable power of attorney or health care surrogate may not direct the withholding or withdrawing of life-prolonging treatments under certain circumstances (R. S. Franklin & W. H. Myers, Naples, Florida, personal communication, September 25, 1992).

A durable power of attorney or health care surrogate document is effective indefinitely in Florida unless a shorter time is stipulated in the document. Both documents and living wills can be changed at any time by a patient.

Living will. A living will is a signed document executed while a person is able to make health care decisions. The living will states what medical treatments to provide and withhold at the end of a patient's life. As an example, Florida law permits a person to withhold or withdraw life-prolonging medical treatment if the patient has a nonrecuperative terminal condition or suffers from a permanent vegetative state.

Before withholding or withdrawing life-prolonging procedures, an attending physician and a second physician must examine the person and document in the medical record that to a reasonable degree of medical certainty there is no chance of recovery.

The living will must be signed in the presence of two witnesses, one of whom may not be a blood relative or spouse. Therefore, a nurse can sign the document. If the patient is unable to sign, the patient or family may instruct one of the witnesses to write the patient's signature in the presence of the patient.

A patient may execute documents for a durable power of attorney and a living will, or a health care surrogate and a living will, or all three. In each case, all directives should be consistent in content and intent. Nurses should be aware that living wills or advance directives can be revoked or changed by a patient deleting sections on a document or telling a physician or nurse. Such changes should be well documented in the patient chart, witnessed by another person, and executed on a new or revised document.

Any competent adult over the age of 18 may write a living will. In Florida the legislature revised its living will statute to include provision of nutrition and hydration as a life-prolonging procedure under certain circumstances. Living wills are written in many different forms with many different titles; two titles are "A Christian Affirmation of Life" and "A Will to Live."

A nurse should see that a copy of the living will is attached to a patient's clinical record. Nurses should document any statements regarding a patient's convictions, intentions, and continued desire to refuse treatment. When there is a potential legal concern of the patient and family, observations of the patient's family, which should not be part of clinical documentation, can be noted and kept personally by the nurse, in case a lawsuit is served at a later date (Hall, 1990).

REFUSAL OF TREATMENT

The patient has a right to refuse treatment. Refusal of treatment often involves complex issues such as refusal of blood transfusions for religious reasons or the predetermined decisions regarding the refusal to initiate or maintain life-sustaining measures. Problems arise with emotional decisions family members must make for care of minor children or for care of incompetent parents. Dealing with these complex issues calls for accurate documentation of the patient's condition, level of consciousness, and verbatim expression of the patient's intent and rationale. In many large organizations an ethics committee of physicians, nurses, clergy, attorneys, psychologists, and ethicists is available to make recommendations regarding individual cases of actual or potential refusal of life-sustaining treatment. If a committee is not part of a health care organization, a nurse manager or

executive can consult with the organization's lawyer. A signed release of liability such as a hospital discharge "against medical advice" is evidence that the patient refused treatment or recommended care.

A landmark case has set a legal precedent regarding a patient's right to refuse treatment. The Florida Supreme Court issued a decision *in re Guardianship of Browning* on September 13, 1990, which sets forth a clear description of an individual's rights to accept or refuse medical treatment under the Florida constitutional "right to privacy."

In 1986, Mrs. Browning suffered a stroke, ultimately resulting in a permanent loss of consciousness. Unable to swallow, Mrs. Browning was fed through gastric and nasogastric tubes. She was in what is commonly referred to as a persistent vegetative state. She had executed a living will, almost identical to the statutory form, which also included a sentence (not authorized at the time by the living will statute) stating her desire that food and water be withheld or withdrawn under these circumstances. There was also other evidence that Mrs. Browning would not have wanted to be maintained through artificial feeding. The medical evidence established that Mrs. Browning would have died within a few days without the artificially provided sustenance and could live as long as a year if the feeding continued.

The guardian of Mrs. Browning's person petitioned to have the tube feeding withdrawn under the living will statute. Since the case occurred before the legislative changes to the living will statute outlined above, which allow food and water to be withheld or withdrawn when a terminal condition exists, the courts had no choice but to find that no relief could be granted under the statutory framework. Fortunately the courts looked beyond the statute to determine what additional rights an individual has to refuse medical treatment under the "right to privacy" found in the Florida Constitution. In this regard, the Florida Supreme Court found:

1. You have an absolute right to refuse unwanted medical treatment, whether lifesaving or otherwise.
2. If you are incompetent you have the same right to refuse unwanted medical treatment as when you were competent, but certain procedures must be followed to ensure the decision made is the one you would have made if competent.
3. No distinctions are to be made between types of artificial life-support systems.
4. No prior judicial approval is necessary for life support to be withheld or withdrawn, but the courts are always open to adjudicate legitimate questions raised by interested parties.

PRIVACY, ACCESS TO RECORDS

In an increasingly consumer-oriented society, patients are becoming more interested in learning details about the services they receive and rationale for those services.

Although a health care organization's record belongs to the organization, confidential information in a record is accessible by right only to the patient to whom it belongs. Because the record is confidential, the patient or legal guardian must sign a release of information whenever a record or portion thereof will be reviewed outside of direct caregivers of the organization. Release of this information should not be a general release but should specifically state what part of the clinical record or what topic of information is to be released and to whom.

If a health care organization receives patient information or documents from another organization, the second organization may not release the forms to a third party without the first organization's documented approval. Usually, the patient would need to sign another release form from the first agency, documenting specifically to whom the information would be released. For the same reason, telephone calls to staff nurses on the division should be handled with confidentiality of information in mind. No information should be given unless a patient authorizes the release in writing.

Patients have the right to view their own clinical record. Some safeguards, however, are advisable.

> For communication and clarity, a patient's nurse or physician should be in attendance when a patient or family views the record, to explain terms, phrases or rationale. If there is information in the record which the physician determines is injurious to, and should be kept from the patient, the family may review the record, with the permission of the patient. (Fiesta, 1983)

Nursing documentation should be written with the thought that the patient does have right of access to the record. Information that the family determines may be upsetting to the patient should not be included in the chart, especially if it is not significant to patient care.

ABANDONMENT

Abandonment or discontinuance of care to a patient is defined as "the unilateral, nonconsensual termination of care without adequate notice or provision of alternative arrangements. If a physician knows or should have known that a condition needs continuous or frequent expert attention to prevent injurious consequences, physician must render care or see that someone else can and does" (Randall & Pritchard, 1987). Abandonment relates to the ethical principal of beneficence, to do good and prevent harm. The concept of abandonment also has consequences from the law that created diagnosis-related groups (DRGs) and the discharge of patients when reimbursement limits are met. Hospitals and especially home health agencies are careful to give the patient notice of pending discharge, and begin discharge planning from

the time of admission. In discharge planning, communication with the patient, family, caregivers, and community resources should be carefully documented in regard to planning for discharge and notification of a discharge date. The nursing process of assessment, care plan, goals, identification of problems, and progress toward goals creates a means by which the patient can foresee, and the nurse can substantiate and discuss, the expected duration of care until discharge.

Critical Issues in Documentation

This section continues to address the procedure and documentation issues that may create liability. Documentation guidelines are presented to increase supportive information in defense claims and to help protect nurses and the health care organization. The following issues are presented:

▲ Verbal orders
▲ Do not resuscitate orders
▲ Declaration of death
▲ Falls and restraints
▲ Incident reports

Verbal Orders

Verbal orders are medical orders from the physician when the physician is communicating orally, most often by telephone. The purpose of verbal orders is to provide for continuity and update of care according to the patient's needs when the physician is not available to submit written orders. A well-written verbal order should document that it is not an on-site order. The nurse taking the verbal order should document the order, his or her name, the date and the time the order was taken, and the time the order is being written and transcribed. An example follows:

> 11-13-90, 3:00 pm. Verbal order received by telephone from Dr. Jones for Mrs. Joanna Stephens, d/c IV after last ordered bag (4).

The verbal order should be signed by the physician within 24 hours in acute care settings. In the hospital, a physician signs the order at the nurses station. An unsigned medical order can be flagged in the chart to remind the physician that an order needs his or her signature. In home health care, the verbal order should be signed by the physician within 8 days. In this setting, the verbal order form can be mailed to the physician for signature and returned to the home health agency. Facsimile machines and computer networks facilitate this procedure.

A significant problem with verbal orders is the potential for error. After repeating the verbal order to the physician, the nurse (according to the American Medical Association's Council on Ethical and Judicial Affairs statement of 1986) has an obligation to challenge questionable orders. (This obligation also refers to written medical orders.) This does not mean to document the questionable orders in nursing notes. This does mean to verbally seek information, clarification, and satisfaction before documenting and executing a medical order.

Do Not Resuscitate Orders

Do not resuscitate (DNR) orders are written by a physician to withhold cardiopulmonary resuscitation (CPR) in the event a patient experiences cardiac or respiratory arrest. DNR orders are usually written for terminally ill patients, severely debilitated elderly patients, and dying patients.

It is difficult to talk to the patient, family, or physician about a DNR order. But there is a liability risk if a medical DNR order is not documented on the chart. A DNR order cannot be just an informal or verbal directive. If a nurse does not initiate emergency CPR when a DNR is not written, the nurse would be making a medical decision and would be practicing medicine without a license (Fiesta, 1983).

> In 1974 and 1980, the American Medical Association proposed that decisions not to resuscitate be formally entered in the patient's progress notes and communicated to all staff:
>
> Orders Not to Resuscitate
>
> The purpose of CPR is the prevention of sudden, unexpected death. CPR is not indicated in certain situations, such as in cases of terminal irreversible illness where death is not unexpected or where prolonged cardiac arrest dictates the futility of resuscitation efforts. Resuscitation in these circumstances may represent a violation of an individual's right to die with dignity. When CPR is considered to be contraindicated for hospital patients, it is appropriate to indicate this on the physician's order sheet for the benefit of nurses and other personnel who may be called on to initiate or participate in cardiopulmonary resuscitation. (Creighton, 1986)

Declaration of Death

With technological advances in cardiopulmonary maintenance, a traditional definition of death (pulse and respiration absent) has become debatable. A faculty committee at Harvard Medical School defined death in terms of a **comatose**, permanently nonfunctioning brain:

▲ Unreceptivity and unresponsivity
▲ No movements of breathing

▲ No reflexes
▲ A flat **electroencephalogram** (Creighton, 1986)

At death, the nurse cannot document that the patient was pronounced dead unless a physician is present to perform that medical responsibility. Nurses are directed, however, to document the time of death, patient condition including signs and symptoms observed, and nursing interventions. For example:

3:08 am. Respirations ceased, no carotid or apical pulse.

3:10 am. Pupils dilated. Dr. John Parson notified.

3:20 am. Dr. John Parson pronounced the patient dead.

Falls

Ethical and legal guidelines indicate hospitals have a duty to take reasonable precautions to provide safety to patients who are likely to injure themselves. Nursing facilities have taken the lead in developing organized alert systems to identify elderly residents who have potential to fall or have fallen recently. In some organizations, ribbons or stickers are used to identify patients likely to fall, by placing these indicators on the door, chart, bed, and wheelchair or walker. Risk assessments are done routinely, and all workers from charge nurse to housekeeper are to observe and assist in preventing falls. Recent research (Johnston, 1988) has identified the following significant risk factors for falls:

▲ Decreased level of mobility
▲ Three or more medical diagnoses, especially cardiovascular or musculoskeletal disease
▲ Use of three or more drugs daily, particularly cardiovascular, antihypertensive, tranquilizer, or antidepressant drugs

Documentation in the patient record should include an assessment of a patient's level of consciousness, balance, and mobility and precautions taken to prevent falls–by assistance or restraints. Further, documentation should also include any declarations of intentions to assist a patient made by family members or other caregivers. In documenting what the family says they will do, the family members have accepted some responsibility for care of the patient, at least in preventing falls. The following situation is an example.

> This author was called to be an expert witness in a negligence suit brought against a home health agency who provided two private duty nurses to a frail husband and wife who lived with their daughter and son-in-law. After alternating day and night 12-hour shifts, the two nurses stated they were asked to both provide daytime care on a one-to-one basis, so each patient had a daytime nurse. The nurses further stated the daughter and son-in-law

agreed they would care for the parents if the parents awoke during the night, giving both nurses adequate sleep time. Because the mother's condition had improved, her previously raised side rail was lowered at night so that she could walk to the bathroom unattended. Within a week after the nurses' schedule change, the mother awoke during the night, called out for help, then tried to ambulate to the bathroom by herself. She fell and broke her hip. During hospitalization, after hip surgery, the patient contracted pneumonia and died. The daughter filed suit, claiming that her mother's condition did not warrant having the side rail down the night she fell at home; that she had not agreed to assist her mother at night; and that the fall precipitated the pneumonia that eventually was the cause of death.

The documentation to support the nurses' position and nursing notes from the 4 days before the fall were "lost" according to the daughter. (Private care notes are left in the home for continuity of care.) Had they been available, the nurses state that documentation would have verified the mother's improved condition and ability to ambulate alone and verified the daughter's offer to get up at night to care for her parents. When the mother fell, a bed restraint was on the chair in the patient's room. With lack of supporting documentation, the lawsuit was settled out of court, in favor of the patient's family.

A key point in this case was the responsibility of the nurse to maintain possession of the clinical record to prevent the record from becoming lost. Civil cases have set precedents that those who lose a chart can be investigated for fraud or covering up negligence. In this case, the missing chart was detrimental to the defense of the nurses and health care organization. Possibly personal notes kept at home by the nurses could have supported their contention. Key points on those notes should be the condition of the patient before the fall and the responsibilities the family had agreed to accept in care of the patient.

Restraints

Accidents and injuries occur even when a patient is restrained. Physical and chemical restraints impose an obligation on nurses to carefully and frequently monitor a patient's condition. Restraints should be used judiciously and according to the health care organization's policy and procedure. Restrained arms and legs should be assessed routinely for circulation and skin condition and release from restraints should allow periodic, routine exercise.

Nursing documentation should reflect patient observations. Documented actions should reflect state law and the health care organization standards regarding restraints—their application, duration, and observation frequency. It should also include the reasons the patient is restrained, what method of restraint is used, the patient's response, outcome, safety, and assessment of the continued need for restraint.

Long-term care facilities, in accordance with new federal and state laws, have developed stringent policies regarding the use of physical and chemical restraints on residents. Using clinical judgment to decrease physical and chemical restraints is closely related to potential for injury assessments and risk management.

PHYSICAL RESTRAINTS

Physical restraints refer to the use of straps or safety vests to maintain a resident's position in bed or in a chair.

> While the belief that it is essential for residents to maintain dignity and independence by being permitted to take "normal risks of daily living," restraints used in an attempt to remove these normal risks violate the rights of residents, reduce their quality of life, and present significant physical and psychological risks. Restraints used at a long-term care facility are considered to treat medical symptom/condition that endangers the physical safety of the resident or other residents and under the following conditions: (1) as a last resort measure after a trial period where less restrictive measures have been undertaken and proven unsuccessful; (2) with physician order; (3) with the consent of the resident (or legal representative); and (4) when the benefits of the restraint outweigh the identified risks. (L. L'Esperance, Naples, Florida, personal interview, September 22, 1992)

Residents are assessed at admission and periodically throughout residency at a long-term care facility. Assessments include the reason for restraints, if the patient can safely and independently get out of a chair, whether the resident has fallen within the past 6 months, and whether the patient is receiving any medication that affects balance or alertness. When restraints are needed, the least restrictive type for the shortest period of time is implemented.

Information is carefully documented in the chart for clinical judgment to initiate restraints and for documentation support for continued restraint use. Documentation of assessment, frequent reassessment, intervention, and resident response to restraints is important because this is a high-risk area of care.

CHEMICAL RESTRAINTS

Chemical restraints refer to the use of medication, such as sedatives and tranquilizers, which alter a resident's emotional state and behavior. Another program that relies on accurate documentation is a long-term care program to reduce the amount of drugs needed to be prescribed for a resident. Certain medication is decreased in dose and frequency, and the resident is assessed to see if the behavior that prompted the order for the medication is still present. If the behavior reappears, as evidenced by documentation, a low-maintenance dose is ordered. In the same way, a physician decreasing the dose of a medication like haloperidol (Haldol) takes nursing observation and documentation of resident response to further assess and use clinical judgment to decide on the effectiveness of a lower dose, considering the comfort and rest of the resident. In the above situations, only consistent, timely, and concise nursing documentation can show patterns of behavior, cause and effect of medication, and patient response.

Incident Reports

An incident report is a form used for documentation of any unusual occurrence in hospital routine or in patient care (see display, Healthcare Personnel Patient Incident

Report). The occurrence may have resulted in an actual injury to a patient (or employee or visitor) or a situation that may potentially cause injury. This report can be used for any injury, errors in treatment or medication administration, or loss or damage to a patient, nurse, or organization's property. Falls, burns, and medication errors are the most common incidents in a hospital (Fiesta, 1983). Nurses have a contractual responsibility to complete incident reports for any incident in which they are involved. Further, insurance companies often have the contractual policy with a health care organization that unless they are given an incident report in a timely manner regarding an incident, they will not insure the resulting litigation expenses.

For legal reasons, the existence of the incident report should not be mentioned in nursing documentation in the chart. Further, these reports should not be attached to the chart. This procedure assists the health care orga-

---

PATIENT INCIDENT REPORT

HEALTHCARE PERSONNEL
PATIENT INCIDENT REPORT

To Be Completed By Employee:

Patient name _____ Social Security number _____

Address _____

Diagnoses _____

Incident date _____ Day _____ Hour _____ am/pm

Witnesses _____ Address _____ Phone _____

Necessary to notify family? Yes _____ No _____ If yes, whom_____

Other notified and when _____

Exact location of incident _____

Patient condition prior to accident/injury _____

_____

How injury/accident occurred _____

_____

Type of injury (include nature of injury and body parts affected) _____

_____

_____

_____

Treatment received including where, doctor's name, date and time (attach treatment report).

_____

_____

If patient has insurance:

Carrier _____ Policy No. _____

Employee's Signature _____ Today's Date _____

(continued)

PATIENT INCIDENT REPORT *(Continued)*

PATIENT INCIDENT REPORT, page 2

To Be Completed By HP Office Staff:

Incident was reported to (office person) _____

Indicent was reported by (employee or family) _____

Incident was reported at (time and date) _____

Report received by HP office (use words of employee or family); *include* treatment stated:

_____

_____

_____

_____

_____

_____

_____

_____

_____

Comments of HP staff _____

_____

_____

_____

If patient has insurance (verified by HP office)

Carrier _____ Policy No. _____

Any follow-up needed:

This section completed by:

HP staff name _____ Title _____ Date _____

Courtesy of Healthcare Personnel Inc, Naples, FL.

nization in keeping the information nondiscoverable from attorneys for the potential **plaintiff** (the suing patient).

The incident report is an internal device for the health care organization. It is considered necessary for the internal use in the quality assurance program and is only available on a confidential basis to the committee during quality assurance meetings. Under these conditions, the incident report is deemed privileged information, which prevents its release to a plaintiff's attorneys.

The patient condition before the accident or injury is an important focus of information, especially as it relates to the possible cause of the injury. Any action the patient engaged in or any refusal of medical or nursing direction before the incident should be documented if it appears that patient behavior contributed to the incident. For example, documentation in the nurses notes before a fall states a nurse instructed the patient to call for help with the call bell the nurse put within reach. This information can be repeated on the incident report. If the patient sues, a judge or jury may determine the patient contributed to the injury by not following the nurse's direction. Therefore, the nurse and hospital would not be liable.

A second focus of information is the condition of the patient after the incident. Assessment should be thorough, concise, and focused on objective and subjective signs and symptoms related to the site(s) of actual injury or potential injury. Absence of pertinent symptoms or complaints of pain are important to document. In an incident in which a patient fell and injured one knee, the assessment portion of the note could read: "R knee slightly red, no induration, skin intact. Pt has full ROM of joint without complaint of pain. Able to continue ambulation with no pain per patient."

A third important focus of information is the nursing intervention after the incident. After a fall in which a patient complains of pain in her upper arm, for example, documentation could read: 'Pt assisted back to bed. Skin and ROM of R upper arm inspected, vital signs checked, assessed situation precipitating fall, reinstructed patient to prevent further incidents."

The first page of the incident report is completed by the nurse who was in attendance during an incident or who first saw the patient after an incident. If a nurse is not in attendance when an incident or accident occurs, the nurse's documentation must clearly show the patient was found *after* the accident. For example, a nurse found a patient sitting on the floor and the patient stated she fell trying to walk to the bedside commode. The nurse does not document that the patient fell because the nurse did not see the fall. The nurse documents the condition of the patient when first observed after the accident. The nurse assesses and documents the patient's condition and complaints of pain and documents the patient's statement regarding how the accident occurred. Also the nurse documents any interventions the nurse performed after the incident and to whom the incident was reported.

The second page of the incident report allows additional documentation of a witness's objective description of an incident. The space may also be used to document additional statements made to the nursing supervisor at the time of the incident or after the incident by the patient or other caregivers.

Although many nurses try to avoid writing incident reports, reports are actually helpful in defense of nurses, as a protection of rights for patients, and as tools to improve quality of care.

KEY POINTS

▲ Nurses are legally responsible to document the following: observations and assessments; interventions; and communications with other caregivers regarding patient data and care, actual and potential problems of the patient, patient responses to treatment, and unexpected or untoward outcomes in condition or care.

▲ A general principle in legal aspects of documentation is "If it isn't documented, it wasn't done."

▲ When documentation follows policies and procedures and is written with legal issues in mind, the law can protect nurses and health care organizations from charges of negligence and malpractice.

▲ In negligence and malpractice cases, four elements decide the merits of a case: legal duty, breach of duty, proximate cause, and damage. Documentation is used to support or refute a case on these merits.

▲ The most frequent documentation problems in malpractice cases are omissions and alterations in a chart. What and how a nurse documents are important aspects in legal risk.

▲ Law and ethics together influence behavior. Law and ethics are two forces that help people ensure rights, minimize potential harm, and guide human behavior. Laws are mandatory guidelines people must follow under obligation of fines or incarceration. Ethics are guidelines based on how we wish people would act, under obligation of consciousness.

▲ The four principles of ethics are autonomy, beneficence, justice, and fidelity. Autonomy and beneficence involve interaction between two people and are intertwined with the law to establish guidelines for informed consent, advance directives, refusal of treatment, privacy, and access to records.

REFERENCES

A Christian Affirmation of Life (1974). St. Louis: Catholic Hospital Association of America.

Creighton, H. (1986). *Law every nurse should know* (pp. 54, 146, 165, 210, 277, 280, 283, 285). Philadelphia: W. B. Saunders.

Fiesta, J. (1983). *The law and liability: A guide for nurses* (pp. 67, 138, 148, 163, 280). New York: John Wiley & Sons.

Hall, J. K. (1990). Understanding the fine line between law and ethics. *Nursing '90, 20*(10), 36–37.

Johnson, S. H. (1988). Who sets the standards for home health care? *Health Progress, 69*(11), 20–21.

Johnston, J. E. (1988). The elderly and fall prevention. *Applied Nursing Research, 1*(3), 140.

Modell, W. (1974). A will to live. *New England Journal of Medicine, 290,* 907–908.

Myers, Krause, & Stevens, Chartered, Attorneys at Law (1990). *Health care decisions* (p. 1). Naples, FL: Personal interview with William H. Myers, October 30, 1990. Communication with Richard S. Franklin of Myers, Krause, & Stevens, and William H. Myers, September 25, 1992.

President's Commission for the Study of Ethical Problems in Medicine and Biomedical and Behavioral Research. (1982). *Making health care decisions* (p. 57). Washington, DC: U.S. Government Printing Office.

Randall, D. A., & Pritchard, M. L. (1987, October 10). *The risk management dilemma: Legal and management questions arising from changing, narrowing or eliminating home care services.* Presentation at the National Association for Home Care Annual Meeting, Washington, DC.

Regan, W. A. (1967). Nursing liability for restraint accidents. *Regan Report on Nursing Law*, 8(6), 1.

Report of the Ad Hoc Committee of the Harvard Medical School to Examine the Definition of Brain Death: A Definition of Irreversible Coma. (1968). *Journal of the American Medical Association*, 205, 337–340.

Salgo v. Leland Stanford Board of Trustees, 317 P.2d 170 (Cal., 1957).

Standards for Cardiopulmonary Resuscitation (CPR) and Emergency Cardiac Care (ECC) (1980). *Journal of the American Medical Association*, 244(5), 453–509.

Stead, E. A., Jr. (1970). If I become ill and unable to manage my own affairs. *Medical Times*, 98, 191–192.

United States Catholic Conference (1971). Ethical and Religious Directives for Catholic Health Facilities, Washington, DC.

CASE STUDY REFERENCES

Battocchi v. Washington Hospital Center 581 A. 2d 759 (D.C. App. 1990). (1990). Cited in Loeb, Stanley. (1992). *Nursing handbook of law and ethics* (p. 245). Springhouse, PA: Springhouse.

In the Guardianship of Browning 568, So 2d 4 (per in Fla, 1990), aff'g, 543 So 2d 258 (per in Fla 2d DCA 1989).

Darling v. Charleston Community Memorial Hospital, 33 Ill.2d 326, 211 N.E.2d 253, (1965), cert. den'd. 383 U.S. 946 (1966). Cited in Guido, G. W. (1988). *Legal issues in nursing* (p. 99). Norwalk, CT: Appleton & Lange.

Engle v. Clarke, 346 S.W.2d 13 (Ky. 1961). Cited in Guido, G. W. (1988). *Legal issues in nursing* (p. 99). Norwalk, CT: Appleton & Lange.

Hiatt v. Grace, 215 Kan. 14, 523 P.2d 320 (1974). Cited in Guido, G. W. (1988). *Legal issues in nursing* (p. 100). Norwalk, CT: Appleton & Lange.

Maslonka v. Herman et al, 414 A.2d 1350 (N.J. 1980). Cited in Cournoyer, C. P. (1989). *The nursing manager and the law* (p. 181). Gaithersburg, MD: Aspen Publications.

Pisel v. Stamford Hospital et al, 430 A.2d (Conn. 1980). Cited in Fiesta, J. (1983). *The law and liability: A guide for nurses* (p. 144). New York: John Wiley & Sons.

Quintal v. Laurel Grove Hospital, 397 P.2d 161,41 Cal. Rptr. 577 (1965). Cited in Fiesta, J. (1983). *The law and liability: A guide for nurses* (p. 144). New York: John Wiley & Sons.

Rogers v. Kasdan 612 S.W. 2d 133 (KY. 1981). Cited in Loeb, Stanley. *Nursing handbook of law and ethics* (p. 244). Springhouse, PA: Springhouse.

Sheppard v. Kimbrough, 318 S.E.2d 573 (S.C. App. 1984). Cited in Guido, G. W. (1988). *Legal issues in nursing* (p. 100). Norwalk, CT: Appleton & Lange.

St. Paul Fire and Marine Insurance Co. v. Prothro 266 Ark. 1020, 590 S.W. 2d, 35 (Ark. Ct. App. 1979). Cited in Loeb, Stanley, *Nursing handbook of law and ethics* (p. 244). Springhouse, PA: Springhouse.

Washington Hospital Center v. Martin, 44 A.2d 306 (D.C. 1982). Cited in Feutz, S. (1989). *Nursing and the law* (3rd ed., pp. 114–115). East Claire, WI: Professional Education Systems.

BIBLIOGRAPHY

Bandman, E. L., & Bandman, B. (1990). *Nursing ethics through the life span*. Norwalk, CT: Appleton & Lange.

Beauchamp, T. L., & Childress, J. F. (1989). *Principles of biomedical ethics* (3rd ed.) New York: Oxford University Press.

Calfee, B. E. (1991). Protecting yourself—nursing negligence. *Nursing '91*, 21(12), 34–39.

Cushing, M. (1988). *Nursing jurisprudence*. Norwalk, CT: Appleton & Lange.

Easterling, M. (1990). Which of your patients is headed for a fall? *RN*, 53(1), 56–58.

Feutz-Harter, S. A. (1989). Documentation principles and pitfalls. *Journal of Nursing Administration*, 19(12), 9.

Fletcher, K. (1990). Restraints should be a last resort. *RN*, 53(1), 52–56.

Haddad, A. M., & Kapp, M. B. (1991). *Ethical and legal issues in home health care: Case studies and analyses*. Norwalk, CT: Appleton & Lange.

Iyer, P. W. (1991). Six more charting rules to keep you legally safe. *Nursing '91*, 21(7), 34–39.

Maher, V. F. (1989). Your legal guide to safe nursing practice. *Nursing '89*, 19(11), 34–41.

Northrop, C. (1987). A question of restraints. *Nursing '87*, 17(2), 41.

Nurses should know charting techniques, hospital policy. (1988). *Hospital Risk Management*, 10(7), 85–87.

Uustal, D. B. (1992). *Values and ethics in nursing: From theory to practice* (4th ed.). East Greenwich, RI: Educational Resources in Nursing & Holistic Health.

▰ PRACTICE SESSION ▰

FILL IN

1. Two of the most common types of litigation are _____

and _____ .

2. _____ are responsible for offering information to patients regarding informed consent.

3. A _____ must be signed by the patient if a patient decides to refuse treatment.

4. If a mistake is made in an entry, the way to correct this is _____

_____ .

5. Once a living will is developed and signed, it _____ be changed.

6. A do not resuscitate order is documented on the _____ .

7. If a nurse recalls information at a later time, an _____ is appropriate.

8. Discharge summaries can be transferred to nursing homes if the nurse obtains a

_____ .

9. The most significant problem associated with verbal orders is _____ .

10. From a malpractice standpoint, most frequent problems with charting involve

_____ and _____ .

MATCHING

Match the problem in Column A with the legal term in Column B.

1. _____ failure to provide care   **a.** commission

2. _____ providing care below standard   **b.** omission

3. _____ professional misconduct   **c.** malpractice

4. _____ deviation from professional standard of care

5. _____ improper performance of professional skill

MULTIPLE CHOICE

1. _____ Elements included in reporting a verbal order include the following aspects:
   a) specific time call received and by whom
   b) to whom information was given
   c) specifics of information
   d) all of the above

2. _____ In terms of consent, an explanation of a procedure should include these elements: benefits and risks, alternative treatments, probable success of various treatments or procedures, and
   a) what medications will be prescribed after treatment
   b) the cost of the procedure
   c) what to expect if a procedure is not performed
   d) all of the above

3. _____ A nurse can detect a problem regarding a patient's understanding of an upcoming procedure/surgery when the patient does not understand the procedure and/or associated risks; signed the consent more than a month ago; had an unauthorized person sign the consent; and

    a) patient does not remember signing a consent form
    b) the family objects to the procedure/surgery
    c) a & b
    d) none of the above

4. _____ Patients who are at risk to fall out of a chair should always be put in

    a) restraints
    b) a recliner
    c) a chair pushed up to a table
    d) none of the above

5. _____ The four elements that decide the merits of negligence and malpractice are:

    a) extent of injury, cost of medical attention, proximate cause, and damage
    b) legal duty owed a patient, breach of duty, proximate cause, and damage
    c) both of the above
    d) none of the above

CHALLENGE FOR CRITICAL THINKING

1. Discuss the difference and similarities between law and ethics. List the four principles of ethics and the relationship of two elements to legal issues of documentation.

2. Describe when and when not to document additional information on a clinical record.

3. What factors have been associated with incidence of falls? What measures would you use to minimize these factors and to minimize legal risk concerning falls?

4. List three characteristics of documentation content that pose a legal risk, and describe three situations that are examples of those three characteristics.

5. List two common characteristics of documentation mechanics that pose a legal risk and give examples to illustrate potential problems.

LEARNING TO DOCUMENT

1. Correct these documentation examples to minimize legal risk.
    a. Patient discharged at 10 am.
    b. Dressing changed per order.
    c. Patient has a stomach ache.
    d. Patient refused medications.
    e. Blood pressure stabilizing.
    f. Appetite poor. Patient ate a little breakfast.
    g. Patient ambulating OK.
    h. Doctor came to visit.
    i. Patient going home tomorrow, needs help at home.
    j. Patient very demanding.

2. Mrs. Mona Jilko, S.S. 123 45 6789, of 111 Bellbottom Lane has a diagnosis of CVA, R sided hemiparesis. While at home, she has been ambulating with a cane from bedroom to kitchen. On Saturday May 1, 1993 she told Virginia Fleck, LPN, that she felt dizzy and her stomach was a little upset. At noon, Virginia told Mrs. Jilko to stay in the bedroom chair and she would bring her lunch in at noon, instead of Mrs. J. walking to the kitchen as she normally did. When

Virginia carried in the lunch, she found Mrs. J. on the floor near the door. Mrs. J. said she was okay, nothing was hurt except her R wrist was a little stiff and sore, and she didn't want her out-of-state daughter to be told. Virginia checked Mrs. J. and found no reddened areas, and Mrs. J. was able to move all extremities and walk assisted back to the chair. She ate with her left hand because of her sore right wrist; but at 2:00 she was able to knit without any pain. The home health agency was celled at 12:10, and a nurse said she would visit this afternoon. Should an incident report be written? If not, why not? If so, why, and how would you complete the form, using the first page of the Healthcare Personnel Patient Incident Report below.

PATIENT INCIDENT REPORT

HEALTHCARE PERSONNEL
PATIENT INCIDENT REPORT

To Be Completed By Employee:

Patient name _____ Social Security number _____

Address _____

Diagnoses _____

Incident date _____ Day _____ Hour _____ am/pm

Witnesses _____ Address _____ Phone _____

Necessary to notify family?   Yes _____   No _____   If yes, whom_____

Other notified and when _____

Exact location of incident _____

Patient condition prior to accident/injury _____

_____

How injury/accident occurred _____

_____

Type of injury (include nature of injury and body parts affected) _____

_____

_____

_____

Treatment received including where, doctor's name, date and time (attach treatment report).

_____

_____

If patient has insurance:

Carrier _____ Policy No. _____

Employee's Signature _____ Today's Date _____

CHAPTER

8

Documenting Continuity of Care

LEARNING OBJECTIVES

After studying this chapter, the learner should be able to:

▲ Define and state the purpose of four types of continuity of care forms.

▲ Describe information that should be documented on teaching records.

▲ Explain information that should be documented on progress summaries.

▲ Identify information that should be documented on transfer forms.

▲ List information that should be documented on discharge summaries.

KEY TERMS

Affective learning outcomes
Cognitive learning outcomes
Community resources

Continuity of care
Discharge summary
Learning outcomes

Psychomotor learning outcomes
Referral
Transfer form

Eggland ET, Heinemann DS. NURSING DOCUMENTATION:
CHARTING, RECORDING, AND REPORTING.
© 1994 J.B. Lippincott Company.

Continuity of care refers to the smooth transition of care from one caregiver or group of caregivers to another. Continuity is accomplished by effectively communicating information and responsibility for health care services.

Teaching records, progress summaries, transfer forms, and discharge summaries contribute to continuity of care. Whereas teaching records and progress summaries communicate information among caregivers currently providing care, transfer forms and discharge forms communicate between caregiving groups (such as another nursing unit or health care organization) who will be providing care.

Teaching, progress, transfer, and discharge forms include information regarding the needs of a patient, interventions performed to date, outcomes of those interventions, and patient status at the time of documentation.

The purpose of these forms is to establish communication and continuation of quality care by providing a concise data base about identified needs, care received, and patient outcomes. By including patient outcomes, these forms provide an overview for evaluating effectiveness of care, which becomes a basis for consideration in further assessment and planning for care. Including patient outcomes in documentation along with the patient's condition is also a basis for legal protection for care during the time service was provided and for care during transition to another caregiver.

Patient Teaching

Patient teaching by a nurse contributes to continuity of care. During hospitalization a patient and family can learn about an illness, its treatment, caregiving skills required, and rationale for care. After discharge they can continue at home the care regimen prescribed according to the mutually established teaching and care plan. Patient teaching assists patients and caregivers to become knowledgeable about their health care, to make informed decisions, and to move toward independence in their health care management.

Health Care Delivery Factors Affecting Patient Teaching

A government prospective payment program for hospitals and development of increasing regulations and standards for health care have emphasized the importance of patient teaching and the necessity of patient teaching documentation.

PROSPECTIVE PAYMENT

In 1983 the federal government began a prospective payment system to hospitals, which resulted in patients being discharged "quicker and sicker." Care a patient needed at home after discharge became more complex for the sicker patient. Patients were often faced with the need to continue wound care and injections, even high-technology care such as intravenous therapy and complex respiratory therapy.

Patient and family teaching in the hospital became critical for patients to be able to continue appropriate care at home after discharge. Home health care nurses are requested more frequently now to continue teaching in the home while they provide skilled care. Nurses teaching patients in the hospital or at home assist the patients to recuperate, prevent complications, prevent rehospitalization, and develop independence in care.

REGULATIONS AND STANDARDS FOR HEALTH CARE

Governmental regulations for the federally funded Medicare and Medicaid programs require that patient teaching be documented. State nurse practice acts and state home health agency licensure laws require that teaching be performed and documented. Standards of nursing and specialty organizations are an indication of a minimum performance or description of responsibility for which a practitioner is responsible. The American Nurses Association (ANA) states that nursing practice includes teaching, and each registered nurse is directly accountable to the consumer for the quality of nursing care rendered. Documentation of teaching is a record for that accountability.

Standards can exhibit a level of attainment. A standard of documenting teaching is one minimum performance required to become accredited by organizations such as the Joint Commission on Accreditation of Healthcare Organizations (JCAHO), National Association for Home Care (NAHC), or National League for Nursing Community Health Accreditation Program (CHAP). In each case, documentation standards must be met for accreditation from that organization.

Where to Document Teaching

Depending on the health care organizations, teaching may be documented on a care plan and nursing notes or on a separate teaching record.

DOCUMENTING TEACHING ON A PATIENT CARE PLAN

In some health care organizations teaching needs and planned teaching interventions are documented within the main nursing care plan. An advantage of this method is that all planning is documented together, so a nurse can quickly see that all aspects of a problem have been considered and interventions are planned and coordinated.

Another advantage is less paper volume. If a patient is knowledgeable about an illness and treatment, learning needs will be few. The method eliminates one sheet of paper on which little would be written.

When teaching is documented on an initial nursing care plan, teaching interventions can be written in clinical progress notes. The advantage here is that all interventions are documented together according to problem topic, so a better evaluation of patient outcome can be made.

DOCUMENTING TEACHING ON A TEACHING RECORD

Some organizations by policy and procedure direct nurses to document teaching in a separate teaching plan or teaching record. An advantage is that if a patient has many or complex teaching needs or difficulty in learning, a nurse may detail the information on a teaching record and could be reluctant to do so on a care plan. Another advantage is that a teaching record form cues a nurse for all aspects to be considered while developing a teaching plan. Another advantage is that a teaching record is readily retrievable for nurses to determine what teaching has been done and what yet has to be taught.

Teaching Records

In general, teaching records are forms on which nurses document an outline of information a patient will be (or was) taught, special patient needs and considerations, and patient outcomes of the teaching sessions (see display, Documentation for Patient Teaching).

Teaching records may have different names according to an organization and different purposes according to design. Teaching records may be called patient education records, patient teaching flow sheets, or standardized teaching plans.

There are two types of teaching records: a teaching plan and a combined teaching plan and summary.

TEACHING PLAN

Sometimes teaching records consist of teaching plans only and do not include space to document teaching interventions performed. Teaching plans are detailed

DOCUMENTATION FOR PATIENT TEACHING

Documentation for patient teaching includes the following:

1. Patient learning needs and requests ranked in priority
2. Weaknesses or problems in learning
3. Teaching interventions planned
4. Teaching interventions implemented
5. Patient outcomes of learning
6. Revisions, if any, on teaching plan

forms designed to outline learning needs and goals, planned interventions, teaching tools and teaching methods, identified strengths for learning, and barriers to learning. Strengths and barriers are special learning considerations that include past education, experience, culture, and patient and family learning priorities. Depending on what these considerations are, they can be identified strengths or they can be barriers to learning. Documentation of strengths and barriers in care plans facilitates interventions to enhance strengths and minimize or overcome barriers.

Developing a teaching plan. Planning for patient teaching is similar to the procedure for care planning. Developing a teaching plan includes:

▲ Identifying patient needs or caregiver needs
  • The nurse assesses what a patient does not know.
▲ Ranking learning needs in priority of importance
  • A patient needs to learn about oxygen therapy to maintain life, then diet and techniques to lose weight.
▲ Ranking needs in sequence of learning
  • A patient needs to learn about a disease before learning about its treatment to better understand rationale of care.
▲ Determining a patient's strengths and weaknesses in learning
  • A patient may have poor reading skills due to limited education; a video with simple language may overcome this learning weakness.
▲ Mutually agreeing on goals or expected outcomes
  • If a patient is involved in planning, motivation is enhanced.
▲ Establishing a teaching plan
  • Use resources to gather patient education materials, such as pamphlets, audiovisuals, and computer programs.

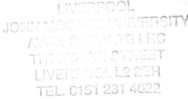

Teaching plan expected outcomes. Teaching plan principles are similar to care plan principles in setting goals called expected outcomes. An expected outcome statement for care plans or for teaching plans is written in patient-oriented measurable terms. An example of an expected outcome statement from a teaching plan follows. The patient will:

▲ Verbalize the purpose of each medication, the dose and schedule of administration, and the side effects of each
▲ Return demonstrate how to read a thermometer correctly
▲ Describe a sample plan in compliance with pre-scribed diet

Teaching plan interventions. In teaching plan interventions, actions are sequential, similar to a nursing care plan. Sequence of information in a teaching plan is from simple to complex and documented accordingly. For example, the care plan states to teach a patient sterile technique, then teach how to irrigate a urinary catheter. The nurse should outline the main points and supplement with supporting information. For example, a care plan lists the principles of sterile technique, and during teaching the nurse supports the information by teaching rationale.

Give a patient written information for easy reference to reinforce what was taught to improve understanding and retention. Besides written information such as lists, reminder tips, or pamphlets, audiovisual materials are sometimes available through health-related organizations. Audiovisual aids are particularly helpful for visual learners who learn better by seeing than reading. When possible, include the family or caregivers in learning. Even if a patient is to learn to provide self-care, a spouse or caregiver can learn and be a knowledgeable, physical, and emotional support during learning and after a patient is discharged.

Implementing and evaluating the teaching plan. After the teaching plan is implemented, the nurse asks the patient for feedback, clarifies any misconceptions, reinforces what a patient has learned, asks for a return demonstration if appropriate, and praises the patient for learning. Then:

1. Teaching interventions are documented, usually on a flow sheet, as interventions are performed or as specific knowledge and skills are learned by the patient.
2. An evaluation is made based on comparison of patient outcome to expected outcomes.
3. Any necessary revisions are made to the teaching plan if desired outcomes are not achieved or interventions cannot be implemented effectively.

TEACHING PLAN AND SUMMARY FORM

Most teaching records are a combination of teaching plan and summary format, on which the teaching plan is outlined and space is available to check off that teaching was performed. A column on the form is also designated to document patient outcomes or progress in learning. Patient teaching documentation should always include teaching interventions implemented and patient outcomes of learning. Additional helpful information to include is methods used in teaching, patient response to learning, and any plans for future teaching.

Patient outcomes. With increased attention to outcomes, regulatory organizations (for Medicare) and accrediting organizations (JCAHO and CHAP) not only focus on the documentation of patient teaching but also on documentation of teaching outcomes. Documentation of these outcomes focuses on a patient's and family's comprehension and compliance to what was taught and ability to perform learned skills. Comprehension and ability to perform skills can be determined by having a patient verbalize what has been taught, demonstrate skills learned, and answer questions regarding what to do in different circumstances.

When an outcome is not achieved, new or revised interventions to meet patient needs must follow a documented outcome. An example is the referral to a home health agency for insulin injections because the patient and family have not met the expected outcome of administering injections appropriately. A nurse should document on teaching records if and why further teaching intervention is necessary. In addition, if teaching or a portion of teaching was not performed, a nurse should document that fact, the reason not performed, and future plans for that teaching.

Patient response. A response to teaching is also important to document. Responses can be patient or family comments during a learning experience, feelings and attitudes expressed during or after a learning experience, and observed behavior during the learning experience or later when asked about learned information. The following are examples of patient responses: a patient feels confident in what was learned; anxious about remembering how to perform skills learned; or apprehensive about being able to perform care without supervision.

Special Considerations in Teaching Plan Documentation

In developing teaching plans and designing teaching record formats, three special considerations are beneficial: consideration of cognitive, psychomotor, and affective learning; consideration of individualizing the teaching record; and consideration of standardizing teaching plans.

COGNITIVE, PSYCHOMOTOR, AND AFFECTIVE LEARNING

Learning outcomes can be documented in the three domains in which learning occurs: cognitive, psychomotor, and affective. **Cognitive learning outcomes** include knowledge learned; **psychomotor learning outcomes** include the ability to perform a skill taught; and **affective learning outcomes** include attitudinal changes that reflect the value a patient puts on skills learned. Examples below show correctly documented interventions with outcomes in each learning area:

> *Cognitive learning outcome*: Instructed pt in purpose, side effects, and administration regimen of ampicillin. Pt able to verbalize correct information; written information provided to pt and family.

> *Psychomotor learning outcome*: Demonstrated H_2O_2 wound cleansing, application of Neosporin and dry sterile dressing. Pt able to verbalize rationale and demonstrate procedure correctly.

> *Affective learning outcome*: Wife expressed concern about being responsible for IV therapy of spouse after discharge; stated she doesn't feel prepared to provide care and needs more practice. Pt referred to home health agency; will continue patient and spouse teaching tomorrow.

Documenting **learning outcomes**, what the patient has learned as shown above, can involve cognitive and psychomotor evaluation areas of learning. Some teaching records differentiate these types of learning (see display, Cognitive and Psychomotor Skills Checklist).

What a patient or caregiver can verbalize (cognitive learning) and what a patient or caregiver can demonstrate (psychomotor learning) may be different because of a physical handicap. Perhaps a learner needs to understand concepts before being able to learn skills correctly. Psychomotor and cognitive learning are differentiated on some teaching records to determine if a patient is having difficulty with the concept or content of information (cognitive learning) or the physical ability to perform a skill (psychomotor learning).

Boxes to write in data or enter check marks provide a fast way to document teaching and a patient's progress in learning. In the IV Caregivers Skills Checklist, both cognitive learning (can verbally repeat) and psychomotor learning (can demonstrate) are assessed and documented. Affective learning is a more difficult area to assess and document, other than by using subjective statements made by the patient or family.

INDIVIDUALIZING THE TEACHING RECORD

A patient's clinical record should include special learning considerations that individualize the teaching plan. Considerations include completed level of schooling (grade school, high school, college), past education regarding pertinent health care information, ongoing learning needs assessment, and patient or caregiver learning priorities. It is helpful to have this information included on a patient teaching record because it individualizes the teaching record, centralizes information helpful to the teaching process, and influences choices of individualized teaching expected outcomes and individualized teaching interventions (see display, Patient Education Form).

STANDARDIZING TEACHING PLANS

The purpose of a standardized teaching plan is to organize information to be taught to a patient. Standardized plans often specify what teaching methods and media to use, based on audiovisual materials available and proved effective. It also establishes standards for evaluating patient learning by standardizing teaching expected outcomes.

Advantages. With standardized teaching plans nurses save composing and writing time. Through careful design development and evaluated use, plans are complete and contain cues for important data to document. Having a mutually agreeable standardized plan provides communication, continuity, and coordination among all nurses who teach the patient, evaluate the teaching, and evaluate the learning.

Flow sheets. Standardized patient teaching flow sheets speed the process of patient education planning and documentation of implementation. Add the flexibility of computerization or teaching plan stickers and individualized standardized patient teaching flow sheets become fast and complete. Teaching plan stickers are preprinted teaching plans for various topics such as postoperative teaching, wound care, and revascularization of lower extremities. Printed as a label, a nurse pulls off the backing from a teaching plan, and the sticky side is attached to the goal and approach area of the teaching plan (see display, Patient Teaching Flow Sheet).

Progress Summaries

Progress summaries are brief narrative reports regarding a patient's health status and needs, nursing care received, and patient outcomes and response.

COGNITIVE AND PSYCHOMOTOR SKILLS CHECKLIST

IV CAREGIVER SKILLS CHECKLIST

Patient _____ Client # _____ Therapy

Caregiver _____

RN _____

Skills	Cognitive Learning *Can Verbalize*	Psychomotor Learning *Can Demonstrate*	Needs Reinforcement	Can Perform Independently	Learning Completed	Initial and Date
Understanding of IV's purpose and rational						
Knowledge of appropriate aspetic technique with IV supplies and procedures:						
attaching tubing and filters						
changing tubing and solutions						
discontinuing infusions						
Identification and safe-guarding of medicine and supplies						
Ability to inventory, order, and store supplies						
Medications administration procedure						
Dressing change procedure						

(Reprinted/adapted with permission from J. B. Lippincott Co., July-August, 1988 issue of Home Healthcare Nurse, "Nursing Implications for Home Parenteral Therapy" by Sr. Theresa Bontempo and Ellen Eggland.)

Progress Summaries in Home Health Care

Progress summaries are especially important in home health care and are used in two ways. First, progress summaries are sent to a patient's primary physician on a routine basis with a request for signed medical orders to continue treatment. A summary provides a picture of a patient's status and needs so that the physician can determine continued medical orders for treatment, be apprised of any new health or treatment problems, and monitor patient progress.

Second, progress summaries are sent to third-party payers (Medicare or insurance companies) to establish · the continuing need for home health care. A release of information signed by the patient or authorized representative is required before sending a progress summary to an insurance company or other entity not a direct caregiver.

Medicare regulations for home health care require that progress summaries be written every 60 days. Medicare auditors assess these summaries to determine if a

(text continues on page 168)

PATIENT EDUCATION FORM

THE CLEVELAND CLINIC FOUNDATION
PATIENT EDUCATION RECORD

Focus: **Knowledge Deficit of**
                          Surgical Experience

Special learning
considerations: _____
_____

Past education experience (identify where, formal,
informal, classes or individual and date completed)
_____
_____

Patient & family/significant other learning priorities
_____
_____

LEARNER ABBREVIATION KEY

NA—Not Applicable

PT—Patient

SO—Significant Other
   (specify in comments)

INCLUDE DATE, INITIAL, AND LEARNER ABBREVIATION UNDER COLUMN

LEARNING OBJECTIVES/CONTENT *TEACHING TOOLS	LEARNING NEEDS ASSESSED	CONTENT PRESENTED	CONTENT REVIEWED	OBJECTIVES ACHIEVED	**EVALUATION OF LEARNING OBJECTIVES** **COMMENTS/PATIENT RESPONSE**
I. The patient describes the necessary preoperative activity and procedures.					
A. Food & fluid restrictions					
B. Lab studies/x-rays					
C. Preps: (evening before)					
1. Shave					
2. Shower					
3. Enemas					
4. IV therapy					
5. Nighttime medication					
6. _____					
D. AM activities					
1. Wake-up time					
2. Appropriate OR attire					
3. Preop medication and effects					
E. Family information					
1. Visiting time					
2. Patient valuables/belongings					
3. Family lounge/purpose					
II. The patient describes the necessary intraoperative environment.					
A. Holding area					
B. Preparation: IV and monitoring lines					
C. Operating room environment					
D. Comfort measures					
E. Induction					

(continued)

PATIENT EDUCATION FORM *(Continued)*

INCLUDE DATE, INITIAL, AND LEARNER ABBREVIATION UNDER EACH COLUMN

LEARNING OBJECTIVES/CONTENT *TEACHING TOOLS	LEARNING NEEDS ASSESSED	CONTENT PRESENTED	CONTENT REVIEWED	OBJECTIVES ACHIEVED	EVALUATION OF LEARNING OBJECTIVES COMMENTS/PATIENT RESPONSE
III. The patient describes the postanesthesia activities and procedures.					
A. Environment/noises					
B. Vital signs/neuro checks					
C. Respiratory care					
D. Stir-up regime/exercises					
E. Comfort measures					
F. Length of time in unit/routines					
G. Visiting					
IV. The patient describes the postoperative activities and procedures.					
A. Diet					
B. Nursing activity					
1. Vital signs/neuro checks					
2. Dressings/drains					
3. IVs					
4. Pain control					
5. Comfort measures					
6. _____					
V. The patient will be able to perform postoperative procedures and exercises.					
A. Turning (self or assisted)					
B. Leg exercises					
C. Ambulation (progressive)					
D. Coughing/deep breathing/splinting					
E. Spirometer					
F. _____					
G. _____					
Refer to surgical patient information brochure.					
Refer to patient teaching picture books as available.					

SUMMARY:

_____

_____

_____

_____

Courtesy of Cleveland Clinic Foundation, Cleveland, Ohio.

PATIENT TEACHING FLOW SHEET

**SAINT VINCENT CHARITY HOSPITAL
AND HEALTH CENTER
PATIENT TEACHING FLOW SHEET**

PARTICIPANTS IN INSTRUCTION

_____ Patient

_____ Family (specify): _____

_____ Other (specify): _____

_____

PROBLEMS AFFECTING LEARNING

Communication skills:

_____ reading   _____ hearing

_____ vision   _____ writing

Language spoken/read:

_____ English

_____ Other (specify): _____

Other impairments (mental/physical):

_____

_____

_____

_____

_____

PATIENT LEARNING NEEDS OR DESIRES

_____ Disease process (specify)   _____ Diet

_____   _____ Activity

_____   _____ Rehabilitation

_____ Signs/symptoms   _____ Psychosocial
                                               adjustment
_____ Medications
                                         _____ Community
_____ Diagnostic tests   resources

_____ Special care procedures

_____ Preventive health practices

_____ Other: _____

_____

_____

Inits.	Name	Inits.	Name

Objective/Goal _The patient/learner will be able to:_	Approach	Date Achieved	Learner Progress/ Comments
By _____, patient will be able to: Identify ways to prevent postop infection: 1. Cough/deep breathe q2h while awake. 2. Use incentive spirometry as instructed. 3. Increase activity as tolerated. 4. Maintain sterile/clean technique during wound care. 5. Avoid touching wound unless completely healed. 6. Drink at least 10 glasses of fluids/day. 7. Maintain balanced nutritional intake. 8. Maintain proper balance of rest and activity. 9. Maintain good personal hygiene. 10. Decrease or stop smoking. Postop 4/90	☐ Discussion ☐ Demonstration ☐ Redemonstration ☐ Other:_____ _____ _____		

Courtesy of St. Vincent Charity Hospital and Health Center, Cleveland, Ohio.

patient meets Medicare requirements. These requirements must be documented in the summary:

1. A patient is homebound and still needs skilled nursing care.
2. Rehabilitation potential is good (or patient is dying).
3. Patient status is not stabilized.
4. A patient is making progress in expected outcomes of care.

Insurance companies usually require the same type of information as described above.

Suggested topics for composing a summary include:

▲ Clinical data
  • Includes the last reported vital signs, signs and symptoms, and complaints of the patient
▲ Current problems
  • Nursing diagnoses or identified patient care needs
▲ Data ranges for vital signs and other measurements
  • Lowest and highest blood pressure, pulse, fasting blood sugar, degrees of peripheral edema, or other measurements pertinent to the patient's health problems
▲ Wound/decubitus specifics
  • Characteristics of any skin lesion: size, description, drainage, odor, related pain
▲ Treatment/interventions/instructions
  • Care the patient is receiving for primary problems
▲ Physician contact/orders
  • Is documented for information sent to other disciplines or to insurance companies or other third-party payers
▲ Reason for change in intensity or frequency of nursing care
  • Health care reasons for a higher level of care, such as personal care to skilled nursing care because vital signs are unstable or the patient's condition is worsening. Less frequent visits or shorter duration of care can also occur due to an improving condition.
▲ Involvement of other disciplines
  • Involvement of other therapists or medical social service (MSS) showing holistic and coordinated care
▲ Patient outcome or response
  • Is important to evaluate patient progress, patient care, and influence on future care planning and clinical decisions

Patient identification information is documented at the top of the progress summary note. An example of a 30-day progress summary follows:

Clinical data: Vital signs on visit of 8-25-92: BP150/90, P95, R18, T98.6°F. Apical pulse strong with regular rate. Heart sounds within normal limits (WNL). Neck veins flat. No cyanosis, no edema, no syncope. No c/o palpitations nor chest pain. Breath sounds clear on auscultation. *Current problems*: Pt initially presented need for assessment of cardiopulmonary status, due to primary hypertension. Current problems are unstable blood pressure and knowledge deficit related to arteriosclerotic heart disease (ASHD) and medication administration. *Data range for VS*: Consistent for pulse and respiration, but BP ranged from 200/120 to 130/90 within past 30 days. *Interventions/instructions*: Assessed cardiopulmonary status each visit. Instructed patient in ASHD and purpose of medications, including side effects, symptoms to report to physician, and administration schedule and charting. *Frequency of nursing care*: Visits increased from weekly to twice weekly due to unstable blood pressure. RN to continue skilled nursing visits to provide ongoing assessment of cardiac status and to continue teaching pt and spouse. *Other disciplines involvement*: MSS visited ×2 to evaluate home management and support of caregiver and investigate financial resources for buying medication. *Pt outcome/response*: Pt able to verbalize information taught regarding medication and return demonstrate charting of medications. Pt states she understands now the importance of taking medication on time and will follow instructions of MSS in obtaining resources for meds. A. Nagle, RN, MSN

Progress Summaries in Long-term Care

Some long-term care facilities require weekly summaries of a patient to reflect their current status, daily functioning, and progress toward expected outcomes. Current status includes information about a patient's admitting diagnoses; vital signs, mental status, and behavior; skin condition; and response to medication. Daily functioning includes personal care and dressing, feeding and nutrition, mobility including assistive devices, and elimination and sleep patterns. Progress toward expected outcomes includes progress related to goals of identified nursing diagnoses, with focus on restorative care and preventive measures.

Progress Summaries in Acute Care

In some hospitals, progress summaries are documented on a routine basis for a fast reference to patient status, patient needs, and most importantly patient outcomes. Summary outlines are based on the expected outcomes on the patient care plan. Progress is written based on those goals for care, as they compare to actual patient outcomes of care.

Transfer Form

A **transfer form** provides transition of care information as a patient moves from one level of care to another or from one specialty unit to another within the same health care facility. An example would be a patient moving from intensive care to a stepdown unit or transferring a patient into or out of a psychiatric unit or rehabilitation unit. A transfer form is also used for transferring a patient between health care settings. Examples include transferring a patient from a short-stay health care setting, such as an emergency department, which transfers a patient to another hospital; transferring a patient from a hospital to a long-term care facility; or transferring a patient to a hospital's affiliated home health care agency (see display, Nursing Transfer Summary). Depending on the policy and procedure of a health care organization, a discharge summary is sometimes used instead of a transfer form.

The 1985 Consolidated Omnibus Budget Reconciliation Act (COBRA) requires Medicare-reimbursed hospitals to stabilize the condition of any patient who seeks care in the emergency department. If a burn patient arrives at an emergency department, the patient must receive treatment to stabilize the condition. The emergency department personnel can call a burn hospital and transfer the patient to that hospital where facilities are available for care, but the law requires a transfer form be sent with the patient to the receiving hospital.

When a transfer form is used for a patient being transferred from one organization to another, information includes patient identification information and the following documented data:

▲ Diagnosis
▲ Physician who provided care
▲ Person contacted in the receiving organization
▲ Dates of care (admission to unit and discharge from unit)
▲ Reasons for care
▲ Services provided
▲ Reason for transfer (can be patient preference or unavailability of necessary treatment)
▲ Type of reimbursement (such as Medicare or insurance)
▲ Allergies
▲ Current medications
▲ Current therapies with regimen schedule including last administration time
▲ Patient status at departure from originating point of service
▲ Needs and goals achieved
▲ Needs and goals still unmet
▲ Time and method of transportation, including interventions to maintain patient status during transport

Whether a patient is being transferred to a unit within the same hospital or between health care organizations, communicating accurate and complete transfer information contributes to the quality of health care delivery and continuity of care.

Discharge Form

A discharge plan or discharge summary is a documentation form used when a patient is discharged from a health care organization. A **discharge summary** cites services provided before discharge and delineates plans recommended for further care.

Services provided before discharge include goals achieved; progress attained toward unmet goals; and equipment, supplies, or community resources needed, obtained, or contacted. **Community resources** are services that support patient care in the home, such as Meals on Wheels, or support groups, such as cancer support groups. Services also include patient teaching, patient's comprehension of information taught, and ability to perform health care skills and health care management.

Plans for further care include identification of the setting to which a patient is going, caregivers available and capable to provide care, recommendations made to the patient and family if they agreed, and additional plans stated by the patient or family.

Discharge planning should begin on admission. Some hospitals include discharge planning in the care plan and identify discharge planning in the nursing diagnosis of Impaired Home Maintenance Management or Altered Health Maintenance (see display, Discharge Planning Form). Discharge planning documentation is required by standard-setting organizations, such as the Joint Commission on Accreditation of Healthcare Organizations (JCAHO), governmental agencies supervising reimbursed care such as Medicare and Medicaid, and professional organizations such as ANA.

Some discharge summary forms, especially those for home health, include the reason for termination of service. In a hospital or nursing home, care is discontinued or the patient is discharged because needs have been met, a lower or higher level of patient service is needed, or the patient no longer qualifies for reimbursed care. In home health, the reason for termination of service includes other variables, such as no capable caregiver to assume ongoing care, home situation is unsafe for patient's care, or relocation to a nonservice area (see display, Healthcare Personnel Discharge Summary).

The "summary of services provided" on this form is required by the state of Florida in their home health *(text continues on page 172)*

NURSING TRANSFER SUMMARY

DUKE UNIVERSITY MEDICAL CENTER
Department of Nursing
NURSING TRANSFER SUMMARY

Patient Data

Admission date _____ Age _____ Diagnosis _____

Transfer from _____ to _____ Date_____
                   (unit & MD/Service)   (unit & MD/Service)

Reason for transfer _____

Pertinent medical history _____

_____

Allergies _____ Current vital signs _____

I & O summary _____ Precautions _____ Current weight _____

                             Signature _____

Review of Systems

Cardiovascular

Respiratory

Neurologic
(Include all sensory
and motor deficits)

Skin & Musculoskeletal
(Include self-care ability)

Gastrointestinal
(Include nutrition/
elimination info.)

Genitourinary

To be used for patients discharged to/from Duke Rehabilitation and Psychiatry

(continued)

NURSING TRANSFER SUMMARY *(Continued)*

Endocrine/
Reproductive

Pain

Psychosocial/
Emotional

Hematology,
Oncology,
Infectious Disease
Information

Interventions (Attach current Care Plan)

Treatments

Medications/IVs

Teaching/discharge planning

Other Information? Pertinent Medical History (Continued)

Signature

Transfer Checklist

_____ Currrent care plan   _____ Old and current chart

_____ Medication plan   _____ Addressograph plate/ID bracelet

_____ I & O, log sheets, flow sheets   _____ Eggcrate mattress

_____ Belongings/valuables, including   _____ Equipment needed (specify below)
       x-rays, personal medications

Disposition of belongings if not sent with patient _____

                            Phone number
_____ Family notified   Family contact _____ Nurse signature _____

Report called to _____ by _____

Signature _____ Date _____ Time_____

Courtesy of Duke University Medical Center, Durham, NC.

DISCHARGE PLANNING FORM

DISCHARGE PLANNING
HOME OR HEALTH MAINTENANCE, IMPAIRED

Assessment	Plan	Interventions	Evaluation
Summary of Discharge Planning Sessions: Date:	Consult: ☐ Social Service ☐ Home Health Care ☐ Nutrition Services ☐ Physical Therapy ☐ Occupational Therapy ☐ Pastoral Care ☐ ☐ ☐ Patient Education Re: ☐ ☐ ☐ Family/Significant Other Education: ☐ ☐ ☐	Consult/Services Scheduled: ☐ Home-Going Equipment: ☐ See Patient Education Record/Progress Notes	☐ Patient Ready for Discharge To _____ On _____ ☐ Patient/Family able to manage care. Understand care instructions and follow-up plan. ☐ _____ RN Signature

Courtesy of Cleveland Clinic Foundation, Cleveland, OH.

agency licensure rules. The summary of services also indicates the type and intensity of care that was given. This indicates to the next caregiver how ill the patient is and the health care services the patient continues to need.

Special Considerations in Discharge Planning Documentation

A discharging nurse is the last nurse to provide care to a patient, to document on the clinical record, and to assess health status before the patient leaves a hospital or stops health care services. A discharging nurse always signs the discharge summary.

A patient will also be asked to sign a form when it is designed to be a patient's copy of a record of service. A record of service includes documentation of care a patient received and a list of discharge instructions, which are reminders of what the patient needs to do to continue appropriate care in the next health care setting. The patient's signature follows a statement that indicates the patient received a copy of the form and understands the contents of the record and discharge instructions.

Discharge instructions should be written in clear and simple language. Instructions should be concise and complete, with steps of each treatment in sequence of how and when it is performed. Precautions should be explained and written for a patient, with instructions of whom to call in any untoward or emergency situation. Telephone numbers should be listed with instructions to a patient to post the information by the telephone.

A patient discharge summary designed for patient

HEALTHCARE PERSONNEL DISCHARGE SUMMARY

HEALTHCARE PERSONNEL DISCHARGE SUMMARY

Date: _____ / _____ / _____   Client number: _____

Patient name: _____

Address: _____

Date of first visit: _____ / _____ / _____   Date of last visit: _____ / _____ / _____

Date of notification to discontinue services _____ / _____ / _____

     _____ Identified goals have been met

     _____ Expired   Date of death: _____ / _____ / _____

     _____ Admitted to inpatient facility _____

     _____ Relocation to nonservice area _____

     _____ No capable caregiver to assume ongoing care

     _____ Patient/family request discharge reason: _____

     _____ Home situation is unsafe for patient's care

     _____ Other (specify) _____

Additional comments:

_____

_____

_____

Condition of the patient on discharge (including goal outcomes):

_____

_____

_____

_____

_____

_____

Recommendations or patient plans for future care:

_____

_____

_____

Primary physician notified of patient discharge?   ☐ Yes   ☐ No

Summary of services provided

	Hours
HHA/CNA	_____
LPN	_____
RN	_____
Therapists	_____
Total hours	_____

RN Signature: _____

Copyright 1986. Healthcare Personnel, Inc.

instructions includes teaching about diet, medications, treatments, physical activity limitations, signs and symptoms to report to a physician, follow-up medical care, equipment, and appropriate use of community resources and support groups. This summary should include specific plans for future care and the setting in which it will be given. Intended caregiver and support systems should be noted. Actual or potential barriers to future care should be discussed with a patient and documented. Any **referral**, which is telling a patient about another agency that can provide assistance, should be written. Referral information should include whether a referral contact was made by a the discharge nurse or social service or is to be made by a patient or family.

Regardless of the discharge summary format, at discharge a patient should be given an instruction sheet to reinforce what was learned and what was told at discharge. Written reminders facilitate planned, follow-up care for high quality continuity of care.

KEY POINTS

▲ Teaching records and progress summaries contribute to continuity of care among caregivers.

▲ Transfer forms and discharge summaries contribute toward continuity of care between health care organizations as a patient moves from one health care organization and level of care to another.

▲ Continuity of care forms include (but are not limited to) information regarding the needs of a patient, interventions performed to date, outcomes of those interventions, and present status of a patient at time of documentation.

▲ Special learning considerations or barriers to learning, past educational experiences, and patient and family learning priorities are important and helpful in planning care.

▲ A transfer form provides transition of care information as a patient moves from one level of care to another or from one specialty unit to another, within the same health care facility. Depending on the circumstance, a transfer form is also used when transferring a patient between health care settings.

▲ A discharge plan or discharge summary is the documentation form used when a patient is discharged from a health care organization. A discharge summary cites services provided before discharge and delineates plans recommended for further care.

REFERENCES

Licensure Rules for the State of Florida, Chapter 10D-78, Florida Administrative Code, Minimum Standards for Home Health Agencies (10D-68.021 1 through 5).

Omnibus Reconciliation Act of 1987 (OBRA '87) Pub. L. 100–203 in Federal Register Feb 2, 1989 in US Government Part 483 Condition of Participation and Requirements for Long Term Care Facilities.

BIBLIOGRAPHY

Alfaro, R. (1994). *Applying nursing process: A step-by-step guide* (3rd ed.) Philadelphia: J. B. Lippincott.

Esper, P. S. (1988). Discharge planning—a quality assurance approach. *Nursing Management, 19*(10), 66–68.

Potter, P. A., & Perry, A. G. (1993). *Fundamentals of nursing: Concepts, process, and practice* (3rd ed.). St. Louis: Mosby–Year Book.

Timby, L. W. (1992). *Fundamental concepts and skills in patient care*. Philadelphia: J. B. Lippincott.

PRACTICE SESSION

FILL IN

1. Key purposes for transfer, discharge and progress summaries, and teaching forms discussed in this chapter are _____and _____

   _____ .

2. A _____ form provides transition of care information as a patient is moved from one level of care to another within the same health care facility.

3. A _____ summary cites services provided before discharge and delineates plans recommended for further care.

4. Two types of teaching records are _____ and _____

   _____ .

5. The first step in developing a teaching plan is _____

   _____ .

6. To better understand the rationale for care, a patient first needs to learn about

   _____ .

7. _____ reinforces learning.

8. Sequence of information in a teaching plan should be from

   _____ to _____ .

9. A major factor influencing patient teaching was enactment of_____

   _____ .

10. The federal government's prospective payment program has caused patients to be

   _____ .

MATCHING

Match domain in Column B with outcome phrase in Column A.

1. _____ planned a correct meal
2. _____ gave an injection
3. _____ accepted advice
4. _____ identified 3 resources for help
5. _____ did not participate in counseling session
6. _____ changed dressing to wound
7. _____ took pulse before taking Digoxin
8. _____ joined a support group
9. _____ listed side effects of medication
10. _____ walked with 3-point gait with cane

a. cognitive
b. psychomotor
c. affective

MULTIPLE CHOICE

1. _____ Continuity of care forms should include
   a) met and unmet patient needs
   b) interventions performed to date
   c) patient outcomes
   d) patient status at time of documentation
   e) all of the above

2. _____ Well-written reports regarding a patient are a basis for
   a) evaluating effectiveness of care
   b) protection in case of legal action
   c) consideration in further assessment and planning
   d) a & b
   e) all of the above

3. _____ Before sending patient information to someone who is not a direct caregiver, the patient or authorized representative must sign a form for
   a) informed consent
   b) release of information
   c) shared governance
   d) transfer

4. _____ In developing a teaching plan, a nurse should consider
   a) special learning considerations or barriers to learning
   b) past educational experiences and effective mode of learning
   c) strengths in learning
   d) patient and family learning priorities
   e) all of the above

5. _____ At discharge the patient should be given a
   a) list of unmet needs
   b) care plan for the next level of care
   c) instruction sheet to reinforce what was learned
   d) phone number of the nursing division in case she has any questions after discharge
   e) all of the above

CHALLENGE FOR CRITICAL THINKING

1. Discuss advantages and disadvantages to standardize teaching plans.

2. List different types of patient education materials and different methods of teaching. Do the different resources or different methods affect how the teaching plan or teaching summary is written?

3. Discuss at least four reasons why an intended teaching plan may not work. How could you avoid these pitfalls?

4. This discharge summary was sent to a home health agency:

   Mrs. J. Lives at 1234 Hickory Lane. She was hospitalized on 3/14/92 and discharged 4/2/92 following bilateral mastectomy. Her course of treatment was unremarkable. On antibiotic following surgery. Please visit her at least twice a week to assess wound sites and healing process. Instruct her on dressing changes. Her return visit to the surgeon is scheduled for 10 am on 4/15/92.

   What referral and teaching information would have been helpful to a nurse visiting Mrs. J.?

5. This transfer information was sent from an acute-care facility to a long-term care facility:

Mr. W. was admitted on 5/23/92 and discharged 6/4/92 following a right-sided CVA. He has received physical therapy daily and will need continued assistance. A speech therapist saw him three times. An occupational therapy evaluation was completed. His Foley catheter was changed before discharge.

What additional information *should* have been communicated in the transfer to help long-term caregivers provide assistance in activities of daily living?

LEARNING TO DOCUMENT

1. Formulate a cognitive, psychomotor, and an affective learning outcome for a patient learning self-injection of insulin for diabetes.

2. Document a discharge summary based on a hospital discharge, using the Discharge Planning form on page 182 and the following information. Nancy Jones, RN, met with Mrs. R. on March 29, 31, and April 2 to plan for discharge to home on April 4, 1993. Mrs. R. has cancer of the pancreas and is receiving IV therapy: TPN (total parenteral nutrition) and PCA (patient-controlled analgesia). A referral to XYZ Home Health Care and TQI IV Therapy Company was made on March 31. The client intake coordinator was told that the patient and husband are receiving education on TPN, PCA, medications, and dressing changes. The report given was based on the patient education record and progress notes for Mrs. R. Both companies will send patient care coordinators to meet with family on April 1. Mr. R. requested pastoral care on March 29; a social service consult is scheduled for March 31 to coordinate, educate, and determine financial resources for patient to procure necessary medication, supplies, and equipment in the home. Those meds and supplies include insulin, analgesia, syringes, dressing change supplies, wheelchair, hospital bed, and bedside commode. At discharge on April 2, Mr. and Mrs. W. could explain care instructions and follow-up plan, but were relieved that home health care nurses would continue education until they felt comfortable about performing procedures at home without supervision.

3. If a patient was discharged from home health care due to patient improvement, what key points do you think would need to be documented? How would you document them in the patient's chart?

DISCHARGE PLANNING FORM

DISCHARGE PLANNING
HOME OR HEALTH MAINTENANCE, IMPAIRED

Assessment	Plan	Interventions	Evaluation
Summary of Discharge Planning Sessions: Date:	Consult: ☐ Social Service ☐ Home Health Care ☐ Nutrition Services ☐ Physical Therapy ☐ Occupational Therapy ☐ Pastoral Care ☐ ☐ ☐ Patient Education Re: ☐ ☐ ☐ Family/Significant Other Education: ☐ ☐ ☐	Consult/Services Scheduled: ☐ Home-Going Equipment: ☐ See Patient Education Record/Progress Notes	☐ Patient Ready for Discharge To _____ On _____ ☐ Patient/Family able to manage care. Understand care instructions and follow-up plan. ☐ _____ RN Signature

CHAPTER
9

Comparing Documentation Methods

LEARNING OBJECTIVES

After studying this chapter, the learner should be able to:

▲ Define the advantages and disadvantages of narrative charting.

▲ Outline the problem-oriented medical record system with SOAP format clinical notes.

▲ Describe Focus Charting® and DAR clinical notes.

▲ Explain the PIE charting format and its advantages.

▲ Describe charting by exception.

▲ Compare the different formats in structure, content, and application to clinical settings.

▲ Identify components of the case management system.

▲ Explain the purpose of guidelines and protocols.

KEY TERMS

Case management	DRG	Narrative nursing progress	Problem-oriented medical
Critical pathway	Focus Charting®	notes	record (POMR)
Charting by exception	Guidelines	PIE	SOAP notes
Data base	Initial plan	Problem list	Variations
DAR			

Eggland ET, Heinemann DS. NURSING DOCUMENTATION:
CHARTING, RECORDING, AND REPORTING.
© 1994 J.B. Lippincott Company.

This chapter compares the different formats and develops a base for learning key documentation techniques in different methods of charting. This is important in learning clinical practice skills. Learning different formats also prepares a nurse to knowledgeably contribute to the process of revising and streamlining nursing documentation systems. When a nursing documentation committee reviews and revises documentation formats, input is requested from all nurses involved in documentation.

A health care organization defines in its policy and procedure manual what format or documentation method(s) nurses are to use in documenting patient care. Although a hospital prefers to use the same method of charting throughout the facility, some specialty areas may have specific needs requiring a different method. Because of different documentation needs in different nursing specialty areas, a hospital conducts different pilot projects in different care units to determine the appropriate format for a unit or entire organization.

Earlier chapters show the narrative charting and flow sheets used in documenting nursing interventions. Some of the different formats in this chapter include narrative charting or the use of flow sheets within a documentation method. For the purpose of comparison, this chapter defines and compares five different methods or formats of nursing documentation:

▲ Narrative progress notes
▲ Problem-oriented (medical) records (POR/POMR)
▲ PIE (problem, intervention, evaluation)
▲ Focus Charting® format
▲ Charting by exception (CBE)

Finally, three of the newest documentation methods are presented:

▲ Case management with critical paths
▲ Guidelines
▲ Protocols

These presentations include a discussion of basic components, mechanics, and unique features of each format. To learn more about each method, refer to the bibliography at the end of the chapter for further reading.

Several advantages and disadvantages of each format are briefly discussed. Most of the formats were created to save charting time, decrease chart bulk, and facilitate retrieval of information, so these factors will not be repeated when listing each format's advantages. Accurately measuring these factors is difficult, but ongoing research in nursing information systems may eventually provide the tools to measure and compare these aspects within different formats.

Presentation of formats in this chapter is in chronologic order according to the year of development. It is interesting to note all of these formats, new and old, are in use at various health care organizations. It attests to the variety of documentation needs and preferences in different nursing units and health care settings.

Narrative Progress Notes

Narrative nursing progress notes are phrases, sentences, and paragraphs a documenting nurse writes without any standardized structure, content, or form. Narrative notes are the most traditional type of documentation.

Since its inception, nursing has used narrative charting, but nurses have not always used it effectively. Nursing notes were often long, convoluted sentences that did not focus on the actual condition of the patient or response to treatment. Ambiguous and unimportant phrases like "good day," "patient sitting in chair," and "no complaints voiced" caused physicians and other disciplines to view nursing narrative notes as unimportant. For years, in fact, narrative nursing notes were not even kept as a permanent part of the clinical record. They were thrown away when the patient was discharged. As the definition and scope of nursing practice progressed through the decades, however, nursing documentation became more formalized. Nursing narrative documentation became important to physicians and other caregivers in communicating the condition of the patient, care interventions, and patient response to illness and treatments. Additionally, documentation of patient status, interventions, and outcomes became important for reimbursement, quality assurance, regulatory, and legal reasons. As a result, nursing notes became an important source of that information. Nurses became more focused on criteria to be included in nursing progress notes, as defined by government, accrediting agencies, and professional organizations.

Advantages of Narrative Progress Notes

Writing narrative notes gives nurses the advantage of describing a condition, situation, or response in their own terms, as they understand it. A nurse can document notes as long, short, broad, or focused as the nurse prefers or the situation demands. Also, learning to write narrative notes is easier than learning a structured note format.

The quality of the narrative note has improved over the years, but certain problems remain.

Disadvantages of Narrative Progress Notes

It is time-consuming and difficult to peruse days and weeks of narrative notes to find a specific problem, its treatment, and the patient's response. No keys, labels, or structures quickly indicate where any particular information can be found. In addition, because narrative notes have no real framework, nurses sometimes write lengthy nonrelevant information, inappropriate personal opinions, and repetitive information found on other forms in the chart.

Despite the inherent problems in narrative progress notes, they are still an important part of documentation within portions of contemporary formats. Even with carefully structured flow sheets, nothing can replace a concise description in narrative form, when a description of condition or patient response is needed. Narrative notes as the only form of documentation, however, offer little more than a chronologic, story format of occurrences during a particular time frame or at a particular time during a patient's day (see display, Sample Narrative Nursing Note).

Problem-Oriented Medical Records (POMR) and the Problem-Oriented Record (POR)

In 1969, Dr. Lawrence Weed at Case Western Reserve University in Cleveland introduced the **problem-oriented medical record** (**POMR**). His intent was to focus documentation on patient problems and interventions to address those problems. The original POMR model was for physicians, but the advantages of the system caused health care organizations to eventually apply the problem-oriented record (POR) format to nursing and multidisciplinary documentation as well. After more than 20 years, Dr. Weed's unique contribution can still be seen in many health care organizations. Some organizations continue to use the entire Weed problem-oriented system, whereas some organizations have incorporated only a portion of his system into their own documentation program. A portion often used is the problem list. Another portion used is the POMR progress note format called SOAP. The SOAP acronym is for note parts labeled subjective, objective, assessment, and plan.

Components of the Problem-Oriented Record

The POR has four components, including:

▲ Data base
▲ Problem list
▲ Initial plan
▲ Progress notes, written in SOAP format

The **data base** is a compilation of organized information from all disciplines, which focuses on present complaints and illnesses. Information is derived from a patient history and assessment, physical examination, and admission laboratory test results. The information identifies patient problems and is a basis for comparison to later evaluate a patient's condition.

The **problem list**, derived from the data base, is used as an index of patient problems or needs. It consists of both active and inactive problems, which are titled and numbered. It is placed at the beginning of the chart as a starting point for patient status review, intervention planning, and outcome evaluation. In some facilities, only problems that exist for more than 72 hours can be included on the problem list, and only actual problems, not questionable problems, can be listed. All problems are listed and labeled acute, chronic, active, and inactive.

The problem list is maintained in chronologic order instead of priority of need. Problems are listed sep-

▲	SAMPLE NARRATIVE NURSING NOTE

NARRATIVE NURSING NOTE	
Date/Time	**Nursing Notes**
3-1-90 8 am	Patient c/o burning on urination, frequency and urgency, and L flank pain. Pt voided "small
	amt" x 6 from 11 pm to 7 am. Notified Dr. Thomas of symptoms. Encouraged pt to increase fluids
	10 - 8 oz glasses of H_2O. 100% of breakfast eaten.
10 am	Pt sleeping. Temp and U.S. WNL (see flowsheet) Taking fluids well (see I & O) No voiding
	since 8 am. Dr Thomas to visit this a.m. E. Eggland, RN

arately. Medical problems include diagnoses, secondary complications, symptoms, abnormal laboratory results, and socioeconomic problems related to health and health care. A problem-oriented medical sample is shown below to differentiate it from a nursing problem-oriented sample.

Case example: Mr. Dustin is a patient who was admitted with diagnoses of asthma, emphysema, and an upper respiratory infection. He was short of breath (SOB), anxious, and withdrawn. His wife states he complains of always being tired and has lost all interest in activities since his respiratory condition caused him to quit work. On examination the patient complained of fatigue and left flank pain for the past 4 days. The physician would write the following medical problem list for this patient.

Problem #1

Acute respiratory distress

Problem #2

Chronic obstructive pulmonary disease (COPD)

Problem #3

Chronic depression

Problem #4

Persistent L flank pain of unknown etiology

Medical problems in the problem-oriented system are written as medical diagnoses. When a diagnosis is not made, the physician writes the problem as a symptom, as in problem #4.

In nursing documentation, the above patient would exhibit the following problems in terms of nursing diagnoses:

Problem #5

Ineffective Airway Clearance related to tenacious secretions

Problem #6

Ineffective Breathing Pattern related to decreased energy and fatigue

Problem #7

Impaired Adjustment related to disability requiring change in life-style

Problem #8

High Risk for Infection related to stasis of body fluids (urine)

An **initial plan** is developed for each problem cited. A medical plan of treatment, written for each listed prob-

lem, includes all diagnostic tests, treatments, medication, and teaching.

In Mr. Dustin's example the medical plan would read:

Problem #1

COPD

a. Arterial blood gases, immediately (stat)

b. Oxygen per nasal cannula, 3 L/min

c. Teach breathing and relaxation techniques

Medical orders written by a physician on the orders sheet are similarly identified by the corresponding problem number. For example a medical order would read: "Problem #1: b. O_2 per nasal cannula 3 L/min.

Nursing orders written by a nurse on the care plan are also identified by the corresponding problem number. One intervention could be: "Problem #8: Instruct pt in s/s of UTI to report to MD." (Instruct patient in signs and symptoms of urinary tract infection to report to physician.)

In other documentation systems, when a nurse implements planned interventions documented on the care plan, actual interventions and outcomes are documented on nursing notes. With SOAP notes, additional components that reflect the nursing process are presented in the note.

SOAP Notes

Problem-oriented record progress notes are organized into a framework called **SOAP notes**:

S: Subjective data

What the patient verbally expressed

O: Objective data

What the nurse observed regarding patient behavior, clinical test results, and so forth

A: Assessment

Conclusion reached regarding a patient's condition, based on subjective and objective data presented; can be written in nursing diagnoses form

P: Plan

Planned course of interventions to address the problem; can be modified at a later date

Later modifications to the SOAP note, made by other individuals, are the following:

SOAPE

E: Evaluation

Reflects patient response to illness, medical treatment, or nursing interventions

SOAPIE

I: Intervention

Reflects a particular action by a discipline

E: Evaluation

Reflects patient response to illness, medical treatment, or nursing interventions

SOAPIER

I: Intervention

E: Evaluation

R: Revision

Reflects change prompted by the evaluation; can be made in outcomes, intervention plans, or target dates (see display, Sample Problem-Oriented (SOAPE) Notes).

Flow sheets are used within a POR system to record intake and output, daily activities, diabetic interventions, vital signs, and other measurements, assessments, or interventions.

Within this system, discharge summaries are also written in the same problem-oriented manner in a SOAP format. These summaries appear the same as nursing notes but are final comments and discharge plans regarding problems identified throughout the time care was provided.

Advantages of the Problem-Oriented Record

An advantage of the POR is the location of the problem list at the front of the chart, alerting all caregivers to ongoing problems and patient needs. It directs care focused on problems and similarly directs documentation of care. Listing and labeling problems with numbers makes it easier to retrieve them to follow a patient's progress in resolving a problem. Easy retrieval facilitates monitoring by quality assurance and accessibility for nursing research.

The use of SOAP and especially SOAPIER notes establishes a note structure that reflects elements of the nursing process. This format is effective in reflecting goal-oriented care and is especially important in documenting patient outcomes. The progression of documentation according to the nursing process supports how patient outcomes are achieved.

Disadvantages of the Problem-Oriented Record

A disadvantage, however, is the level of ability and the consistency of caregivers in organizing information into the SOAP format. Often, the assessment portion of the note creates problems. Nurses are reluctant to make assessment decisions for fear of inaccuracy and for concerns of making a medical diagnosis. Assessing for nursing diagnoses has helped to decrease this problem and concern. Another problem with POMR is that maintaining a neat, up-to-date problem list takes constant vigilance and routine review.

PIE—Problem, Intervention, Evaluation

The **PIE** charting system was instituted in 1984 at Craven Regional Medical Center in New Bern, North Carolina. This system is unique within the collection of documentation methods in that it does not develop a separate care plan. Instead, the care plan is incorporated into the progress notes, in which problems are identified by number.

Another feature of the PIE system is that a complete patient assessment is written at the beginning of each shift, on a preprinted fill-in-the-blank assessment form.

From these assessments, problems are identified and written in nursing diagnoses form. A problem number is assigned, and an entry is structured to label a *P* for problems, *I* for an intervention, and *E* for evaluation (see display, Sample PIE Charting).

Each identified problem is evaluated at least once every 8 hours. After the completion of three shifts, the nurse reviews the notes from the previous 24 hours to ascertain the patient's current problems and responses to interventions. Continuing problems, along with relevant interventions and evaluations are redocumented and renumbered daily. Resolved problems are dropped from the daily documentation. This review promotes continuity of care from day to day (Siegrist, Dettor & Stocks, 1985).

A modification of the PIE system incorporates a nursing diagnosis/problem list and the addition of *A* in numbered problems (eg, AP1), to designate abnormal or "new-problem" assessments. Another variation is identifying an intervention or evaluation with the numbered problem. For example, EP1 means evaluation for problem #1. This variation allows evaluation or intervention to be written at any time regarding a problem, without PIE being written together as a unit. This variation is especially helpful when results, outcomes, or evaluations are carried out later, after an intervention or when additional interventions are ordered to approach a particular problem.

Again, in this adapted system, "evaluation statements are required every shift for each nursing diagnosis (which) . . . encourages nurses to collaborate and consult with each other when planning, delivering, and evaluating nursing care" (Buckley-Womack & Gidney, 1987).

▲			SAMPLE PROBLEM-ORIENTED (SOAPE) NOTES	
Date	**Time**	**No.**	**Problem**	**Patient Progress Notes**
3-2-88	8 am	3	Potential for infection R/T alteration in kidney function	S: Pt c/o burning on urination, frequency & urgency. c/o Ⓛ flank pain.
				O: Pt voided "small amt" x 6 from 11 pm – 7 am. Observed crying on commode "because of pain." Urine amber & cloudy.
				A: Alteration in kidney function. Potential UTI. Pt has history of recurring UTI (see assessment)
				P: Notify Dt T of symptoms. Encourage fluids to 10 – 8 oz glasses H_2O. Take temp & v.s. q 4 h Encourage bed rest Maintain accurate I & O Observe urine for color & odor. Observe for symptoms of hypertension or renal failure. E. Eggland, RN
				E: Pt sleeping. Temp & V.S. WNL (see flow sheet). Taking fluids well (see I & O). No voiding since 8 am. Dr T to visit this am ——————E. Eggland, RN

Teaching, along with other interventions, is also documented on the progress notes. Teaching plans are written in a similar manner to care plans with nursing diagnoses of Knowledge Deficit.

Advantages of PIE

Without a formal, separate care plan, the PIE format saves documentation time because a nurse does not have to create or frequently update a plan. Outcomes can be documented on the initial plan or can be documented in the evaluation portion of the nursing note for quality assurance. It takes time to write assessments as frequently as the beginning of each shift. But when nurses using the system were queried, they reported that after becoming accustomed to the format, they found it to be a timesaving system.

Disadvantages of PIE

Nurses admitted that they "tended to revert to a narrative style when pressured for time, (or) when they were unable to locate an identified problem on the accepted list of nursing diagnoses" (Siegrist, Dettor & Stocks,

---

▲	**SAMPLE PIE CHARTING**

P: Spiritual distress, related to separation from religious/cultural ties, and impending death.

I: Acknowledged the patient's spiritual concerns (regarding death) and encouraged expression of thoughts and feelings; assisted in helping the patient arrange for clergyman's visit tomorrow 9/25 at 12:30; obtained Bible for patient to continue customary daily prayers.

E: Patient verbalized a feeling of spiritual comfort and anticipation about talking with his clergyman.

A more detailed version below, identifying patient problem numbers works well when data is collected sporadically over a period of time. Here again P, I, and E are problem, intervention, and evaluation. IP#1 means intervention for problem #1.

P#1: Spiritual distress, related to separation from religious/cultural ties . . .

IP#1: Acknowledged the patient's spiritual concerns (regarding death) and encouraged expression of thoughts and feelings.

IP#1: Assisted in helping the patient arrange for clergyman's visit tomorrow, 9/25 at 12:30.

IP#1: Obtained Bible for patient to continue customary daily prayers.

EP#1: Patient verbalized a feeling of spiritual comfort and anticipation about talking with his clergyman.

Amended from Taylor, C. L. & Cress, S. (1986). Nursing diagnosis cards (p. 806). Springhouse, PA: Springhouse.

1985), or when they had difficulty separating data into problems, interventions, or evaluation.

Because there is no formal care plan, the nurse preparing to provide care will need to read all the nursing notes to determine problems and planned interventions and evaluations to see if those interventions were effective. This process involves some time. Based on this nursing note review, the nurse will plan her interventions, according to current problems cited and past effective interventions.

Many health care organizations state that PIE is an effective, efficient system that concisely reflects all components of the nursing process.

Focus Charting

Focus Charting® format has its origins in 1981 at Eitel Hospital in Minneapolis. Focus Charting® has since been trademarked by Creative Nursing Management of Minneapolis. The method was further developed by Susan Lampe, former chairperson of the documentation committee at Eitel Hospital.

Focus Charting® format for progress or nurses notes uses a focus column to include topics that involve many aspects of a patient and patient care. These topics include patient behavior; therapy and response; concerns; change of condition; and significant events such as teaching, physician's visit, monitoring, chemotherapy, activities of daily living, or functional health patterns. The focus can present positive occurrences or patient strengths, not just negative problems or needs. The focus can be presented as a nursing diagnosis and include problem and etiology. Defining a focus moves away from a problem statement and avoids the temptation to identify a medical diagnosis rather than a patient response to a health situation.

The words or phrase identified in the care plan under "problem/need" or "nursing diagnosis" can be entered in the focus column when documenting about progress toward the care plan goal. The use of the same word or phrase in the focus column promotes continuity between the care plan and the documented care.

Focus Charting® effectively brings the focus of care back to the patient and patient concerns. This method is accomplished in the choice of "focus" over "problem" and in the identification of "patient care notes" instead of the traditional title "nursing notes."

Focus DAR Progress Notes

The narrative portion of Focus Charting® is organized into data, action, response (**DAR**) (Eggland, 1988). Focus progress notes are easy to learn because they are a logical sequence:

▲ What is the area of concern? (focus)
▲ What is the data base? (data)
▲ What action did a nurse take? (action)
▲ What is the patient outcome from actions? (result)

Documenting a result is important in reflecting the nursing process because it involves evaluation of patient outcomes following the nursing interventions (see display, Sample Focus Patient Care Notes).

▲	SAMPLE FOCUS PATIENT CARE NOTES	

Date/Time	Focus	Patient Care Notes
3/2/88 8 am	Pain	Data: Pt crying when voiding c/o burning on urination and Ⓛ flank pain.
		Action: Dr. T notified. Pyridium 200 mg po administered as ordered
	Potential for	Data: Frequency, urgency. Voided x 6 on night shift.
	infection R/T	Urine amber & cloudy
	alteration in	Action: Urine culture sent
	kidney function	Monitor TPR q 4 h
		I & O recorded
		Pt instructed in force fluids & bed rest
	Elevated temp	Data: Oral temp 39.5
		Action: Oral antipyretic given as ordered ——————————E. Eggland, RN
10 am	Pain	Response: Voided x 1 s̄ c/o pain
		Response: Oral temp 39.3 ——————————E. Eggland, RN

(Reprinted with permission from the November issue of Nursing 88. Copyright 1988 Springhouse Corp., 1111 Bethlehem Pike, Springhouse, PA 19477. All rights reserved.)

Advantage of Focus DAR Progress Notes

Ease of charting with DAR is an advantage because categories of data, action, and response are not required for each focus cited. Components of DAR can be charted alone or out of sequence. For example, a nurse can document:

Data alone

D: Patient complains of +3 dull constant pain in right ankle

Data and action

D: Patient complains of +3 dull constant pain in right ankle

A: Administered two Tylenol with codeine

Data, action, response, and action

D: Patient complains of +3 dull constant pain in right ankle

A: Administered two Tylenol with codeine

R: Patient states no relief

A: Elevate ankle

"In Focus Charting® . . . the progress notes reflect analysis and conclusions" (Lampe, 1989). Important content and interrelationship of details are enhanced with this practice, and unnecessary repetition of data is avoided.

Disadvantage of Focus DAR Progress Notes

As in most structured progress notes, many nurses have difficulty in documenting information by separating the data into categories (in this case, DAR). The result portion of the note seems to be a particularly difficult area for accurate use of focus notes. Some nurses relate the result portion to the resulting problems identified from the assessment data. This is incorrect because the result represents the patient outcome of care following nursing intervention.

Charting by Exception

Charting by exception (CBE) originated in 1983 at St. Luke Medical Center in Milwaukee. The main premise of CBE is exactly what it implies: normal findings and standards of practice are the norms, and only items outside the norm are charted in narrative form. CBE changes the philosophy of "if it isn't documented, it hasn't been done," to "all standards have been met with a normal or expected response unless documented otherwise" (Murphy & Burke, 1990). In simplest form, check marks on a flow sheet format indicate the norms were observed, and brief narratives explain any exceptions to the norm.

The CBE format is a complete system, using the following forms:

▲ Nursing data base (history and physical)
▲ Nursing/physician order flow sheet, also called assessment/intervention flow sheet
▲ Graphic record (flow sheet for vital signs and other parameters)
▲ Patient teaching record
▲ Patient discharge note
▲ Nurses note form (uses SOAPIER format)
▲ Nursing diagnosis list
▲ Nursing diagnosis-based standard care plan
▲ Profile of patient care in Kardex (Burke & Murphy, 1988)

In this system the SOAPIER format is used for notes, and the patient teaching record is a separate yet integral part of a patient chart. The most unique, identifying characteristic of CBE is the nursing/physician order flow sheet, also referred to by CBE authors as the assessment/intervention flow sheet.

Nursing/Physician Order Flow Sheet

The nursing/physician order flow sheet excerpt used as an example shows an interesting adaptation of flow sheet concepts.

The examples shows a nursing order of respiratory assessment, the next columns are horizontal, corresponding boxes for charting by asterisk (*) or check mark (✔) according to the time of the assessment. An asterisk indicates an abnormal finding, an exception, which is described in narrative significant findings portion at the bottom half of the sheet. A check mark indicates an assessment was within the norm (or an order for intervention was completed).

Order or Assessment		Time	
	2:00 pm	6:00 pm	10:00 pm
Respiratory assessment	✔	✔	*

Significant Findings
10:00 Rales and rhonchi in right lower lobe, (etc.)

In the above example, at 2:00 pm and 6:00 pm the respiratory assessment performed by the nurse was normal according to the agency's normal parameters for respiratory status (usually printed on the reverse side of this form). Again, normal is indicated by a check mark, so a check mark is made at the 2:00 and 6:00 time frames. At 10:00 pm, however, the respiratory assessment was not normal, so this time frame was marked with an asterisk to note an exception to the norm. The exception, a narrative note indicating only the problem, was then documented on the lower, narrative portion of the flow sheet. The narrative shows that instead of a normal respiratory status, crackles and rhonchi were found in the right lower lobe.

In another example, if an abnormal finding was discovered at 2:00 pm and again at 6:00 pm, documentation on the nursing/physician order flow sheet could look like this:

Respiratory assessment	2 pm	6 pm	10 pm	2 am
	*	→	√	√

The arrow at 6:00 indicates that the abnormal deviation previously described in the asterisked note continues to be unchanged. A narrative note is not required for an arrow; this saves rewriting time, yet indicates the patient status. The arrow serves as a horizontal ditto mark only for abnormal findings, repeating what was said from the left of the arrow. The frequency of orders, in this case how often to do a respiratory assessment, is directed by the care plan and a nurse's clinical judgment considering the patient's condition.

The nursing/physician order flow sheet is used for a 24-hour period. At the beginning of each day, a new order flow sheet is printed with orders written and numbered. Some preprinted forms are available, however, and are specific to the nursing unit and patient diagnosis.

An important part of the order sheet is the guidelines for use located on the reverse side of the order flow sheet. These guidelines include a protocol for each type of assessment and parameters that indicate normal findings (Burke & Murphy, 1988). These guidelines create the basis for normal comparison against exceptions. An adapted order flow sheet and an assessment/intervention sheet are shown in the display, Charting by Exception, Sample Assessment/Intervention Flow Sheet.

CHARTING BY EXCEPTION, SAMPLE ASSESSMENT/ INTERVENTION FLOW SHEET

DATE ① _____   PATIENT NAME _____

NSG DX	ORDERS										
		②									
		③									
			④								

SIGNIFICANT FINDINGS ▼   NURSE INITIALS ▶   ⑤

NSG DX	TIME	SIGNIFICANT FINDINGS	INIT

INIT	RN SIGNATURE	INIT	RN SIGNATURE	INIT	RN SIGNATURE

⑥ See reverse side

① Each flow sheet is used for 24 hr.

② If an order or assessment results in no significant findings (a "normal" result), place a check mark in the corresponding box to indicate the order was completed.

③ If an order or asessment deviates from normal, place an asterisk in the box to signal a problem. The asterisk directs the reader to a corresponding narrative entry in the "Significant Findings" section below. Because abnormalities are the only narrative entries, they stand out.

④ If, on reassessment, an abnormality remains the same, don't write another narrative entry. Simply place an arrow in the next box to indicate that abnormal findings remain unchanged from the last documentation. This eliminates repetition and gives information at a glance.

⑤ If an order is discontinued, write "D/C" in the appropriate box, and draw a line through the remaining boxes.

⑥ Assessment protocol and criteria for normal results are clearly defined on the reverse side of the flow sheet to ensure consistent evaluations among all nurses. (Nonassessment interventions are defined in the patient's care plan.)

Reverse Side

When completing a nursing assessment, use the following protocol and criteria to confirm a normal assessment with no significant findings.

NEUROLOGIC ASSESSMENT includes orientation, pupils, movement, sensation, quality of speech, swallowing, memory.
Normal: Alert and oriented to person, place, and time. Behavior appropriate to situaton. Pupils equal and reactive to light. Active range of motion of all extremities with symmetry of strength. No paresthesia. Verbalization clear and understandable. Swallowing without coughing or choking on liquids and solids. Memory intact.

NEUROVASCULAR ASSESSMENT includes color, temperature, movement, capillary refill time, peripheral pulses, edema, patient description of sensation affected

SOAPIER Notes

Charting by exception can be combined with any type of care planning system that generates nursing orders, Focus Charting®, POR, and even PIE charting. The CBE authors are currently exploring ways to combine it with a critical pathways system as well.

In CBE, using problem-oriented systems, nurses chart each SOAP component in sequence for every entry. If SOAPIER notes are used, however, *I*, *E*, and *R*, can be used separately as needed. They are used to document additional interventions, evaluation, and revision (change in care plan, expected outcome, or evaluation date; Burke & Murphy, 1988).

The CBE originators recommend bedside chart accessibility with their system for saving time and providing accurate data. Bedside accessibility of charts was a popular practice decades ago, but the following reasons influenced many administrators to relocate all patient charts to nursing stations: concerns of confidentiality, patient access to records, and physician/nurse convenience in reviewing and writing progress notes. In CBE, however, nursing segments of the charts are at the bedside. To facilitate interdisciplinary access to essential patient data, certain forms are printed on carbonless copy forms in order that copies of data are available both in the bedside chart and central station chart.

Advantages of CBE

The CBE format has many advantages:

▲ Abnormal status can be seen immediately with narrative easily retrieved.
▲ The flow sheet format shows overall trends in the patient's condition.
▲ Guidelines provide specific but concise standard information regarding "normal" assessments and expected outcomes.
▲ Documentation time is decreased because standard care is not written in narrative and duplication of charting is eliminated.

Disadvantages of Charting by Exception

A disadvantage of CBE is that preventive and wellness-promoting functions of a nurse are not documented on this format because they do not address problems. Documentation focuses instead on problem identification and problem-solving care.

Documentation in CBE requires predictable defined patient outcomes. Outcomes are difficult to predict in home care because of variables found in different families and home environments. In ambulatory care, expected outcomes are sometimes difficult because of the problem in defining what is normal in patient outcomes for patients at different stages of aging and chronic illness.

Until technology makes progress in computer software, CBE will continue to be more difficult to computerize than other documentation formats. Table 9–1 compares the documentation formats.

Case Management Model

Case management as discussed in this chapter is specific to the hospital setting. For this presentation, it is defined as managed care that is focused on quality but cost-effective care within an established length of stay (LOS). LOS is the period of time a patient stays in the hospital. Case management in home care is different. In that setting, case management is the coordination and procurement of care for cost-effective home health care. Definition and functional differences exist between these two models. Do not confuse the home care model with the hospital model information within this chapter.

Development of Case Management

In 1983, the government introduced prospective payment to hospitals for care provided to Medicare patients. Instead of Medicare paying retrospectively for services provided to a patient while in the hospital, payment to hospitals became prospective and based on defined diagnosis-related groups (**DRGs**) of illnesses. Under the prospective system, Medicare pays the hospital a predetermined rate based on the patient's diagnoses. This payment does not consider the length of inpatient stay or what services are provided to the patient. These set rates are a strong incentive for the hospital to decrease the patient's LOS in the hospital. Nursing interventions to stabilize and improve patient conditions and prevent complications help to decrease the patient LOS. With the DRG system, most patients who stay in the hospital are sicker and, at the same time, hospital reimbursement is decreased. Because of the loss of money by the hospital, nursing staff is often kept to a minimum. The result for nurses is acutely ill patients requiring increased nursing time, with a minimum number of nurses to provide care.

One way to have more time for nursing care is for nurses to document more concisely and efficiently. However, at the same time, documentation requirements for Medicare increased and required more specific detail. Finally, overall, the hospital wanted every day planned for patient interventions to help decrease LOS. The solution to the dilemma is managed care, in which interventions are scheduled and implemented within a set time frame. Using a time frame creates a total plan of patient care based on an efficient day-by-day series of short-term goals or outcome criteria.

TABLE 9-1. COMPARING FORMATS

	Source-Oriented Narrative	PO(M)R Problem-Oriented (Medical) Record	PIE Problem, Intervention, Evaluation	Focus Charting®	CBE Charting By Exception
Initial nursing assessment	Nursing history Nursing admission note	Data base	Patient assessment sheet (done every shift at beginning of shift)	Patient information Nursing admission assessment	Nursing data base/Physical assessment form
Ongoing assessment	Nursing/progress notes	Progress notes	Patient assessment sheet	Patient care notes (D-data)	Nursing–physician order flowsheet
Care plan	Nursing care plan	Problem list (problems numbered) Problem/care plan	No care plan separate in nursing notes under P#1 problem number 1, etc.	Focus list (optional) Patient care plan	Nursing diagnoses based standard care plan
Update care plan	Initial nursing care plan	Initial nursing care plan	Nursing notes written p#2, p#3, etc.	Initial patient care plan	Nursing notes under P–plan R–revision
Nursing note format	Narrative time entry or shift entry or day entry	S–subjective data O–objective data A–assessment P–plan E–evaluate	P–problem I–intervention E–evaluation P#2 = Problem No. 2 IP#2 = Intervention for Problem No. 2 EP#2 = Evaluation for Problem No. 2	Patient care notes Focus column D–data A–action R–response (of patient)	S–subjective data O–objective data A–assessment P–plan I–intervention E–evaluation R–revision (in outcome care plan or target date)
Evaluation documentation	In nursing note and discharge summary, no designated place.	Nursing note S O A P E–Evaluation	Nursing note P I E–Evaluation EP#2	Patient care notes D A R–Response	S O A P I E–Evaluation R
Unique features	Nursing notes separate or in interdisciplinary progress notes	Problem list Numbered problems	No care plans No outcomes No target dates	Focus = Patient care, significant events Nursing notes renamed patient care notes	Documents adherence to standard of care, policies, procedures, and protocols.
Usable in H–hospitals N–nsg, homes HC–home care A–amb. care	H, N, HXC, A	H, N, C In A, assessment may be difficult due to short term data collection.	H In N, HC, and AC daily assessment redundant because patient status doesn't change	H, N, HC, A	H, N Need predictable defined patient outcomes. May be difficult in HC & A due to home variables and problem establishing norms.

The categorization of the above formats is for fast comparison only. It is not intended to show that one format is better than another. For detailed, thorough accounts and applications systems, refer to the references at the end of the chapter.

Case Management Process

Case management, sometimes called managed care, is a process, not an outcome. To understand the documentation of case management, it is important to first understand the process. Presented here is a brief description of case management with a focus on nursing care and nursing collaboration within case management. This explanation will make it easier to understand the content and rationale for case management documentation.

> **Case management** or managed care is defined as a methodology for organizing patient care through an episode of illness so that specific clinical and financial outcomes are achieved within an allotted time frame. Nursing focus is identifying and specifying critical care events in the usual hospital episode for a medical diagnosis/DRG case type. (Del Togno-Armanasco, Olivas, & Harter, 1989)

This means that for each type of patient, on every day during their hospitalization, certain events should happen that will allow them to be discharged within a certain expected period of time based on their diagnosis.

Case management is a process in which the nurse, as case manager, collaborates with the physician to establish patient outcome criteria for a patient with a particular (DRG) diagnosis. The outcome criteria are generally standardized for that particular DRG. For example, a postsurgical patient on the third day should show no signs of incision infection and should be able to walk 30 feet without pain.

Interventions to achieve those outcomes are plotted on a schedule to anticipate early discharge or at least discharge within an average LOS. Depending on the system, care plotted on the schedule includes medical and nursing interventions or multidisciplinary interventions.

The managed care concept includes daily assessment documentation, care plan individualization, care plan revisions, outcome-oriented interventions, teaching, and discharge planning. At admission, a nurse case manager and attending physician individualize the daily care plan schedule, called a critical pathway, to meet each patient's specific needs. The pathway is reviewed and updated every 24 to 48 hours to meet a patient's changing needs. The pathway can be kept with the patient's Kardex and used as a basis for shift report.

The nurse case manager or a collaborative team reviews the patient's progress on the critical path to see if interventions are performed on time and patient outcomes are met on time, according to the pathway expected time frames. The case manager documents any individual patient exceptions (called variations) in outcomes, care processes, or timeliness of outcome achievement. The case manager documents patient needs and responses, evaluates and revises expected outcomes, and plans further interventions. The case manager observes for duplication in services or medical orders when more than one discipline and more than one physician is involved in care. The case manager begins discharge planning at patient admission and follows through to discharge. During development, evaluation, and revision of pathways, a nurse case manager and the collaborative team make clinical decisions to maximize coordinated care, continuity of care, and efficient and appropriate use of resources.

Case Management Models and Adaptations

Several different models of case management and numerous adaptations of models have been reported in the literature and in hospital pilot projects. As hospitals conduct projects to revise and refine models of care and documentation, they most frequently pattern a case management program based on the model developed at the New England Medical Center (NEMC). Hospitals use the NEMC model as a starting point, then adapt the model and documentation system to respond to their particular needs, current system of care delivery, current documentation method, and philosophy of care.

CASE MANAGEMENT TOOLS

The tools used in most case management systems are patterned after the NEMC model tools called the case management plan and critical path. These tools direct and evaluate patient progress and outcomes. The NEMC tools identify patient problems (nursing diagnoses) as the bases of care. The tools focus on nursing and medical interventions scheduled within a day-by-day time frame.

Case management plan. The case management plan is a detailed, standardized care plan that is documented for a patient population with a designated diagnosis or group of diagnoses. The case management plan includes lists of interventions to be performed and the sequence and timing of those interventions. Generally, expected patient outcomes are also listed on the case management plan. The plan designates who will perform which interventions and sometimes the qualifications of those who will perform certain procedures. Procedures are often listed in detail, or reference is made to protocols that list procedures in detail on a protocol form.

Critical pathway. A **critical pathway**, sometimes called a critical path, in case management is an abbreviated summary of key information taken from the more detailed case management plan. The path serves as a quick reference for medical and nursing actions planned for specific hospital days. The critical path helps a case manager monitor care by specifying important incidents or activities according to categories of care such as nursing assessment data, medications, tests, treatments, diet, activity, teaching and discharge planning (see display, Sample Critical Pathway Outline).

Variations. **Variations**, sometimes called variances, are goals not met or interventions not performed according to the time frame. They are exceptions to what is planned on the critical pathway. Variations are unexpected occurrences that affect the planned care and planned timing of care. A nurse documents variations on the back of critical pathways. A nurse documents the

SAMPLE CRITICAL PATHWAY OUTLINE

CRITICAL PATH

Primary Diagnosis _____

DRG Code _____

LOS _____

	Day 1–Date:	Day 2–Date:	Day 3–Date:
Consults			
Tests			
Patient activities			
Teaching			
Treatments			
Medication			
Diet			
Discharge planning			

VARIATION	CAUSE	ACTION TAKEN

unexpected event, the cause for the event, actions taken in response to the event, and discharge planning when appropriate. These notes identify what factors affect the expected course of treatment and expected LOS. For example, a patient is admitted for hip surgery. The hip is healing well, but the patient develops pneumonia, and develops a pressure sore. The variance could be written in the following manner:

Variation	Cause	Action Taken
Airway clearance	pneumonia 10/9	10/9 increase fluids to 2 L/day 10/10 Proventil (aerosol) for wheeze 10/11 instruct pt to cough and deep breathe every hour while awake 10/15 instruct wife in oxygen admin 10/18 XYZ contacted for home oxygen
Impaired skin integ	pressure sore on sacrum 10/20	10/20 Position on sides; turn patient q2h while awake; apply Duoderm every am

MULTIDISCIPLINARY MODEL

Another type of critical pathway includes interdisciplinary case management and patient/family responsibilities (see display, Cleveland Clinic Coordinated Care Format for Partial or Total Parotidectomy). This portion of the recovery path presents the nursing process from preoperative teaching through postoperative day 2.

Advantages of Case Management

Case management makes efficient use of time because each day has planned interventions and patient expected outcomes documented on the plan. With the series of daily expected outcomes on the plan, case management increases the probability that a patient will be discharged in a timely manner. With the expected outcomes on the plan, care remains goal focused, which increases the level of quality of care.

Case management promotes collaboration, communication, and teamwork among caregivers as pathways are reviewed on a routine basis and meeting outcomes are a patient and team success.

Disadvantages of Case Management

The case management system is effective for patients with one or two diagnoses and few complications. A patient who presents many variances because of complications makes documentation lengthy and sometimes complicated in terms of LOS and revising the critical

path. A patient who has an unpredictable course of symptoms and interventions is the most difficult to document on a critical path. An example is a neurologic patient with seizures. A critical path is developed with interventions and expectations toward diminishing or eliminating seizure activity. When seizures still occur, each seizure adds additional daily planning and documentation and extends the LOS. Preprinted pathways do not include additional days of care nor accommodate many changes of care within a day.

Space to document is limited on critical pathways. Too much writing in a space causes illegibility. The number of interventions and outcomes on any one day may be too much for the space available. Space for individualization is limited.

Separate narrative notes must be used for documentation of care. With flow sheets to document care, documentation of implemented nursing care in case management is on three forms, rather than two forms. Those three forms are the intervention flow sheet, nursing notes, and critical path. All must be reviewed to get a picture of a patient's condition, care, and outcome of treatment on a day.

Guidelines and Protocols

Guidelines and protocols are the newest innovative methods of nursing documentation. Depending on the health care organization, guidelines and protocols are defined in different ways, are used for different purposes, and are labeled with different names. Standards of care and clinical practice guidelines are two of those names. The concept for all these methods is the same. Care management problems are written in a standardized manner for use as a reference to outline how care should be delivered.

Guidelines

Guidelines, sometimes called clinical practice guidelines, are outlines of sequential interventions to manage a particular patient problem. They include detailed standardized interventions generic to any patient who has a particular condition or symptom or is receiving a specific treatment. For example, a guideline can be written for pain management, for postoperative care for a hip replacement or other care management problems (see display, Guidelines for Care of Patient with Urinary Tract Infection).

Nursing practice guidelines are specific to a clinical condition (eg, pain, urinary incontinence, pressure ulcers), and assist a nurse and others in clinical decision-making by describing recommended courses of action for var-

CLEVELAND CLINIC COORDINATED CARE FORMAT FOR PARTIAL OR TOTAL PAROTIDECTOMY

Case Type: Partial or Total Parotidectomy

DRG LOS: 2.3 days

Actual LOSE:

Patient Goals to be Achieved Prior to Discharge

The patient will be able to...

1. explain pain management measures
2. perform suture line care
3. maintain nutritional status
4. demonstrate eye care measurs (if applicable)
5. be afebrile and vital signs consistent with preadmission values
6. explain possible complications, trouble-shooting measures and appropriate resources

Hosp. Day	Physician	Nurse	Patient/Family	Other Services	Progress Analysis
Pre Op	PE ▲ Special studies ▲ Blood work ▲ EKG ▲ Chest X-ray Anesthesia clearance	▲ Assessment ▲ Pre-op teaching ▲ Explain CM model and recovery pathway ▲ Communicates assessment & possible D/C needs to G81 Case Manager ▲ CM communicates A71-G81	▲ Routing = 6 hours		

OR	▲ VS
	▲ Activity
	▲ Labs
	▲ Meds
	▲ Chest X-ray
	▲ drain suture
	▲ IVs
	▲ I & O
	▲ Suture line care
	▲ Incentive spirometry
	▲ Diet, as tolerated
	▲ Humidity-cool mist
	▲ assess facial nerve function & flap assessment
	▲ Lacrilube & moisture chambers (if applic.)
	▲ Isotears q1–2h w/a (if applicable)
	▲ Foley
		▲ PACU—G81
		▲ Initiate recovery path
		Major Aspects of Care
		a. Airway management
		  ▲ pulmonary assessment
		  ▲ incentive spirometry
		  ▲ C & DB
		  ▲ cool most
		b. Pain management
		c. Circulation
		  ▲ positioning
		  ▲ VS
		  ▲ flap assessment
		  ▲ activity
		d. Hydration
		  ▲ IVs
		  ▲ POs
		  ▲ Voiding/Foley
		  ▲ I&O
		e. Skin integrity
		  ▲ flap assessment
		  ▲ suture line care
		  ▲ drain
		f. Nutrition
		  ▲ abdominal assessment
		  ▲ diet
		  ▲ assess swallowing
		g. Alteration in mucous membrane
		  ▲ assess vision
		  ▲ moisture chambers
		  ▲ eye drops
		h. Facial nerve/neuro-assessment
			▲ Family lounge during OR
			▲ Visit patient on G81
			▲ Bring dentures, hearing aid, glasses, slippers, robe
			▲ meet with social worker (if applicable)
			▲ Demonstrate incentive spirometry
			▲ Perform oral hygiene
			▲ Drink full to clear liquids
			▲ Void
				▲ Respiratory therapy	

(continued)

▲ **CLEVELAND CLINIC COORDINATED CARE FORMAT FOR PARTIAL OR TOTAL PAROTIDECTOMY** *(Continued)*

Hosp. Day	Physician	Nurse	Patient/Family	Other Services	Progress Analysis

		i. Verbal communication
		j. Coping/body image
		k. Alteration in oral mucous membrane
		  ▲ oral hygiene
		l. Knowledge deficit
		  ▲ mouth care
		  ▲ incentive spirometry			

POD 1	▲ Labs
	▲ Advance diet as tolerated
	▲ IV—heparin lock
	▲ Ophthalmology consult re: tarrsophhy if approp.
	▲ Radiation Therapy (if applicable)
	▲ Dental consult (if applicable)
		▲ Am care in BR
		▲ IV—heparin lock
		▲ Monitor diet
		▲ Encourage activity
		▲ Knowledge deficit
		  ▲ suture line care
		  ▲ eye care
		  ▲ drain care (if applicable)
		  ▲ review drain care instruct. (if applicable)
		  ▲ initiate PERS			

POD 2		Continue to teach suture line care/eye care; drain care if applicable.	▲ AM Care—self
			▲ Demonstrate
			  a. oral hygiene
			  b. incentive spirometry
			  c. suture line care
			  d. eye care
			▲ Swallowing and nutrition instructions if applicable
			▲ Drain care if applicable
			▲ Ambulate
				▲ Nutritional services assessment
				▲ Speech pathology if swallowing difficulties occur	

Courtesy of Cleveland Clinic Foundation, Cleveland, OH.

ious clinical situations or specific client conditions or populations. Guidelines provide linkages among diagnoses or clinical conditions, interventions, and outcomes. They also describe alternatives available to each client or client population and provide a basis for the evaluation of care and allocation of resources. (American Nurses Association, 1991, p. vi)

A contemporary way of including detailed expected outcome criteria and detailed interventions in care planning is to develop guidelines. Guidelines are used four different ways to document planned care: as care standards, as basis of a care plan, as nursing orders, or as implemented interventions.

Using guidelines with a care plan results in a shorter, individualized patient care plan. The care plan does not repeat basic information presented in the guideline, and care plans focus on individualized patient needs. A care plan can include references to many different guidelines, instead of writing out planned interventions, which lengthen the care plan.

When a guideline is used as the basis of a patient's care plan, a copy of the guideline should be attached to the individualized patient care plan. When a guideline is used as a standard for care in place of a care plan, it should be available in a nursing manual on the unit.

GUIDELINES FOR CARE OF PATIENT WITH URINARY TRACT INFECTION/UTI

Interdependent

1. Keep pt/SO informed of hospital routines and patient status to decrease anxiety and knowledge deficits related to being hospitalized.
2. Monitor complaints of dysuria.
*3. Explain importance and reason for increasing PO fluid intake unless contraindicated.
*4. Explain to pt the reason to void as soon as the urge is felt.
*5. I&O q8h × 25 h continue while IV infusing.
*6. Record color of urine q shift while on I&O.
*7. Temperature q4h until afebrile for 24 h and then as specified in hospital policy.

Frequently Associated Independent Nursing Diagnoses

1. Comfort, Alteration in
2. Body Temperature, Alteration in
3. Urinary Elimination, Alteration in
4. Knowledge Deficit

* = Record on chart
Courtesy of Lee Memorial Hospital, Ft. Myers, FL.

GUIDELINES USED AS CARE STANDARDS

Guidelines as standards are used in place of a care plan. If guidelines are used to replace a care plan, they are used in a system that has no "formal" separate care plan. The information in guidelines is used as minimum performance measurement, which must be performed to reach a minimum level of quality of care.

For example, the PIE system uses no formal care plan, yet a PIE note could have the intervention of "implement pain management guideline."

P: Pain related to invasive procedure

I: Implement pain management guideline

E: Patient verbalizes relief from pain 30 min after Demerol injection

There is no care plan, so the pain management guideline lists what interventions a nurse should perform when a nursing diagnosis of pain is identified.

GUIDELINES USED AS BASIS OF CARE PLAN

A guideline can be a supporting document for an individualized nursing care plan. Interventions generic to a specific patient population are detailed on the guideline and not repeated on the shorter, individualized care plan. The individualized care plan is used for planning care for other nursing diagnoses.

The top of the care plan has an area where guidelines are listed. (See display, Care Plan).

In this care plan for a patient who underwent surgery, the primary interventions are those listed in generic guidelines of pain management and postoperative course. Constipation is a problem this particular patient has and the interventions are individualized to this patient.

GUIDELINES USED AS NURSING ORDERS

Guidelines can also be listed as interventions on a care plan. The care plan would have the following appearance:

In this example, the nursing actions that constitute interventions for pain management, impaired physical mobility, and stress incontinence are listed in generic guidelines, separate from the care plan. The guideline list of actions does not need to be repeated on the care plan.

GUIDELINES USED AS IMPLEMENTED INTERVENTIONS

Guidelines can represent planned care when no separate care plan is used. A protocol or nursing/physician order flow sheet will list protocols to be implemented,

---

▲ **CARE PLAN**

PATIENT NAME _____

Implement: Pain management guideline
            Posteroperative course guideline
            Guideline for impaired physical mobility

Nursing Diagnoses	Expected Outcome	Interventions
Constipation R/T anesthesia and immobility	The patient will resume regular pattern of elimination by discharde	Auscultate bowel sounds q8h Establish regular time for elimination. Patient states is usually 9–10 am Observe for adbominal distention, tenderness Record stool characteristics 6 oz prune juice every am per patient request
Pain R/T invasive procedure	The patient will verbalize relief from pain 30 min after Demerol injection	Pain management guideline
High Risk for Injury R/T immobility	The patient will not fall during hospitalization	Risk for falls guideline
Stress Incontinence R/T overdistension of bladder between voidings	The patient will be continent of urine within 6 days	Bladder training guideline

---

for checking off when completed. This method can be used with PIE, SOAP, and CBE clinical progress note documentation.

Protocol	12/4	12/5	12/6	12/7
Respiratory assessment	√	√	√	
Surgical wound protocol	√	√		
Pain management	√			

In this example, a respiratory assessment, as defined on the back of the form, was performed on December 4, 5, and 6. Surgical wound protocol was completed on December 4 and 5, and pain management was implemented on December 4.

Protocols

Protocols are different from guidelines because protocols traditionally combine nursing, medical, and multidisciplinary interventions. Guidelines list specific interventions for a nursing diagnosis or patient care management problem. Depending on the health care organization or health policy agency developing the protocol, informa-

tion on protocols can be categorized into various topics. Some of the most common topics in protocols include:

▲ Subject of the protocol (eg, home heparin infusion therapy)
▲ Brief background data or statistics regarding problem
▲ Purpose of the protocol
▲ Agency-specific recommendations and equipment
▲ Qualified personnel responsible to perform interventions
▲ Factors to identify at-risk individuals
▲ Preventive measures of problem or complications
▲ Expected outcomes
▲ Interventions
▲ Patient education
▲ Emergency treatment or follow-up care
▲ Monitoring and evaluation

Protocols are written by the health care organization to define therapy and its purpose. A shorter category format can include purpose, responsible parties, general information, patient/caregiver education, treatment (including emergency treatment), and monitoring. Some protocols even include competencies or qualifications defined as knowledge and skills a professional must have demonstrated to perform certain procedures. Protocols are often used as a policy and procedure rather than a tool in documentation. Regardless of its direct use, when protocols are written, they should be used as a standard reference by which all patients' care should comply. It can be written in a format of principles and considerations or step-by-step procedures to follow in giving care.

Using Guidelines and Protocols

Case management and standardized formats have the advantage of incorporating protocols and guidelines into documentation, which facilitates thorough care and accurate and complete documentation. Nurses in continuous quality improvement (quality assurance) can use protocols and guidelines as a basis for evaluation. A quality assurance nurse can check the quality of documentation by comparing the actual documentation to guideline or protocols, to ensure that key elements in the guideline or protocol are included in documentation. These key elements are criteria for quality improvement and for accrediting and reimbursement purposes, and are therefore essential in documentation.

Guideline and protocol documentation makes coordination of interdisciplinary care, planned sequential procedures, and outcomes more apparent. This gives a more definite, tightly monitored time frame for a totally planned series of interventions. A result is that the patient care process remains dynamic and goal oriented.

Successful use of guidelines or protocols is important in establishing appropriate care for a patient. Actions that can prevent or resolve difficulty in documenting with guidelines and protocols include individualizing guidelines and protocols, keeping guidelines and protocols current, and using guidelines and protocols appropriately.

Individualize guidelines and protocols. If a care plan is used with a guideline, the care plan's purpose is to document care individualized to that patient. On the care plan a nurse documents additional diagnoses, outcomes, interventions, and more detail regarding a patient's specific care. The care plan should not repeat information already on the guideline.

If a care plan is not used, the guideline or protocol should be individualized to reflect specific outcomes or interventions to meet an individual patient's needs.

Keep guidelines and protocols current. Guidelines and protocols need to be reviewed routinely and updated immediately to reflect the current standard of the health care organization. If a standard affecting a guideline or protocol is changed, and a nurse gives care according to an outdated guideline or protocol format, the nurse is liable for not following the standard or protocol of the facility.

Use guidelines and protocols as intended. In using guidelines, protocols, and care plans, a nurse needs to completely understand how the form is intended to be used according to the health care organization's policy and procedure on documentation. In orientation a nurse learns if a guideline is used as a standard, as a basis for a care plan, as a nursing order, or as an implemented intervention. Also important for communication is whether the guideline or protocol should be filed in a patient's record or kept in a reference manual.

KEY POINTS

▲ Contemporary charting formats were created to save charting time, to decrease chart bulk by fewer narrative notes, and to structure information for better retrieval for review or audits.

▲ The components of a problem-oriented record are a data base, problem list, initial plan, and progress notes. The problem list, derived from the data base, is used as an index of patient problems or needs. It consists of both active and inactive problems, which are titled and numbered.

▲ SOAPIER notes are an acronym for subjective data, objective data, assessment, plan, intervention, evaluation and revision.

▲ In the CBE method, SOAPIER can be documented out of sequence, such as SOAPIEIER. The SOAP should be in sequence, however.

▲ In the PIE format, there is no separate care plan. Outcomes are written in the evaluation portion of the clinical note. A problem number can be added to the P, I, or E if a problem list is used. In the PIE system, an assessment is completed at the beginning of every shift.

▲ DAR is the Focus Charting® clinical progress note charting format that stands for data, action, response. Categories of data, action, and response are not required for each focus cited. Components of DAR can be charted alone or out of sequence.

▲ Case management is a documentation format that uses a critical pathway to outline care by time frame in an attempt to control and decrease LOS. The critical pathway is an abbreviated version of the case management plan. The critical pathway includes daily expected outcomes, including patient outcomes and multidisciplinary interventions.

▲ Guidelines and protocols are the newest innovative methods of nursing documentation. Care management problems are written in a standardized manner for use as a reference to outline how care should be delivered.

▲ Guidelines and protocols should be individualized; kept current; and used appropriately, according to the intended purpose.

REFERENCES

American Nurses Association. (1991). *Standards of clinical nursing practice*. Washington, DC: Author.

Buckley-Womack, C., & Gidney, B. (1987). A new dimension in documentation: The PIE method. *Journal of NeuroScience Nursing, 19*(5), 259.

Burke, L., & Murphy, J. (1988). *Charting by exception* (pp. 11, 51). New York: John Wiley & Sons.

Del Togno-Armanasco, V., Olivas, G. S., & Harter, S. (1989). Developing an integrated nursing case management model. *Nursing Management, 20*(10), 27.

Eggland, E. T. (1988). Charting: How and why to document your care daily–and fully. *Nursing '88, 18*, 83.

Lampe, S. S. (1989). Nursing documentation: A new perspective. *Journal of Nursing Administration, 19*(3), 3.

Murphy, J., & Burke, L. J. (1990). Charting by exception: A more efficient way to document. *Nursing '90, 20*, 68.

Siegrist, L. M., Dettor, R. E., & Stocks, B. (1985). The PIE system: Complete planning and documentation of nursing care. *Quarterly Review Bulletin, 11*, 6, 186–189.

Taylor, C. L., & Cress, S. (1986). *Nursing diagnosis cards* (p. 806). Springhouse, PA: Springhouse.

BIBLIOGRAPHY

American Nurses Association Task Force on Case Management in Nursing. (1988). *Nursing case management*. Kansas City, MO: Author.

Cline, A. (1989). Streamlined documentation through exceptional charting. *Nursing Management, 20*(2), 62.

McKenzie, C., Torkelson, N. G., & Holt, M. A. (1989). Care and cost: Nursing case management improves both. *Nursing Management, 20*(10), 30–34.

Owen, L., Bojanowski, C., & Vermillion, C. (1988). A process to improve the documentation of nurses' notes. *Journal of Nursing Staff Development*, Summer, 104–111.

Sinha, H. L., & Driedger, M. (1988). Patient focused charting. *Canadian Journal of Nursing Administration, 1*(2), 20–22.

Weed, L. (1971). *Medical record, medical education and patient care*. Cleveland: Press of Case Western Reserve University.

NOTE: Focus Charting® information can be obtained by contacting Susan Lampe, Creative Nursing Management, 614 East Grant Street, Minneapolis, MN 55404, 612-339-7766. Other formats can be found in reference information.

Ferszt, G., & Taylor, P. (1988). When your patient needs spiritual comfort. *Nursing '88, 18*, 48–49.

Focus Charting®. (1988). Minneapolis, MN: Creative Nursing Management, Inc.

Halloran, E. J. Kiley, M., & Nosek, L. J. (1987). Nursing complexity, the DRG and length of stay. In A. M. McLane (Ed.). Utilization Studies: Paper presentation section of *Classification of nursing diagnoses: Proceedings of the Seventh NANDA Conference*. St. Louis: C. V. Mosby.

Lampe, S. S., & Hitchock, A. (1987). Documenting nursing diagnosis using Focus Charting®. In A. M. McLane (Ed.). *Classification of nursing diagnoses: Proceedings of the Seventh NANDA Conference* (pp. 377–382). St. Louis: C. V. Mosby.

Matthewman, J. (1987). Combining care plan and Kardex. *American Journal of Nursing, 87*(6), 853.

PRACTICE SESSION

FILL IN

1. The most traditional method of documenting nursing care is writing

   _____.

2. A compilation of organized information about a patient's present condition and past health

   care history is called a _____.

3. A_____ is derived from a data base and consists of
   active and inactive components, which are titled and numbered.

4. In POMR format, a problem list is maintained in

   _____ order.

5. Case management is not an outcome but a _____.

6. Nursing notes and _____ are documented in SOAP
   format in a problem-oriented system.

7. SOAPIER notes establish a note structure that reflects elements of the

   _____.

8. The PIE charting system does not include the use of a

   _____.

9. In the Focus Charting™ format, the_____ column identifies topics
   that involve many aspects of a patient situation, condition, and care.

10. DRGs in prospective payment stands for _____.

MATCHING FORMAT AND RULE

Match documentation format in column A with rule for clinical note in column B.

1. _____ Problem-oriented record (SOAP)

2. _____ Problem, intervention, evaluation (PIE)

3. _____ Focus (DAR)

4. _____ Charting by exception (SOAPIER)

a. Must document acronym components of
   nursing note in sequence

b. Can alter sequence of acronym components in intervention and evaluation part
   of clinical note

MATCHING CHARACTERISTIC AND FORMAT

Match documentation characteristic in column A with format in column B.

1. _____ Problem list

2. _____ Patient assessment made at beginning of each shift

3. _____ Data, Action, Response

4. _____ Assessment/intervention flow sheet

5. _____ Critical pathway

a. PIE

b. Charting by exception

c. POMR

d. Case management

e. Focus

MULTIPLE CHOICE

1. _____ Reasons for using documentation formats are
    a) saves time
    b) decreases chart bulk
    c) faster information retrieval
    d) all of the above

2. _____ Disadvantages of narrative charting include
    a) potential for redundant information
    b) time consuming to read
    c) no flags to find important information quickly
    d) all of the above

3. _____ Flow sheets are used for recording the following types of information
    a) intake and output, vital signs, daily activities
    b) characteristics to assess for a particular condition
    c) teaching interventions for a specific knowledge deficit
    d) all of the above

4. _____ In Charting by exception
    a) a check mark indicates an exception to the normal range
    b) narratives are written as a daily routine
    c) an asterisk and narrative indicate an abnormal finding
    d) a & b

5. _____ Outcome criteria in case management are
    a) generally standardized for a particular diagnostic group
    b) appear in documentation only at the end of care
    c) established and revised every day by the health care team
    d) a trend no longer required

CHALLENGE FOR CRITICAL THINKING

1. Why is it important to have nurses involved in determining documentation methods?

2. Why might it be reasonable for a health care organization to use several methods of documentation?

3. List advantages and disadvantages of formats discussed in this chapter.

4. Which format(s) do you prefer? Why?

5. What factors influence changing documentation methods?

LEARNING TO DOCUMENT

1. At 8:30 am, 30 minutes after eating, your patient with esophageal hiatus hernia complains of "heartburn." When asked for details she says it is a burning sensation in her upper abdomen, constant, dull +6 pain, and feels worse when she lies down. When asked, she says she has no nausea or vomiting. Her body language is consistent with pain as she grimaces, leans forward and hold her hand against her upper abdomen. You give her Mylanta 30 mL PRN as ordered and elevate the head of the bed to a 45° angle. Half an hour later she says the pain is +2.

    Using this information, write a nursing note in four different formats: narrative, problem-oriented (SOAPE), PIE, and focus (DAR). See forms on following pages.

2. What could be a likely variation in the critical pathway for a patient who had a knee replacement? Using the sample critical path outline, briefly plot a critical pathway for this patient and document the variation on the bottom of the pathway.

SAMPLE NARRATIVE NURSING NOTE

NARRATIVE NURSING NOTE	
Date/Time	**Nursing Notes**

SAMPLE PROBLEM-ORIENTED NOTES (SOAPE)

Date	Time	No.	Problem	Patient Progress Notes

SAMPLE FOCUS PATIENT CARE NOTES

Date/Time	Focus	Patient Care Notes

SAMPLE CRITICAL PATHWAY OUTLINE

CRITICAL PATH

Primary Diagnosis _____

DRG Code _____

LOS _____

	Day 1–Date:	Day 2–Date:	Day 3–Date:
Consults			
Tests			
Patient activities			
Teaching			
Treatments			
Medication			
Diet			
Discharge planning			

VARIATION **CAUSE** **ACTION TAKEN**

The Reporting Process

LEARNING OBJECTIVES

After studying this chapter, the learner should be able to:

▲ Apply the principles of communication to the process of reporting.

▲ Explain steps and rationale in preparing for presenting reports.

▲ Identify the role of participants in the reporting process.

▲ Compare the types and advantages of different methods of reporting.

▲ Identify legal and ethical considerations in reporting.

▲ Describe essential information to document after completing a telephone report.

KEY TERMS

Confidentiality	Nursing rounds	Reporting	Veracity

Eggland ET, Heinemann DS. NURSING DOCUMENTATION:
CHARTING, RECORDING, AND REPORTING.
© 1994 J.B. Lippincott Company.

Reporting is the verbal communication of information regarding a patient's health status, needs, treatments, outcomes, and responses. The purpose of reporting is continuity of care and problem-solving. Whereas nursing documentation is the recording of the pertinent and significant aspects of daily care, reporting summarizes communication to facilitate the daily continuity of care among caregivers. In this aspect, reporting is the supplement of fast transmission of data, which ensures current information. This current information is critical for all caregivers to make appropriate clinical decisions for care.

Reporting is also an important component of patient care problem-solving among nurses and other disciplinary caregivers. Reporting provides a better opportunity than recording for explaining the details of a problem. Verbal communication is more timely in relaying information to key decision-makers in care and receiving a timely response so that care can be provided without undue delay. Through reporting, nurses and other caregivers solve problems while minimizing the documentation of those problems. Clinical judgments are documented as such, and alternatives considered during the process are only verbalized. This aspect of communication saves time, minimizes documentation bulk, and contributes to protection from liability.

A complementary relationship exists between reporting and recording, and fundamental similarities are apparent between the two methods of communication. The principles of communication apply to both reporting and recording. The nursing process is an inherent structure in which both reporting and recording can be organized. Legal and ethical principles apply to both means of communication. Finally, standards of care apply to reporting and recording because both reflect the quality of care a nurse provides.

Communication and the Process of Reporting

Although there are similarities in reporting and recording, differences also exist. A major difference is the fact that verbal communication is less likely to be organized in thought before it is spoken. Verbal communication—speaking and listening—often does not allow participants to visually prepare and organize thoughts and check for completeness of information before the verbal exchange is finished. The goal of this chapter is to assist the nurse to apply the principles of communication in what may be termed practical aspects of communication in reporting.

Practical Aspects of Communication

Key to the effectiveness of reporting is the actual exchange of information within the communication of those involved in the reporting process. The effective exchange of information (patient data) requires a focused presentation by a presenter or speaker (nurse) who holds the attention of a receptive participant or listener (another caregiver). To accomplish this, information must be exchanged in the following manner:

1. Those involved in reporting must value the exchange of information as important to the care of patients.
2. Patient data must be pertinent, accurate, thorough, and current.
3. The environment of the verbal exchange must be without distraction and must be comfortable to all involved.
4. The timing and duration of the reporting should be acceptable to those involved.
5. Participants in reporting should feel personally involved and accountable for transmitting and receiving information.
6. All participants in the reporting process should exhibit communication behaviors that show interest, attentiveness, respect, professional demeanor, sensitivity, and acute perception.
7. Information should be personalized in the reporting process by calling patients by name, not by room number or diagnosis. Similarly, participants should be addressed by name to promote professional familiarity and teamwork.

To communicate well verbally and to give efficient reports, nurses must consider what they want to say, why they want to say it, where and when they are going to say it, and how they will say it. It is important to know during a report when to speak and when to listen. Planning is important in giving or receiving reports so that normally informal, spontaneous speech becomes meaningful and concise communication.

Effective Presentation of Information

Planned presentation of patient information is a key to effective reporting. The data must be appropriate, concise, and organized for appropriate use within the nursing process. The data given and received in the reporting session can make a significant difference in the effectiveness of care planned and implemented. Because presentation of information affects the quality and comprehensiveness of care, consider the preparation for reporting and recommended presentation techniques.

PREPARATION

The following information on presenting a report applies to group presentations or one-to-one reports. For ease of discussion, this process is presented below as a group presentation report.

Preparing for report starts with a chart or Kardex review to learn background information on the patient, the chief complaint, the primary diagnoses, and any appropriate and pertinent information related to that complaint. Other diagnoses are considered as well as the patient's past and present response to the diagnoses and treatment. This data review gives the nurse a starting point in focusing on the patient's medical diagnoses, associated and nursing diagnoses, and overall condition.

The nurse then determines the goals for the report and any variation in the type of approach to take, regarding content progression (main complaint first, then related diagnoses and problems) and presentation of continuity of care problems (with empathy and sensitivity to other nurses' concerns).

Further, determining the content and goals for a report depends on the practice setting and the amount and type of information an oncoming nurse needs for appropriate assessment, care planning, and discharge planning for a particular type of patient. For example, presenting a report in home care will require a nurse to obtain and present more detailed information regarding family support systems and home care environment, whereas a preoperative report would have a different focus of patient condition: surgery, physical and psychological preparation for surgery, emotional concerns, and outcome expectations.

For effective reporting, eliminate barriers to communication that can be controlled, such as timing and place. Preparing for report takes planning as well—planning for the best time of day in terms of others' schedule and the participants' alertness, comfort, and attention. If the report is given at the beginning of the shift, give the oncoming staff time to settle in and get oriented. If a special case study report is being scheduled for a nonroutine meeting time, look at the schedule for meetings, peak patient care periods, and physician visiting time, so that the report comes at a time when participants will not be interrupted.

Planning the setting environment is important in reporting to accomplish a pleasant, nondistracting conversation and focused interchange of communication. Participants must be able to hear, see, and make sense of what a presenter is saying for reporting to be effective. Select a quiet room, not a treatment room where nurses will be coming in and out during report. The room a nurse chooses for the interview should provide privacy so that participants feel free to speak confidentially and should be isolated so other persons do not hear the report. It should be comfortable to all the senses, in temperature, lighting, sound, and vision (neat, clean, and nonthreatening), and in touch (comfortable seating) and spatial comfort (seating arrangements in relation to the presenter and other participants). Ideally the room environment should be a pleasant surrounding in which the participants can feel relaxed. It should be free from distractions and interruptions. But if interruptions are unavoidable, the presenter should apologize for the interruptions, express interest in continuing the report, and take steps to minimize or alleviate any further interruptions.

PRESENTATION TECHNIQUES

Putting the participants at ease begins with a pleasant greeting and an approach that shows interest in them and in what they need in a report. Listen carefully for those clues as the report proceeds. Begin with brief, pleasant conversation that sets a professional tone and a positive attitude. While participants are assembling, a conversation beginning with a brief comment on the weather or pretty flowers in a vase may be mundane, but it gives participants the opportunity to establish a mind set for a compatible interrelationship and a mental preparation for the report at hand. Do not prolong small talk, however, because it suggests patient care concerns are not a priority, the nurse is uncomfortable or reluctant to give the report, or the time schedule of participants is not a concern. The presenter begins the report by stating the purpose of the report and mentioning a few of the priority topics to be discussed. If a participant knows what to expect or why something is being done, the person is more relaxed and provides better, more detailed exchange of information.

Talk at the participant's level, avoiding technical phrases and acronyms that may be misunderstood. When reporting to physicians or caregivers of other disciplines, focus on the discipline information they will need to plan and provide their component of care. When reporting to new or novice nurses, focus on tangible facts they can comprehend in a sequence that assists them in applying the nursing process and analyzing clinical decision-making.

Avoid any prejudicial comment, show of judgment of any kind toward patients being reported, or judgment toward participants involved in report. Participants should feel free to express any professional opinion or attitude. If a participant expresses a belief or opinion contrary to the presenter or expresses displeasure at another nurse or physician's care, do not express anger or disagreement, sympathy, or any committing emotion. Do try to get objective information regarding the participant's feelings or behavior. Lead the group to focus on objective data regarding a patient and patient care. Be wary of participants who manipulate or express courteous hostility. Remedy should be timely to promote a collegial, collaborative relationship early in the group dynamic process (see display, Keys to an Effective Presentation).

Be aware of body language so that a hurried or judgmental message is not sent to participants. Do maintain a time limit. Meet that limit by stating "we only have (number) minutes left and I'd like you to tell me (or I'd like to tell you) about (or more about) . . . (subject)."

Be receptive to what the participants say. Ask one question at a time and allow participants adequate time to express a thought completely. Respect for individual input minimizes frustration and makes individuals feel they are an important part of the group with an active voice in planning patient care. More important, effective problem-solving in a group generates creative analysis and innovative ideas in planning, implementing, and evaluating care.

Use a pause in the conversation to allow and encourage the participants to ask questions or give further information or explanation regarding the subject being discussed. Silence can be positive, generating more thought, analysis of data, or concern for a patient or other report participants. A silence, too, can indicate caring about a feeling or concern a participant may have. Even with silences, keep an eye on the objective of the report, set a comfortable pace of conversation, and keep the initiative for questioning, steering the conversation to health care information needed. A presenter should not shy away from asking hard questions or resolving conflicts, but should prepare the participant for them by entering the subject in a logical and progressive way. Repeat questions in different words if a participant does not understand a question, is embarrassed by a question, or needs more information regarding the question. Remember to be unhurried, professional but not too formal, focusing on the participants by making eye contact and acknowledging their responses. Do not prolong the report; keep the presentation concise and limited to the summary information the nurses need to know to provide care and to picture overall patient needs and progress in care. A presenter focuses on giving a report but also must remember to listen.

Techniques When Receiving Information

When receiving information in a report, participants need to ask questions to clarify or add information. Participants should focus on details needed to provide care, assess thoroughly, perform activities, and evaluate effectively. Open-ended questions, requiring more than just yes or no responses, elicit more information and give the presenter or entire group the opportunity to raise topics that are additional priorities or concerns regarding a patient. For example, after a report on Mrs. Jones, a participant may ask for additional information:

"Since Mrs. Jones' mastectomy, she becomes very anxious when her husband comes to visit. What can you tell me about her perception of altered body image?"

By directing and organizing questions a nurse can investigate subjects thoroughly and in the order of investigating or validating nursing diagnoses or patient outcomes. The patient's incision was described, but this participant identified a high-risk psychosocial nursing diagnosis for this condition. By asking an open-ended question, other participants have the opportunity to say they have perceived the anxiety, have talked to the patient about the anxiety, or have other clues or information that will help verify nursing diagnosis and related factors. As in any communication and investigation, a speaker must know what the goal of the communication is, avoid straying from the intended subject, and mentally plan what question to ask next without losing focus on what is being said in response.

THE ART OF LISTENING

Attentiveness along with real interest in patients and their problems sets the stage for an effective report. When participants feel respected and accepted, they are more likely to submit to their true selves and express their true feelings. Listening intently and keeping to a minimum the amount of verbiage used encourages the participants to express themselves and their concerns. Further, a nurse uses body language to encourage the participants to feel comfortable in contributing to the conversation. Face participants squarely, making eye contact and having a relaxed body posture. This will help focus on listening as well.

▲ **KEYS TO AN EFFECTIVE PRESENTATION**

Make people comfortable
Talk at the participant's level
Avoid being judgmental
Be aware of body language
Be receptive
Encourage participation

Listening is an art and a chore. Because most people have a relatively short attention span and because people can think faster than they can speak, listening is an art that can be quickly cut off by external distractions or internal thoughts. Participants can tune in and out of conversations until they realize they cannot grasp the main thought of what is being said, or they hear a key word that quickly brings attention back to the presenter.

As a report participant a nurse needs to learn to concentrate and eliminate distractions. Concentrate on what is being heard, not exclusively on what is being seen. Put other distractions down, such as the forms or memos that are not needed for the moment. Make notes only as needed. Do not assume what a presenter or participant is going to say next in the report; that is just half-listening. Similarly, do not let thoughts race ahead of the speaker because listeners lose what a presenter says while planning on what to ask next.

Learn to hear the feelings and emotions in a participant's comment, not just the content of the message. Also, if the participant makes a comment or uses an emotion with content that sparks an emotional issue, do not stop listening while reacting to what was said and do not mentally formulate a rebuttal, which can or cannot be made. Instead of reacting, try to respond with understanding or tolerance. Listen to the conflict but do not enter into it by taking sides, either by refuting the information or sympathizing with a participant (see display, Effective Listening Behaviors).

Remember—how a nurse presents or participates in a report will make a first impression on professional colleagues. This impression will be a first step in developing rapport and will lay groundwork for confidence in the nurse as a competent and caring person. This reporting process determines to a certain extent the success in gaining colleague cooperation in providing continuity of care. Reporting gives participants pertinent and precise data to begin the nursing process for each patient. In meeting other nurses' needs, the reporting process becomes a component in developing effective interprofessional and intraprofessional relationships that benefit patient care.

EFFECTIVE LISTENING BEHAVIORS

Attentiveness
Interest
Respect
Concentration

Types of Oral Reports

The presentation of information during group reports or one-to-one reports depends on the purpose of the report. One type of a report is a summary report, another type is problem reporting or clinical decision-making.

SUMMARY REPORT

Summary reports are given at the change of shift and at transfers to other health care organizations. The purpose of a summary report is to quickly provide new caregivers a focus of patient needs and details regarding different stages of those needs within the nursing process. Communicating this information from nurses who provided care (to a patient) to those who will be providing care contributes to continuity of care.

A summary report is a brief oral presentation of the following information regarding a patient:

▲ Background data and reason for care
▲ Primary medical and nursing diagnoses
▲ Explanation and status of current priority problems
▲ Changes in condition or in treatments
▲ Effective interventions or treatments of priority problems
▲ Patient outcomes and response to priority problems
▲ Progress toward expected outcomes in discharge planning
▲ Priority interventions of a timely nature

Family needs and interventions are reported within the context of nursing diagnoses. Social support by family and friend visits is the norm. There is no need to report coming and going of visitors unless there are no visitors; visitors have raised a question, a problem, or a concern; or visitors are involved in teaching and referral activities (which is desirable).

Background data and reason for care. Information about a patient should be brief and concise. Identifying information is limited to that which gives personal identity or is pertinent to care. Consider the following two patients:

Juan Sanchez, a 69-year-old patient of Dr. Parsons in 234A, was admitted 12/10 with a duodenal ulcer. He speaks and understands basic phrases in English but reads information only in Spanish.

Jane Sanders, a 30-year-old patient of Dr. Morris in 225B, was admitted today for a fractured shoulder from an automobile accident; she is scheduled for surgery tomorrow. She is a mother of two preschool children at home.

The information about Mr. Sanchez alerts nurses to speak slowly with him, using simple words and asking questions to be sure he understands any directions. Patient teaching regarding diet will require obtaining educational resources in Spanish and talking with a family member who is fluent in English. The background data regarding Mrs. Sanders alerts nurses that the patient is dealing with a number of emotional upsets: trauma from the accident, pending surgery, and concern for care of children at home. The data offer clues for nurses about actual and high-risk nursing diagnoses.

Primary medical and nursing diagnoses. Additional medical diagnoses that affect the reason for care are listed here, as well as nursing diagnoses. Reading a long list of medical and nursing diagnoses is not necessary because the information is written on a Kardex or client profile form. The nurse who will be caring for the patient will read this information more thoroughly early in the shift because this more detailed information is needed for care.

> Mr. Sanchez has a history of labile hypertension and is having upper GI (gastrointestinal) pain. He has a knowledge deficit R/T (related to) bland diet and medication regimen.
>   Mrs. Sanders has acute pain of right shoulder, anxiety regarding surgery, and parental role conflict R/T hospitalization.

This report tells participants that Mr. Sanchez has a medical diagnosis of hypertension and nursing diagnoses are Pain and Knowledge Deficit. Mrs. Sanders has no other medical diagnoses; nursing diagnoses are Pain, Anxiety, and Parental Role Conflict.

Explanation and status of current priority problem; changes in condition or in treatments; effective interventions or treatments of priority problems; patient outcomes and response to priority problems. Summary reports are intended to be a synopsis of problems and not a case study; therefore, not all information about a patient is included in a report. What is included is the priority problem or focus of care for the nurses who will continue care within the next shift or visit. Because care is in accordance with the nursing process, each nursing diagnosis is discussed in terms of brief assessment data, effective interventions, any changes in interventions, patient outcomes, and responses to interventions. Excerpts from various patient reports continue below.

> Mr. Sanchez's pain is +5 today, down from +8 last night. He was awake from 12 am to 2 am complaining of sharp, burning upper GI pain. Camalax 30 mL given with immediate relief. Dr. Parson changed Zantac from 400 mg bid (twice daily) to 300 mg qid (four times daily). Mr. Sanchez napped for approx 4 hours this morning.

> Mrs. Sanders cried intermittently today, concerned about not being at home to care for her children. We discussed present care at home with husband and possible alternatives with family caregivers during her recuperation. She made calls to sister and mother to make plans; states she feels better about situation because children excited about "grandma's visit."

Each nursing diagnosis or care management problem will be handled as a unit, discussing the problem, intervention, and outcome. Mrs. Sanders' next problem would be her anxiety regarding surgery, with interventions of preoperative teaching.

Progress toward expected outcomes in discharge planning. The reason that the day of admission is helpful in a hospital report is the limited length of stay that is reimbursable by Medicare or insurance. Focus of care should be on resolution of problems and expected outcome accomplishment in discharge planning. By reporting progress toward goals in discharge planning, all caregivers can provide teaching or make referrals on a timely basis, with time for patient learning and referral arrangements.

> Mr. Sanchez's daughter Marisa will care for Mr. Sanchez after discharge. Instructed her in diet restriction and medication regimen. She was able to demonstrate meal plan and medication schedule. Pt still needs referral to a community resource for a stop-smoking program.

> Mrs. Sanders scheduled for discharge on 12/18. Healthcare Personnel Home Health Services contacted 12/10 for physical therapy referral and home health aide assistance.

Priority interventions of a timely nature. A nurse providing care to a patient is able to delineate quickly the care that is due within a short period of time in which another nurse provides care. Nurse Emma Moore who cared for Mr. Blanco during the day shift is giving report to Nurse Byron James:

> Mr. Richard Kettle, Room 330, a 50-year-old patient of Dr. Lyte, admitted 12/10 for left renal calculi. Had lithotripsy today 9:00 am. Returned to floor at 2:00 pm. Pt states feels fine; no complaint of pain. Has altered urinary elimination with 18 Foley patent catheter to constant drainage. Output 200 mL since 2:00 pm. Has peripheral IV in right arm running D5W at keep vein open (KVO) rate. Vital signs q2h are stable; last VS measure BP130/90, P98 R12. Vital signs due at 4:00, and IV has 50 mL remaining in bag.

Pointing out that vital signs are due in an hour and the IV bag may need to be replaced within an hour helps the oncoming nurse to remember those interventions when organizing care for a number of patients. Because memory is best for the first and last information given, mentioning the information at the end of that patient's report facilitates mental and written note-taking. Other information preceding that gives rationale for the interventions as a complete sequence of care is presented (see display, Guidelines for Change of Shift Summary Reporting).

REPORTING A PATIENT PROBLEM OR NEED

Nurses use reports to present a patient problem or need to other disciplines or other departments in the hospital. The outline of this report is focused on one problem, or one problem at a time, from greatest to least importance. For each problem the following data are presented:

▲ Patient care problem with medical and nursing diagnoses
▲ Data that substantiate or compound the problem
▲ Interventions performed to date, with degree of success
▲ Target date by which expected outcome should be resolved

An example follows in which a nurse calls the physical therapy department in a hospital and gives the following patient data report:

Mrs. Anna Hopkins, Room 12 Bed 4, is an 83-year-old patient of Dr. Cross; she had bilateral knee replacement 4 days ago on 12/6. Has impaired physical mobility and anxiety. She refuses to get out of bed because she says she does not know how to use her walker. Her sister visits every day and encourages her to stay in bed so she doesn't fall. We've encouraged the sisters to have lunch in the day lounge, but they refuse. Mental health nurse clinician has been called and will visit today at 1:00 pm. Dr. Jones has ordered physical therapy to assess and provide care as needed. Goal is to ambulate 15 feet with walker and assistance before discharge to nursing home on 12/22.

Reporting Changes in Condition

Many reports are for the purpose of reporting changes in patient condition. During the course of a shift, a patient's condition can change and that change needs to be reported to a head nurse or to another nurse who may relieve the assigned nurse during lunchtime.

The basic guideline for reporting changes in condition is to provide measurable data to show the degree of change and descriptive data so that the subject is thoroughly understood. Information should be provided, particularly to the novice nurse, for signs and symptoms to watch for as a patient condition declines or improves. The report could be outlined in the following manner:

▲ Subject of change
▲ Present measurement

 ## GUIDELINES FOR CHANGE OF SHIFT SUMMARY REPORTING

Do

▲ Read the shift nurses' notes and get report from direct caregivers before giving report.
▲ Use concise phrases. Use acceptable terminology that all participants will understand. Allow opportunities for questions.
▲ Be brief. Don't repeat all background data available or routine care.
▲ Conduct the shift report where only caregivers can hear patient information.
▲ Be definite. Avoid "apparently," "appears to be." Substantiate with facts.
▲ Have the Kardex or patient profiles available for more detailed information.
▲ Describe reported symptoms accurately. Use the patient's words in describing symptoms when these words are helpful.
▲ Help incoming staff organize priorities by pointing out interventions due and priority events of the upcoming shift.
▲ Respect privacy of patient's feelings if not related to nursing care.

Don't

▲ Gossip or criticize or make fun of patient, patient behavior, or family.
▲ Give a report by room number only. Do use the patient's name, age, sex, and diagnosis.
▲ Rush through report and rush to leave the unit until all incoming staff has the opportunity for questions of any nurse or caregiver.
▲ Report in advance that a procedure was done.
▲ Wait until the end of the shift to collect data for report or rely on memory.
▲ Make assumptions about patient feelings or family.
▲ State relative statements such as "Wound is healing." Instead, describe the wound.

▲ Prior baseline measurement showing a degree of change

▲ Course of change throughout past 48 hours (acute care) or 2 weeks (home health care)

▲ Signs and symptoms of potential complications

▲ Any current interventions with patient outcomes

Using some of the above topics, the following is an example of a report an experienced nurse may give to a novice nurse:

> George Johnson, 25 years old, in Room 545B, has a sacral pressure sore that is stage 2, 5 mm × 2 mm, red and blistered. Two days ago it was a stage 1, 2 mm × 1 mm. No signs or symptoms of necrotic tissue, drainage, or infection. Dermaplast applied today per physician order. No complaint of pain or discomfort.

With the above data, the novice nurse can measure any further worsening of the pressure sore. Hearing a report of what signs and symptoms to look for provides the novice with a focus of assessment with a negative baseline measurement.

Reporting to Another Nurse

In giving and receiving reports from another nurse, nursing diagnoses terms and nursing process terms should be used with assurance that the information is understood. Because nursing terminology is not yet standardized, a nurse should use terms commonly used on the unit. When introducing new nursing diagnosis labels, for example, a nurse should include pertinent details for description and explanation. In any report, but especially when reporting to nurses with different training backgrounds and nurses with different years of experience, a reporting nurse should always provide an unhurried opportunity for questions.

Reporting to a Physician

In giving patient reports to physicians, nurses should use medical diagnoses and concentrate on objective assessment data. Before giving the report, the nurse should gather objective and subjective assessment data and verify the information. Assessment data should describe the condition of the patient and investigate for potential complications of the illness or injury. Data should be collected with the focus on information that would assist the physician make a medical diagnosis and order appropriate treatment (see display, Data to Include in Reporting).

Methods of Reporting

Intershift reporting allows the transference of necessary information from one shift of nurses to another to provide a summary of nursing care for continuity of care. Methods of reporting between shifts include:

▲ Change of shift report meeting

▲ Audiotape report

▲ Walking rounds

Different units in a hospital often have different methods of reporting. Many hospitals allow each group of nurses to decide which method they prefer for their unit.

Change of Shift Report Meeting

The content of the change of shift or intershift report meeting is described earlier (summary report). Nurses from a prior shift meet with nurses from the next shift to directly share information by means of an oral report on patients. The report meeting can be managed in a number of different ways.

Charge nurse reporter. In the first method, the charge nurse receives report from all the nurses on the floor, and she alone reports to the oncoming shift of nurses. The other nurses on the prior shift continue to provide care during the report meeting. Those nurses are available after report for any questions that the charge nurse may not have been able to answer.

The advantage of this method is that only one nurse is pulled from the floor and other nurses are available for care. Another advantage is the charge nurse reporter gets an overview of care on all patients on the unit and can unilaterally make suggestions for continuing care for all patients. Using just one reporter allows greater control of the report, which usually results in a shorter report period. The disadvantage of this method is that any further information requested about a patient may not be immediately answerable by the charge nurse, who did not provide direct care.

Group shared report. In this report meeting, all the nurses from the prior shift enter the report room and give report to all the nurses on the incoming shift; they individually report on patients for whom they cared during the shift. The various nurses can rotate in, so that nurses are available to answer call lights or provide care during the report time.

The advantage of this method is the ability for nurses to get clarification or additional information directly from the person who provided care. Another advantage is when nurses give a report on their own patients the information is more detailed. With this shared report by direct caregivers, oncoming nurses get a better picture of the patient's condition and a better sense of what stage of the nursing process each diagnosis is in or simply what is going on with the patient (A. Nagle, RN, MSN, Seattle, telephone interview, December 10, 1992).

▲	DATA TO INCLUDE IN REPORTING	

Data Topic	Change of Shift Report to a Nurse	Telephone Report to a Physician
Identifying patient data	Name, sex, age, Room number Physician	Name, sex, age
Diagnoses	Primary Medical diagnoses Nursing diagnoses	Primary medical diagnosis
Patient condition	▲ Data related to primary diagnoses and current problems ▲ Use objective measurements	▲ Data related to current problems only ▲ Objective measurements ▲ Presence or absence of signs and symptoms of potential complications
Interventions	▲ Any new orders or changes in treatment ▲ Teaching plans/progress	▲ Interventions current
Outcomes	▲ Expected outcomes of one or two nursing diagnoses (for that shift's focus for a patient's care) ▲ Patient learning outcomes related to diagnosis mentioned	▲ Patient outcomes of interventions for the stated problem
Discharge plans	▲ Expected date of discharge ▲ Referrals needed/made ▲ Self-care management and readiness to go home	Ask for plans for referral orders if current problem affects care after discharge
Family/care support	▲ Problems and concerns ▲ Positive support as it relates to patient problem	▲ Family problems, concerns ▲ Questions for physician
Timely interventions	Interventions due priority for shift	Request medical orders

Person-to-person report. In this method of reporting, a staff nurse who provided care to a particular patient gives report to the staff nurse who will provide care to that same patient. The theory behind this is that those nurses who will not be providing care to particular patients do not benefit nor do they listen to reports about those patients. The purpose of the method is to save time.

Advantages of the method are the time saving and the ability to learn detailed information usually known only by a direct caregiver. This detailed information can include how much weight bearing a patient has in pivotal transfers or exactly how much assistance a patient needs in activities of daily living, or the stage of grieving in an altered body image. Disadvantages are the other nurses on the floor know nothing about the patient. If those nurses are called in to answer a call light or relieve a nurse going to lunch, they know little about diagnoses, needs, activity restrictions, or prescribed diet (J. Neun-

dorfer, RN, BSN, Houston, telephone interview, December 10, 1992).

Audiotape Report

In taped reports, a charge nurse or each staff nurse records on a tape recorder the information oncoming staff nurses need to provide care. The format is similar to report meetings, but the in-person speaker is replaced by a tape recorder. In this type of report, the quality of the machine and tape, the diction and clarity of the speaker, and the hearing ability of the listener are variables that can affect the sending and receiving of the message.

An advantage of this method is that the report tends to be brief because it is not interrupted with questions or comments. Another advantage is that the nurses from the previous shift can continue to provide care on the floor while the oncoming nurses get report. A disadvantage is the inability to ask questions spontaneously. When report is over, it is sometimes difficult to locate and talk with nurses who are leaving the floor after their shift.

Depending on the quality of the report given, sometimes not enough information is given to provide safe care. Talking into a machine rather than directly to nurses sometimes lulls nurses into reading from the Kardex rather than concentrating on the daily changes in the patients and patient care. With taped report there is little or no opportunity for nursing interaction and exchange of information to contribute to problem-solving. The opportunity to have direct caregivers explain a patient problem during a different time frame or from a different perspective is helpful in viewing a problem and viewing a patient as a multidimensional person. In organizations that employ part-time nurses, those nurses complain of frustration with taped report. Many part-time nurses prefer to have report given by a full-time nurse to get more detailed and comparative daily information about a patient. Finally, use of the machine can also be a problem. Depending on the quality of the machine and the acoustics of the room, the clarity of the transmission can be a disadvantage. Compounding the problem can be cultural accents, which can be more difficult to understand on audiotape.

Walking Rounds

Walking rounds can be **nursing rounds** in which only nurses participate; nurse–physician rounds in which usually the charge nurse and physician(s) make rounds; or multidisciplinary health team rounds in which all disciplines are involved.

Advantages of the nurse–physician or multidisciplinary health team rounds include the enhancement of communication, the view of the whole patient from a comprehensive care viewpoint, and coordination of care. In these walking round models, usually the physician is in charge of rounds. For this chapter discussion, focus will remain on the nursing rounds in which the nurse is the organizer of rounds.

Walking rounds is the report method in which the nurse(s) from the prior shift walk to each patient's room with the nurse(s) from the oncoming shift. Usually one charge nurse from the prior shift makes rounds with the oncoming charge nurse. During the walking rounds, the prior nurse introduces the oncoming nurse to the patient and informs the patient of any plans, appointments, or treatments in the upcoming shift.

Walking rounds are most effective in observing and receiving information from the patient when the patient:

▲ Is not receiving a treatment
▲ Is not experiencing discomfort
▲ Is not eating a meal

▲ Is not mentally preparing for the physician's visit
▲ Feels presentable in terms of appearance
▲ Is not anxious to get to the morning grooming routine

Walking rounds provide the prior shift and incoming nurses the opportunity to observe each patient who is the subject of the report. Although this method may take more time initially, it leaves less to chance about transmitting problem-focused data. This method also provides a unique opportunity to include the patient in evaluation and planning of care. Walking rounds also place full accountability on the departing caregiver for the condition of the unit and its occupant.

An advantage of this method is the symbolism of continuity that is shown to the patient. Another more important advantage is the ability of one nurse to show specific assessment data or demonstrate techniques to the oncoming nurse. A disadvantage is the lack of privacy in discussing patient information. It is difficult to find a quiet place in the hallway to share information the patient or other patients should not hear.

Telephone Reporting

Nurses frequently communicate reports by telephone, in transfers, in obtaining patient data, in referrals, and in problem-solving. Nurses call other nursing divisions, physicians' offices, discharge planning offices, and other health care organizations. Nurses will initiate or receive professional telephone reports and must handle them with courtesy and professionalism.

In giving or receiving a telephone report, some key, standard guidelines are practical for any organization or professional communication.

▲ Organize the information to report.
▲ Identify the caller and nursing division or organization.
▲ State the purpose of the call.
▲ Be brief, avoid redundancy.
▲ Do not talk with others or take other calls during the call.
▲ Listen carefully. Repeat information to verify orders or diagnostic test results.
▲ Take notes to accurately remember important communicated data.
▲ Always write down the name of the person talked with.
▲ Do not make personal remarks. Maintain a professional tone.
▲ Avoid slang. Do not use clinical language that another discipline will not understand.
▲ Maintain courteous demeanor. Stay calm to prevent arguments.

▲ Ask and answer questions after the other party has finished speaking.

▲ End the call pleasantly, allowing the caller to hang up first.

A nurse giving a report should collect information and write down data accurately before making a call. Outlining the information in the order of how it should be said is a helpful tool to use while making a telephone report. Writing the name of the person to whom you spoke and pertinent information from the call facilitates recording pertinent information in an organized, accurate manner.

Reporting During Referrals and Transition of Care

Whereas transition of care is primarily documentation based, referrals are primarily reporting based. Both events use reporting and recording, and information from both sources must be consistent for any patient.

Referrals

Referrals, sometimes called consults, are requests for a specialty professional or agency to intervene with a patient to meet special needs. Health care today is a multidisciplinary endeavor; even within the walls of a single institution, a patient receives services from many departments and different disciplines. This is one effect of continuing specialization in health services. The referral process facilitates communication of special patient needs and promotes continuity of care, an essential element of quality. Because nurses cannot be all things to all people, it is a nurse's ethical responsibility to direct the patient to services that can meet the individual's needs for information, direct care, social services, counseling, and other assistance. Common referrals are to consulting specialty physicians, dietitians, counselors, chaplains, and enterostomal therapists.

Referrals depend on accurate verbal and written communication. The referral should prepare other caregivers for what to expect with regard to the patient's condition and individual concerns. For example, a referral to a counselor (psychologist, psychiatric nurse, or social worker) might initially address the patient's and family's reaction to an illness episode, the patient's support needs, and the technique of intervention the staff has used successfully. A quality referral paints a verbal picture that describes the patient as an individual and gives the receiving professional a head start on establishing a positive relationship with a patient.

Transition of Care

When a patient is transferred from one unit to another within a hospital, a transfer form is completed and a phone call is made to the unit to which the patient will be transferred. An oral summary report is given, including the interventions due within a short period of time, such as medication administration.

Transferring or discharging patients to another health care organization requires a transfer or discharge form, but this communication is sometimes supplemented by a telephone report. The outline of a verbal summary report could be used, with emphasis on information specific to the institution to which the patient is going. For example, for a patient being discharged to a long-term care facility, it would help them to begin care by knowing how much assistance the patient needs in activities of daily living, if the patient is oriented, how the patient has socialized, and what activities the patient enjoys. Another example is a discharge to a home health care agency. Information helpful for continuity of care would be how mobile the patient is; how much help the person needs in daily activities; if a family member or friend may be a reliable caregiver; if there are any treatments or special instructions to the patient; what teaching has been given to the patient; what has been the patient response to learning; what other referrals have been made; and what needs are still unmet.

During discharge of patients, reporting may be from a nurse to a social service or discharge planning department. When giving a report to a social service worker, focus on the information pertinent to that discipline. Concern for financial resources would be an area social services would handle. Specific needs requiring community resource referrals is another area of focus. Patient strengths such as family support and caregiving abilities are important for effective discharge planning. When talking with social service personnel, do not use nursing terminology that might be unclear to them. Be clear, accurate, and concise about patient needs and the progress in meeting those needs.

Appropriate communication between facilities during transfer of care is not limited to helpful information to provide care. Communication should focus on essential information a receiving facility should have to prevent injury, death, and legal action. Allergies, adverse reactions to combinations of drugs, and endangering patient behavior are data that must be communicated. A nurse should not overlook communicating life-threatening information or think that once a patient is discharged responsibility ends. The following case is an example of a preventable death.

In *Krestview Nursing Home v. Synowiec* (1975), a long-term care facility was held liable for the death of a patient they had transferred to an acute care facility. At transfer, the nursing home did not provide information about the patient's diagnosis of organic brain syndrome or that he had a history of wandering. The patient wandered from the hospital and was found dead several days later.

Had the hospital been aware of the patient's secondary diagnosis and consequent tendency to wander, they would have provided special supervision that would have prevented the untimely death.

Legal and Ethical Considerations in Reporting

Health care technology, complexity of coordinated care, and increased transitions of care increase the number of situations in which health care providers need to consider and understand legal and ethical issues.

The laws are clear on certain issues relating to reporting. Legal transgressions are punishable by fine or imprisonment. Ethical considerations in reporting are not as clear, but they provide guidelines to determine what is right or best in a difficult situation. Ethical transgressions are subject to a person's conscience or occasionally to decisions rendered by a professional ethics committee.

Reporting patient health care information involves the ethical principles of truth-telling, veracity, and confidentiality. Closely linked to these principles are professional nursing values that must be considered in the course of delivering care and reporting care.

How you perform as a nurse depends on your philosophy. Values form your philosophy and are the basis for your actions. If you do not take time to examine and articulate them, you will not be as clear or conscious of your beliefs and values and the significant impact they have upon your behavior. The price you pay for value conflicts is often confusion, indecision, and inconsistency. (Uustal, 1992)

Veracity

Does every nurse value truthfulness? Nurses provide services with respect for human dignity and patient rights. Truthfulness is one of those rights. **Veracity**, or the duty to tell the truth, is a value inherent in professional nursing standards. However, truth-telling *does not* obligate the nurse to tell the patient whatever that patient wants to know. As the patient's advocate, however, the nurse can choose to speak to the physician. If the physician and nurse take a different perspective on the divulgence of the truth, the situation can be referred to an organization's ethics committee. The ethics committee does not rule on right and wrong but uses communica-

tion as the heart of the ethics process. The committee will encourage communication so that all participants in a situation operate from a knowledgeable, reasonable, intellectual, and rational basis, weighing all alternatives, benefits, and risks.

Confidentiality

The ethical principle of **confidentiality** is defined as keeping private all information received within the context of a special relationship, such as the nurse–patient relationship. The American Nurses Association Code for Nurses and the Standards of Clinical Nursing Practice address this responsibility to respect privileged information. This means that nurses and the organization as a whole are obligated to keep confidential all the information received by the organization that was attained as a result of the patient–provider relationship. To ignore that obligation can result in a nurse being charged with civil liability for damages or for breach of confidentiality (Haddad & Kapp, 1991).

Law and ethics allow the nurse to share information among caregivers who are providing direct care to the patient. As discussed throughout this book, nursing and multidisciplinary communication is essential among caregivers to plan and coordinate care so that continuity of care is maintained. The sharing of this information must be done carefully, however. Release of information forms should be signed before giving any patient report by telephone or documentation to anyone other than direct caregivers. Idle conversation about patients to people other than direct caregivers can lead to civil lawsuits for breach of confidentiality. Derogatory remarks can lead to charges of slander and defamation of character. Nurses should take special care that discussions regarding patient information be confined to involved caregivers and private places that safeguard patient privacy.

Potential Legal Problems

Change of shift reporting and telephone reporting are methods the nurse uses to fulfill professional responsibility of communicating patient information. Like recording, reporting has obligations for which the nurse is accountable. The nurse can be liable if certain obligations are not met.

Communication among nurses during patient rounds and during the change of shift nursing report is critical because nursing care is based in large part on verbal orders. . . . Liability may be based on the legal theory of delay in communicating or failure to communicate essential patient findings or changes. (Cushing, 1988, pp. 187–188)

Important assessment information or information from a family member can constitute data that would make a difference in diagnoses or planning of care. Situations in which that information is not communicated, or is communicated after a lengthy delay, may be a source of potential negligence or malpractice lawsuits. If a nurse delays or does not communicate information, the nurse and the health care organization can be held liable. Consider the following case in which a change of condition was not reported:

> A 9-year-old boy fractured his left femur and was put in a cast and traction. After 6 days the patient had pain in both legs and an edematous right foot. The nurse's note indicated circulation remained "good." After 6 more days the right foot was swollen and cool. On the 13th day, responding to the boy's complaints, a second physician discovered the problem. Removed from traction, the boy's right leg lacked sensation and movement. The boy's leg had to be amputated due to necrosis. (*Garfield Park Community Hospital v. Vitacco*, 1975)

In this case, the nurse was negligent in not reporting the change of condition to the physician. The nurse should have contacted the physician immediately on observing the cool skin, swelling, and decreased sensation. Measurable data should have been documented, such as capillary refill, or how fast blood returned to the nail after pressure was released with a finger.

In the following case, the nurse did not report bleeding in a timely manner, which resulted in a patient's death. This nurse's report was unduly late, and the court ruled negligence because of it.

> After a woman delivered a baby, the attending nurse reported to the physician at three different times that bleeding was excessive. The physician instructed the nurse to measure the vaginal bleeding. Three hours later bleeding was still excessive but the nurse did not call the doctor because "he would not have responded." An hour later another nurse called the physician. By that time, the patient went into shock and died (*Goff v. Doctor's General Hospital of San Jose*, 1958).

The nurse should have measured vital signs and notified the physician and nursing supervisor of the unusually heavy postpartum bleeding. The delay of reporting contributed to the patient's death. Reports to physicians must be timely and accurate. The health of patients and the legal protection of nurses are critical issues that depend on this timeliness.

When a nurse reports a patient's condition to a physician or nursing supervisor, the report is documented in the patient's clinical record. For example, the following information is what should be documented when a telephone report is made:

The important information to be contained in the entry includes:

- ▲ The specific time that the telephone call was made
- ▲ Who made the telephone call, if other than the writer of that information
- ▲ Who was called
- ▲ To whom information was given
- ▲ All (specific) information given
- ▲ All (specific) information received (Feutz-Harter, 1989)

It is important to note that one phone call in an attempt to contact a physician does not relieve a nurse of liability. Documentation of attempts to call the physician should be noted according to the above guidelines. If a response from the physician is not timely nor deemed appropriate by the nurse, a second phone call should be made to a secondary physician and a nursing supervisor. Careful attention to what time the unavailable physician(s) were called should be equal to the careful documentation of what time the physician(s) returned the call.

KEY POINTS

- ▲ **Communication in nursing includes reporting and recording. Reporting accomplishes fast transmission of specific patient information for continuity of care and problem-solving. A patient's information transmitted by reporting and recording should be consistent.**

- ▲ **To verbally communicate well and to give efficient reports, nurses must consider what they want to say, why they want to say it, where and when they are going to say it, and how they will say it. Planning is important in giving or receiving reports.**

- ▲ **Participants in reporting should feel personally involved and accountable for transmitting and receiving information. All participants in the reporting process should exhibit positive communication behaviors, which include interest, attentiveness, respect, professional demeanor, sensitivity, and acute perception.**

- ▲ **Different methods of in-person change of shift reports include one presenter, group presenters, or person-to-person reports. The advantage of in-person reports is the opportunity for clarification of information and time for questions. Audiotaped reports provide a faster report, allowing nurses from the prior shift to continue to provide care while the oncoming shift attends report. Walking rounds are a longer report but have the advantage of including patients in care planning and evalua-**

tion and demonstrating certain aspects of assessment or treatment.

▲ Veracity and confidentiality are two ethical principals that directly apply to reporting. Nurses have the duty to tell the truth in reporting and recording and the obligation to keep confidential the patient information received by virtue of the nurse–patient or patient–organization relationship.

▲ When a telephone report is made, an entry is placed in the clinical record. Important information to document includes time call was made, who made the call, who was called, to whom information was given, and all information given and received.

REFERENCES

Cushing, M. (1988). *Nursing jurisprudence*. Norwalk, CT: Appleton & Lange.

Feutz-Harter, S. (1989). Documentation principles and pitfalls. *Journal of Nursing Administration*, *19*(12), 9.

Garfield Park Community Hospital v. Vitacco, 327 N.E.2nd 408 (IL, 1975). Cited in Cushing, M. (1988). *Nursing jurisprudence* (p. 189). Norwalk, CT: Appleton & Lange.

Goff v. Doctor's General Hospital of San Jose, 333 P.2nd 29 (CA, 1958). Cited in Cushing, M. (1988). *Nursing jurisprudence* (p. 190). Norwalk, CT: Appleton & Lange.

Haddad, A. M., & Kapp, M. B. (1991). *Ethical and legal issues in home health care: Case studies and analyses*. Norwalk, CT: Appleton & Lange.

Krestview Nursing Home v. Synowiec 317 S. 294 (Fla, 1975). Cited in Cushing, M. (1988). *Nursing jurisprudence* (p. 197). Norwalk, CT: Appleton & Lange.

Uustal, D. B. (1992). *Values and ethics in nursing: From theory to practice*. East Greenwich, RI: Educational Resources in Nursing & Holistic Health.

BIBLIOGRAPHY

Bandman, E. L., & Bandman, B. (1990). *Nursing ethics through the life span* (2nd ed.). Norwalk, CT: Appleton & Lange.

Beauchamp, T. L., & Childress, J. F. (1989). *Principles of biomedical ethics* (3rd ed.). New York: Oxford University Press.

▬▬▬▬▬▬ PRACTICE SESSION ▬▬▬▬▬▬

FILL IN

1. Two purposes of reporting are _____ and

_____ .

2. Four similarities between reporting and recording are

_____ ,

_____ ,

_____ ,

_____ .

3. Three positive communication behaviors of change of shift reporting participants are

_____ ,

_____ , and

_____ .

4. A key to effective reporting begins with _____ .

5. Effective listening techniques include _____

_____ and _____ .

6. Three methods of giving change of shift report include

_____ , _____ , and

_____ .

7. Two determinants of the acoustic quality of an audiotape report are the

_____ , and the

_____ .

8. Three types of walking rounds are _____ ,

_____ , and _____ .

9. Reporting of information for a referral should focus on

_____ .

10. Two ethical principles that directly relate to reporting are

_____ and _____ .

MATCHING

Match the phrase in Column A that matches its definition in Column B.

1. _____ veracity   **a.** recording

2. _____ confidentiality   **b.** reporting

3. _____ guidelines of consciousness   **c.** ethics

4. _____ oral transmission of patient information   **d.** privileged information

5. _____ written transmission of patient information   **e.** truth-telling

CHALLENGE FOR CRITICAL THINKING

1. List the content that should be included in a summary report. Choose two of those components and discuss why they are important in continuity of care.

2. A woman brought her son into the emergency department with a temperature of 103.8°F. She said the boy had been exposed to a friend who had strep throat. She also said that they had been camping on the weekend and she removed a tick from the boy's scalp. The nurse told the physician about the strep throat but forgot to tell him about the tick. The boy died of undiagnosed Rocky Mountain spotted fever. Is this a case where the nurse or doctor would be liable? What would be the legal term for that liability?

3. A nursing supervisor calls your unit. She would like to make walking rounds with you to learn more about the patients on your unit. What factors would you consider before setting the time for the walking rounds? Why?

4. As a treat during the holidays, for each oncoming shift, the head nurse of a hospital nursing unit ordered soft drinks and a party tray of sandwiches and cookies to be shared during report. Is this a good idea? Why or why not?

5. Compare the advantages of the different types of change of shift report: one presenter, group presentation, or person-to-person. Which type would you prefer and why?

6. Discuss the purpose, similarities, and differences in law and ethics.

7. A charge nurse gives report by telling you about the stroke patient in 512, coronary patient in 515, and postop patient in 517. Could this affect the participants in report? If so, how?

8. The ethical content presented in this last section is designed to acquaint the nurse with current ethical principles that serve nurses in the practice setting. Each nurse brings a set of values to nursing practice. Each nurse needs to examine those values to define them in light of law and ethics in the nursing profession. Discuss your thoughts about the following statement: A value all nurses should practice is truth-telling.

9. With a brief introduction to legal and ethical principles in this book, students learn certain facts about the legal system, risk situations, and the parameters of safe practice. What seems to be the best method of protecting yourself from liability as a nurse?

10. Do you think there is a complementary relationship between reporting and recording and that there are fundamental similarities between the two methods of communication? If basic principles of communication apply to both reporting and recording, discuss those basic principles and how they apply to reporting and how they apply to recording.

LEARNING SKILLS IN REPORTING

1. Do you think the reporting process parallels the nursing process? How does that affect the outline of the report you compose? Does a nurse use critical thinking or clinical decision-making during this process?

2. A patient who has had abdominal surgery in the morning is returned to your unit in the afternoon. Medical orders are for nothing by mouth (NPO), but the patient insists he feels fine and needs a glass of water. You give him the water and he vomits. He becomes pale, starts to perspire, and says he feels awful. Should this be reported? To whom? What would you say?

3. Determining the content and goals for a report depends on the practice setting and the information a nurse needs to provide care for particular patients. What practical information would you need to give a friend to care for your 1-year-old niece? What information would you include in a report for a 1-year-old pediatric patient who has a temperature of 103°F?

4. Sarah Sommers is a 20-year-old college student. She was admitted into room 222 at noon with a fractured ulna in her right arm and a concussion. She fell while roller blading. Compared to her left hand, her right hand seems swollen, pale, and cold. She says her R fingers feel "funny," kind of "tingly," and the cast feels tight around her wrist. She has 2+ edema >3 sec capillary refill and the cast is clean and dry. Outline a telephone report you would make to her physician.

5. After you made the telephone call regarding Sarah Sommers, write how you would document the telephone call in the clinical record?

6. Divide into groups of four. Each student writes a brief description of a patient including all the information about that patient that would be given in a report. *Do not use personal or real patient information in this activity*; instead create fictitious patient situations. Combine that information to create a fictitious unit of patients. Role play by giving a change of shift report using a charge nurse presenter, then a group report, then a person-to-person report.

7. Take the patient information created for the last activity and borrow a tape recorder. Audiotape a charge nurse presenter report and a group presentation report.

8. Role play walking rounds by using the patient information collected in the last activities, and visiting patients at various locations in the room.

9. Using sensitivity and *constructive* criticism, analyze each presenter's report in the previous activities. Point out the strengths of the presentation and weaknesses that can be improved.

10. Discuss what type of report is performed at your clinical site. What advantages do you see with that type of report. Compare those advantages to the type of report that you personally prefer.

APPENDIX

A

Joint Commission on Accreditation of Healthcare Organizations' Nursing Care Standards Related to Documentation

Following are selected nursing care standards recently formulated by the Joint Commission on Accreditation of Healthcare Organizations for use in hospital settings. They became effective for accreditation purposes on January 1, 1991, for all settings in which nursing care is provided in the hospital.

The standards and characteristics included in this appendix were chosen because of their relationship to nursing documentation. The standard and required characteristics that relate to information management systems are included because of the evolving and increasing use of computer systems in nursing documentation. A complete listing of nursing care standards and required characteristics can be found in the Joint Commission's 1991 Accreditation Manual for Hospitals (AMH).

Standard

NC.1 Patients receiving nursing care based on a documented assessment of their needs.*

Required Characteristics

NC.1.1 Each patient's need for nursing care related to his/her admission is assessed by a registered nurse.*

NC.1.1.1 The assessment is conducted either at the time of admission or within a time frame preceding or following admission that is specified in hospital policy.*

NC.1.1.2 Aspects of data collection may be delegated by the registered nurse.

---

*The asterisked items are key factors in the accreditation decision process.

(Copyright 1990 by the Joint Commission on Accreditation of Healthcare Organizations, Chicago. Reprinted with permission.)

NC.1.1.3 Needs are reassessed when warranted by the patient's condition.*

NC.1.2 Each patient's assessment includes consideration of biophysical, psychosocial, environmental, self-care, educational and discharge planning factors.*

NC.1.2.1 When appropriate, data from the patient's significant other(s) are included in the assessment.

NC.1.3 Each patient's nursing care is based on identified nursing diagnoses and/or patient care needs and patient care standards, and is consistent with the therapies of other disciplines.*

NC.1.3.1 The patient and/or significant other(s) are involved in the patient's care, as appropriate.

NC.1.3.2 Nursing staff members collaborate, as appropriate, with physicians and other clinical disciplines in making decisions regarding each patient's need for nursing care.

NC.1.3.3 Throughout the patient's stay, the patient and, as appropriate, his/her significant other(s) receive education specific to the patient's health care needs.*

NC.1.3.3.1 In preparation for discharge, continuing care needs are assessed and referrals for such care are documented in the patient's medical record.

NC.1.3.4 The patient's medical record includes documentation of*

NC.1.3.4.1 the initial assessments and reassessments;

NC.1.3.4.2 the nursing diagnoses and/or patient care needs,

NC.1.3.4.3 the interventions identified to meet the patient's nursing care needs;

NC.1.3.4.4 the nursing care provided;

NC.1.3.4.5 the patient's response to, and the outcomes of, the care provided;

NC.1.3.4.6 the abilities of the patient and/or, as appropriate, his/her significant other(s) to manage continuing care needs after discharge.

NC.1.3.5 Nursing care data related to patient assessments, the nursing care planned, nursing interventions, and patient outcomes are permanently integrated into the clinical information system (for example, the medical record).*

NC.1.3.5.1 Nursing care data can be identified and retrieved from the clinical information system.

Standard

NC.5 The nurse executive and other nursing leaders participate with leaders from the governing body, management, medical staff, and clinical areas in the hospital's decision-making structures and processes.*

Required Characteristics

NC.5.5 The nurse executive, or a designee(s), participates in evaluating, selecting, and integrating health care technology and information management systems that support patient care needs and the efficient utilization of nursing resources.*

NC.5.5.1 The use of efficient interactive information management systems for nursing, other clinical (for example, dietary, pharmacy, physical therapy) and nonclinical information is facilitated wherever appropriate.

APPENDIX

B

Glossary of Commonly Used Abbreviations

abd.	abdomen, abdominal	CHF	congestive heart failure
a.c.	before meals	chol.	cholesterol
AC	anterior chamber	cldy.	cloudy
ACTH	adrenal corticotropic hormone	cm.	centimeter
ADL	activities of daily living	CNS	central nervous system
ad lib.	as desired	c/o	complains of
adm.	admission	CO_2	carbon dioxide
AF	atrial fibrillation	cont.	continued
AK	above knee	COPD	chronic obstructive pulmonary disease
alb.	albumin	C + P	cystoscopy and panendoscopy or pyelogram
AMA	against medical advice	CPK	creatine phosphokinase
amp.	amputation; ampule	C + S	culture and sensitivity
amt	amount	CSF	cerebrospinal fluid
ASCVD	arteriosclerotic cardiovascular disease	CT	clotting time
ASD	atrial septal defect	CVP	central venous pressure
ASHD	arteriosclerotic heart disease	cx.	cervix
as tol.	as tolerated	D/C	discontinued
AX	axillary	D + C	dilation and curettage
BCBS	Blue Cross and Blue Shield	decr.	decreased, diminished
b.i.d.	twice a day	Derm	dermatology
bil.	bilirubin	diag.	diagnosis
BK	below knee	dias.	diastolic
bl. cult.	blood culture	diff.	differential (blood count)
BM	bowel movement	disc.	discontinued
BMR	basal metabolism rate	disch.	discharged
BP	blood pressure	DOA	dead on arrival
BPH	benign prostatic hypertrophy	DOE	dyspnea on exertion
BRP	bathroom privileges	DP	dorsalis pedis (pulse)
BSC	bedside commode	drsg.	dressing
BUN	blood urea nitrogen	DSD	dry sterile dressing
Bx	biopsy	DT's	delirium tremens
cc	cubic centimeter	Dx	diagnosis
c	with	E	enema
CA	cancer or carcinoma	ECG, EKG	electrocardiogram
cath.	catheterize, catheterization	ECHO virus	enterocytopathogenic human orphan virus
caut.	cauterize, cauterization	EDC	estimated date of confinement
CBC	complete blood count	EEG	electroencephalogram
CC	chief complaint	EMG	electromyogram

ENT	ears, nose, throat	lymphs	lymphocytes
eos.	eosinophil	meds.	medicines
epith.	epithelium	mEq	milliequivalents
EST	electroshock therapy	mg, mgm	milligram
exam.	examination	MI	myocardial infarction
exp.	expiration	MOM	milk of magnesia
FB	foreign body	multivits	multivitamins
FBS	fasting blood sugar	Na+	sodium
FF	force fluids	neg.	negative
FH	family history	Neuro	neurology
FSH	follicle-stimulating hormone	noc	night
FTND	full-term normal delivery	noct.	nocturnal
FUO	fever of unknown origin	no., #	number
Fx	fracture	NPO	nothing by mouth
GBS	gallbladder series	NS	normal saline
GC	gonococcal, gonococcus	NSR	normal sinus rhythm
gr.	grain	N+V, N/V	nausea and vomiting
grav.	gravity	O_2	oxygen
gtts.	drops	OD	right eye
Gyn	gynecology	oint.	ointment
H_2O	water	o.j.	orange juice
HBP	high blood pressure	OM	otitis media
hct.	hematocrit	OOB	out of bed
HEENT	head, eyes, ears, nose, throat	OR	operating room
hemi	hemiparesis/half	Ortho	orthopedics
hgb.	hemoglobin	OS	left eye
HH	hiatus hernia	OU	each eye
HHA	home health aide agency	oz.	ounce
HOH	hard of hearing	p	after
hr	hour	P	pulse
h.s.	hour of sleep at bedtime	P+A	percussion and auscultation
Hx	history	PAT	paroxysmal atrial tachycardia
I+D	incision and drainage	PBI	protein-bound iodine
IHSS	idiopathic hypertrophic subaortic stenosis	p.c.	after meals
IM	intramuscular(ly)	Ped	pediatrics
incl.	include, including	PERLA	pupils equal, react to light and accommodation
incr.	increase, increasing		
I+O	intake and output	PH	past history
IQ	intelligence quotient	PI	present illness
irreg.	irregular	PID	pelvic inflammatory disease
irrig.	irrigate	p.o.	by mouth
IV	intravenous(ly)	post	after
IVP	intravenous pyelogram	postop.	postoperative
kg.	kilogram	preop.	preoperative
KUB	kidney, ureter, bladder	prep.	prepare (usually refers to skin prep.)
KVO	keep vein open		
L	left	p.r.n.	as needed
lab.	laboratory	prot.	protein (TP = total protein)
lat.	lateral	pro. time	prothrombin time
lax.	laxative	Psych	psychiatry, psychology
LDH	lactic dehydrogenase	pt.	patient
liqs.	liquids	PVCs	premature ventricular contraction
LLL	left lower lobe	PVD	peripheral vascular disease
LLQ	left lower quadrant	q	every
LMP	last menstrual period	q.d.	every day
LOA	leave of absence	q2h	every 2 hours
LOC	level of consciousness	q3h	every 3 hours
LP	lumbar puncture	q4h	every 4 hours
LUL	left upper lobe	q.i.d.	four times a day
LUQ	left upper quadrant	q.n.	every night
		q.n.s.	quantity not sufficient

q.o.d.	every other day	Surg	surgery, surgical
q.s.	quantity sufficient	sympat.	symphathetic
quant.	quantitative, quantity	sympt.	symptom
R	right, respiration, rectal	syst.	systolic
RA	rheumatoid arthritis	Sx	signs or symptoms
reg.	regular	tbs.	tablespoon
rehab.	rehabilitation	TIA	transient ischemic attacks
resp.	respirations	t.i.d.	three times a day
retics	reticulocytes	TO	telephone order
RLL	right lower lobe	tol.	tolerated
RLQ	right lower quadrant	TPR	temperature, pulse, respirations
RML	right middle lobe	tsp.	teaspoon
R/O	rule out	TUR	transurethral resection
ROM	range of motion	Tx	treatment, therapy; transfusion
ROS	review of systems	U	unit
RR	recovery room	ung.	ointment
RRE	round, regular, and equal (pupils)	URI	upper respiratory infection
RUL	right upper lobe	Urol	urology
RUQ	right upper quadrant	UTI	urinary tract infection
Rx	therapy or treatment	VD	venereal disease
s	without	vit.	vitamin
S&A	sugar & acetone	VS, V/S	vital signs
sed. rt.	erythrocyte sedimentation rate	VT	ventricular tachycardia
SGOT	serum glutamic oxaloacetic transaminase	WC, w/c	wheel chair
SGPT	serum glutamic pyruvic transaminase	WDWN	well-developed, well-nourished
SOB	short of breath	WNL	within normal limits
s.o.s.	one if necessary	wt.	weight
spec.	specimen	X	times
sp. gr.	specific gravity	X-match	cross-match
SR	systems review	♀	female
SSE	soap suds enema	♂	male
ST	speech therapy, speech therapist	>	greater than
staph.	staphylococcus	<	less than
stat.	immediately	↑	increase
STD	sexually transmitted disease	↓	decrease
strep.	streptococcus	=	equals
supp.	suppository, suppurative		

PRACTICE SESSION
ANSWERS

CHAPTER 1

1. American Civil War—Called attention to the need to provide humane care in organized settings.

    The Depression—Scarce jobs; underemployment of nurses; decline in private duty work.

    Federal Emergency Relief Act (1933) and Social Security Act (1935)—Increased job opportunities for nurses.

    World War II—Introduction of the LPN and volunteers in hospitals to replace RNs who enlisted; explosion of medical technology and knowledge; increasing use of antibiotics; increased need for nurses. **Functional method** of nursing care delivery.

    Hill-Burton Act (1946)—Increased the number and distribution of hospitals and increased the need for nurses.

    1950s—Development of the associate degree program in nursing by Mildred Montag increased access to nursing education and created another level of nurse.

    Introduction of **team method** of nursing care delivery.

    1960s—Federal legislation creating Medicare and Medicaid increased access to physicians and hospital care for older and disabled Americans.

    ANA position paper—Recommended the baccalaureate degree as the entry level for nurses, creating pressure on hospital nursing programs.

    1970s—ANA *Standards of Nursing Practice* published. AHA publication of the *Patient's Bill of Rights*.

    1980s—introduction of **primary nursing** by Marie Manthey.

    Shortage of RNs.

    Introduction of **prospective payment** for hospital care led to decreased length of stay, increased patient acuity, financial pressures on hospitals, reintroduction of assistive levels of care givers.

    Identification of **magnet hospitals**.

    1990s—Development/resurrection of nursing delivery models. Decentralization of hospital organizations.

2. Late 19th century—Direct reporting to the patient's physician; minimal narrative charting. *Total patient care.*

    Pre World War II—Narrative nursing notes in a separate part of the record.

    1960s—Development of **nursing process** affected the content and organization of documentation.

    1970s—National Joint Practice Commission recommended collaborative nurse–physician practice and joint documentation on progress notes.

    Increasing number of intensive care units led to development of **flow sheets**.

    ANA *Standards* addressed documentation.

    AHA *Patient's Bill of Rights*—addressed privacy and confidentiality.

    1980s—Clinical specialization and development of standards for specialties in nursing.

    1990s—Computerization of hospital systems including the patient's record; bedside entry of data.

    Charting by exception. Increased attention to clinical nursing research dependent on accurate patient data.

4. **Total patient care**—Nurse reports the patient's condition to the charge nurse, who gives report to the oncoming nurse/shift. Report on individual patients may be taped for review by the next shift.

    Functional nursing—The charge nurse receives report on the tasks completed for each patient, patients reactions, etc. Report is received from staff assigned to medications and treatments. The charge nurse reports to the oncoming shift.

    Team nursing—A designated team leader and team members receive report from the charge nurse or team leader of the previous shift and report to the charge nurse at the end of their shift on assignments completed and patient status.

    Primary nursing—Each patient has a primary nurse who gives report to her associate nurses and receives reports from them. All communication involves the primary nurse, who has 24-hour accountability for the care delivered.

    Case management—Extends the communication and accountability pattern of primary nursing to the health care team, who receive and give reports to the case manager who then focuses on the patient's progress toward preestablished goals in a plan of care or "care map" called a "critical path." The care plan is shared with the family.

5. Leadership: the ability to influence others toward a course of action; a process of interpersonal interaction based on communication and the development of mutual goals. Admirable leaders are often described as expert, dependable, respectful of others, open to ideas, autonomous, accountable, responsible, flexible, skilled communicators, effective change agents, likeable, able to bring out the best in people.

One can acquire these attributes through observation, education (formal course work, seminars, reading, preceptorships), mentoring, and experience.

CHAPTER 2

1. Beliefs, values, self-esteem, perception, empathy, attitude, gender
2. Nonverbal communication
3. Spoken or written word, or, a language is used
4. Intimacy and connectedness; maintaining independence
5. Interpersonal communication
6. Professional relationships and collaboration
7. Reporting, recording, interviewing, negotiating
8. Communicate between staff and administration, maintain leadership power, evaluate employee performance, manage conflict
9. Content of the message and the relationship of the individuals involved
10. Communication

CHAPTER 3

Fill in the Blank

1. Kardex
2. Transfer form
3. Outcome sheet
4. Interdisciplinary communication
5. Communication, legal protection, reimbursement, education, quality assurance (or quality improvement), and research
6. Standardized flow sheets
7. Comparison of data to judge indications of improvement or decline or to show data within normal range for that patient
8. Teaching plans
9. Gathering certain information for fast retrieval and comparison
10. Nursing information system

Matching

1. g	9. h
2. b	10. n
3. i	11. c
4. f	12. l
5. k	13. m
6. j	14. a
7. d	15. e
8. o	

Multiple Choice

1. d
2. a
3. c
4. b
5. d

Challenge for Critical Thinking

1. Advantages
   Key words to document specific data
   Easy retrieval, saves time
   Fast comparison of data
   Disadvantages
   No room for patient individualization
   Can be illegible if write outside lines or write too small
   Checklist may cause some nurses not to write descriptive narrative
   To minimize disadvantages: Think about what important and patient–specific observations, descriptions, and explanations should be documented. Make a conscious effort to document important narrative on the back of flow sheets where indicated. Write only between the lines and write legibly.
2. Advantages
   Legibility
   Accuracy
   Timely, updated information
   Fast communication between departments and more than one caregiver can simultaneously see the chart
   Disadvantages
   Computer malfunction (downtime)
   May seem impersonal to patient
   Cost—computers are expensive and can be broken
   Confidentiality can be threatened
   To minimize disadvantages: In advance of a computer malfunction, learn procedures to retrieve data and to document data. Make a concerted effort when interviewing a patient to make eye contact while talking or listening and concentrate on the patient, not on the computer. Learn how to use and handle computers to avoid breakage; for example, always keep food and drink away from keyboards. Never give anyone or allow someone to see your identification code for computer entry.
3. A student can look at the design of the system, what forms are used, and where data are shared into other parts of the clinical record. A student should read how to care for the hardware; learn the software screen progression and how to move from one screen to another; learn what the icons or processing buttons mean; learn how to avoid common errors; watch a demonstration of what to do or whom to call when an error is made or a problem occurs. Learn keyboard skills, participate in a formal training program followed by supervised practice, before using the computer on the nursing unit.
4. More than a task, nursing documentation should be based on the nursing process. Therefore, forms on

which nurses document should parallel or relate to each step of the nursing process (see Figure 3–1). Nursing documentation facilitates effective care because a patient need can be tracked from assessment, through identification of problems, care plan, implementation and evaluation in correlation with the nursing process. Nursing documentation is integral in communication, legal protection, education, research, quality assurance and cost-effective care. The quality of documentation indicates the quality and effectiveness of care.

5. Communication because all clinical decisions (diagnoses, plans, and interventions for care) are based on what is communicated about the patient.

Learning to Document

1. The first and second paragraph of the case study, and the current prescribed insulin and diet.
2. See display, Sample Kardex, on page 242.
3. See display, Sample Vital Sign Graph, on page 243.

CHAPTER 4

Fill in the Blank

1. Assessment documentation
2. Patient is admitted for care
3. Determining a nursing diagnosis
4. Patient acuity
5. Nursing history and physical examination documentation
6. Subjective
7. Objective
8. Nurses may ask different questions
9. Condition
10. Reassessments

Matching Definitions

1. c
2. e
3. a
4. d
5. b

Matching Types of Data

1. b		6. b
2. a		7. b
3. a		8. c
4. b		9. b
5. a		10. a

Multiple Choice

1. d
2. d
3. a
4. c
5. b

Challenge for Critical Thinking

1. The physical examination can verify assessment data to determine health or illness and nursing diagnoses.
2. Important data would be missing for clinical decisions regarding communicable disease risk, appropriateness of level of growth and development, pattern of communication, assistance needed to maintain normal routine in eating and sleeping and toileting, and emotional security needs.
3. By assessing patient and family learning abilities, knowledge of a problem, and emotional state, a nurse can formulate a teaching plan. Some factors to consider are level of education, any trouble with memory or hearing or vision, and any functional disabilities that would prohibit performing a particular skill.
4. Difficulty walking, or difficulty adjusting to walking with a cane or walker; neurologic impairment that affects balance or feeling; dizziness due to medication or alcohol; confusion or agitation; generalized weakness or fatigue from overexertion; previous falls.
5. Distractions in an interview include a noisy setting, people in close proximity who can hear the conversation, unreasonable time constraint, either the interviewer or person interviewed is uncomfortable or distracted, or focus is on a documentation form or computer instead of the person being interviewed.

Learning to Document

1. Criticisms may include not enough focus on patient, or asking closed (yes–no) questions rather than open-ended questions. Some criticisms may include the interviewer taking too long or moving too fast in the interview, interrupting the patient or not giving the patient enough time to organize thoughts, or pausing too long between questions or topics. Finally, not keeping the interview focused on assessment.
2. See display, Skin Risk Assessment Form, on page 244.
3. See display, Neurologic Flow Sheet, on page 245.

CHAPTER 5

Fill in the Blank

1. Care plan
2. Nursing diagnoses
3. An actual health problem
4. Setting appropriate for expected outcomes and criteria
5. Nursing diagnosis, expected outcomes, nursing interventions
6. Nursing interventions
7. Expected outcome; nursing interventions
8. Listing diagnoses in order of importance
9. Medical diagnosis
10. Individualize

Matching

1. b		4. a
2. c		5. e
3. d		

Identifying Nursing Diagnoses

1. yes
2. no, Diarrhea
3. no, Impaired Physical Mobility
4. no, Activity Intolerance
5. no, Altered Nutrition: Less Than Body Requirements
6. yes
7. yes
8. no, High Risk for Infection
9. no, Impaired Skin Integrity
10. no, Altered Thought Processes

Multiple Choice

1. d
2. d
3. d
4. b
5. a

Challenge for Critical Thinking

1. Nursing diagnosis is a clinical judgment identifying a patient's human response to actual or potential health problems, by which nurses can autonomously intervene to achieve expected outcome. Its components include the actual, potential or high-risk health problem as it relates to the patient's response to illness or injury; the etiology or related information; and signs and symptoms, or identifying characteristics of the problem. Nursing diagnosis is the part of the care plan that identifies patient problems, needs, or concerns.

2. Listing nursing diagnoses in priority brings a list of problems organized by most important first to less important needs. High-priority problems must be addressed to meet immediate needs of the patient or needs that must be met before other related concerns can be addressed. Priority can be categorized by: first, urgent or health threat needs, and all physiologic needs; second, psychological, emotional, and social needs; and last but not least, spiritual needs. This priority can change as the physical and psychosocial condition of a patient changes.

3. Because a care plan shows problems and reasons for care, it supports the need for care and level of care that qualifies for reimbursement. For example, many insurance and government-reimbursed programs require that skilled nursing be needed and the patient shows a potential for improvement following nursing intervention.

4. The care plan must be individualized or customized to the patient, both in describing needs and expected outcomes and in establishing interventions to respond to those specific needs and expected outcomes. Modifications to standardized care plans must be documented to support individualization of care.

5. Pro: The care plan is a communication tool that promotes coordination and continuity of care, reflects accepted standards of care, contributes to concise reporting, and is used in patient acuity determination and staffing.

Con: The separate care plan is time-consuming to write. Takes time away from bedside care and is often the same for patients with the same diagnoses. Physicians don't write medical care plans, so should nurses?

Learning to Document

1. Pain; Impaired Skin Integrity; Knowledge Deficit R/T chemotherapy; Body Image Disturbance; Impaired Home Maintenance Management; Anticipatory Grieving; High Risk for (Spouse) Caregiver Role Strain; Family Coping: Potential for Growth.

2. Within 1 hour of therapy pt will
   a. have improved breath sounds as evidenced by absence of wheezing on auscultation
   b. have reduced hypoxemia as evidence by Pco_2 within normal range
   c. exhibit stable vital signs within normal limits for patient
   d. mobilize sputum as evidence by expectorating mucus
   e. exhibit decrease in anxiety as evidenced by relaxed facial expression and posture and as verbalized by patient

   Before discharge pt will
   a. have absence of upper respiratory infection as evidenced by negative throat culture
   b. establish a plan to quit smoking as evidenced by contacting community resources for relevant programs
   c. identify potential precipitators of asthma attacks and demonstrate strategies to prevent and to respond to acute episodes

3. a. Instruct pt in MI disease process and treatment, including diet
   b. Instruct pt in medication purpose, administration, and side effects
   c. Instruct pt in need and rationale for schedule rest periods and avoidance of stress and overexertion
   d. Encourage pt to verbalize concerns and ask questions about disease and treatment
   e. Refer pt to support group
   f. Refer pt to home health agency for skilled nursing and homemaker support

4. Be sure to include nursing diagnoses listed in priority, expected outcomes with time frame or target dates, and nursing interventions that relate to each expected outcome.

CHAPTER 6

Fill in the Blank

1. Care plan
2. Clinical progress notes
3. Nurse-initiated treatment interventions, physician-initiated treatment interventions, and collaborative interventions
4. Patient outcome
5. Nursing diagnosis, what was assessed, clinical data, intervention(s), and patient outcome or response

6. Date, time, and signature of nurse
7. Who, what, why, when, where, and how
8. Target date or time frame
9. Desired behavior or physical improvement, conditions that verify attainment of expected outcome, and time frame
10. MAR (medication administration record)

Matching

1. b	9. a
2. b	10. b
3. c	11. a
4. a	12. a
5. a	13. b
6. b	14. c
7. b	15. a
8. a	

Multiple Choice

1. a
2. d
3. d
4. d
5. c

Challenge for Critical Thinking

1. Reasons for revision include: patient needs or condition changes; updated medical orders restrict achieving initial goals; desired outcomes are not achieved with appropriate intervention. The patient's condition is constantly changing; as needs change, new goals or outcome criteria should be developed. For example, as a surgical patient meets the goal of walking 15 feet assisted to the bathroom, new outcome criteria may be to walk 50 feet in the hall with assistance, then without assistance. If updated medical orders restrict or prohibit achieving outcomes, criteria must change. For example, if that same surgical patient develops an infection and fever, the physician orders bedrest, and the goal of ambulation must be discontinued temporarily. And last, if outcomes are not achieved, criteria may have to be revised. For example, a patient or family is unable to learn a skill for self-care after discharge. Expected outcomes must always be realistic and attainable.

2. Advantages include fast entry, easy retrieval of information, easier visual comparison of data, and standard language for standard comparisons. Disadvantages include less area for descriptive documentation, inability to customize categories of data collection, and potential for poor legibility if not enough area to write or writing crosses over lines.

3. A nurse compares patient outcomes on nursing notes to the expected outcomes on care plans to document what progress the patient has made.

4. Outcomes are documented either on weekly narrative outcome summary notes, nursing plan outcome record, or criteria-based outcome record. Advantages of outcome records are the same as for flow sheets: rapid data entry and information retrieval. Advantages of criteria-based outcome records are more detailed outcomes and comparison of target (goal) date to resolution (date accomplished) date.

5. Nursing interventions for planned care include assessing specific body systems or functions; administering medication or treatments; teaching the patient or family caregivers; assisting in activities of daily living; supporting respiratory and elimination functions; providing skin care; providing nutrition and hydration; referring to appropriate agencies for care. Nursing interventions are called nursing orders on a care plan when they are nurse–initiated treatments and interventions that the nurse can autonomously initiate and provide. Nursing orders relate to the diagnosis and treatment of human response.

Learning to Document

1. See Comparing Clinical Progress Notes on page 246.
2. See display, Daily Observation Record, on page 247.
3. See display, Treatment Flow Sheet, on page 248.

CHAPTER 7

Fill in the Blank

1. Negligence and malpractice
2. Physicians
3. Release of liability
4. 18
5. Can
6. Chart or care plan
7. Addendum
8. Signed release of information
9. Potential for error
10. Omissions and alterations

Matching

1. b
2. c
3. c
4. c
5. c

Multiple Choice

1. d
2. c
3. a
4. d
5. b

Challenge for Critical Thinking

1. Law and ethics are two forces that help people ensure rights, minimize potential harm, and guide human behavior. Laws are mandatory guidelines people must follow, under obligation of fines or incarceration. Ethics are guidelines based on how we wish people would act, under obligation of consciousness. The "force" of

the law and the "persuasion" of ethics are intertwined in legal issues of reporting and recording. There are four principles of ethics:

- ▲ Autonomy
- ▲ Beneficence
- ▲ Justice
- ▲ Fidelity

Autonomy is the respect we have for others as human beings, which allows them the right to make judgments and choose actions. The principle of autonomy underlies legal issues of informed consent, advance directives, refusal of treatment, privacy, and confidentiality in access to records.

Beneficence is the duty to do good to others, to help them, to their interests, while refraining from harming others (nonmaleficence). This principle underlies discontinuing service and abandonment.

2. Document a postscript or an addendum if you've forgotten to document important information after signing your name on a clinical note entry. Do not add information after you've learned that a lawsuit is filed, or another nurse asks you to document for her after she has left the nursing unit after her shift.

3. The following factors pose significant risk for falls: decreased level of mobility; three or more medical diagnoses, especially cardiovascular or musculoskeletal disease; use of three or more drugs daily, particularly cardiovascular, antihypertensive, tranquilizer, or antidepressant drugs; decreased level of consciousness; and a history of falls.

   A measure to minimize legal risk regarding these factors is to document in the patient record an assessment of a patient's level of consciousness and balance, mobility assessments, and precautions taken to prevent falls (assistance or restraints). Measures to minimize the patient's risk of falling include communication among caregivers of a patient's high risk for falls; nurse–physician collaborative assessment of medications and medication interactions that affect level of consciousness; nurse–physical therapist collaborative assessment of assistive devices (cane, walker, wheelchair, restraints) to prevent falls; and patient education in safety measures to assist in preventing falls.

4. Certain characteristics of documentation content that pose a legal risk include the following:
   - ▲ The content is not in accordance with professional or health care organization standards.
   - ▲ The content is not appropriate to patient needs.
   - ▲ The content does not include description(s) of situations that are out of the ordinary.
   - ▲ The content overgeneralizes patient assessment of nursing intervention.
   - ▲ The content is not timely or is chronologically disorganized.
   - ▲ The content is incomplete or inconsistent.
   - ▲ The content does not include appropriate medical orders.
   - ▲ The content implies a potential or actual risk situation.
   - ▲ The content implies attitudinal bias.

   (Answer should indicate two of the above characteristics, with examples.)

5. Certain common characteristics of documentation mechanics that pose a legal risk include:
   - ▲ Lines between entries
   - ▲ Countersigning documentation
   - ▲ Tampering
   - ▲ Different handwriting or obliterations
   - ▲ Illegibility
   - ▲ Dates and time of entries omitted or inconsistently documented
   - ▲ Improper nurse signature or unidentifiable initials

   (Answer should indicate two of the above characteristics, with examples.)

Learning to Document

1. a. 10 am pt discharged via w/c with husband
    b. Wound cleansed with PhisoDerm and DSD applied.
    c. Pt c/o of constant, dull +2 pain in RLQ of abdomen.
    d. Pt refused isoniazid because it "upsets his stomach."
    e. Range of B/P within past week is 140/90 to 120/86.
    f. Pt c/o not hungry. Ate 75% of breakfast.
    g. Patient ambulating 30 ft in hall unassisted without SOB.
    h. Dr. Jones visited at 4:00 pm, ordered stat Percodan for pain.
    i. Pt going home tomorrow, Soc. Serv. contacted for home health agency referral for physical therapist and home health aide.
    j. Pt wants meals delivered at 8 am, 12 noon, and 6 pm; wants pain med within 5 min of ringing call bell; and does not want to be awakened for 7:30 am routine vital signs.

2. Incident reports should be written in any unusual occurrence. A patient can claim permanent damage even years later, long after the details of the incident are forgotten. This incident report protects the nurse and home health agency; most insurance company contracts require documentation of all unusual occurrences, even if no immediate injury is apparent.

3. See display, Patient Incident Report, on page 249.

CHAPTER 8

Fill in the Blank

1. Communication and continuity of care
2. Transfer
3. Discharge
4. Teaching plan and combined teaching plan/summary
5. Identifying patient and caregiver needs
6. The disease and its treatment
7. Written and visual patient education materials
8. Simple to complex
9. Prospective payment
10. Discharged quicker and sicker

Matching

1. a
2. b
3. c
4. a
5. c
6. b
7. a & b
8. c
9. a
10. b

Multiple Choice

1. e
2. e
3. b
4. e
5. c

Challenge for Critical Thinking

1. Advantages include
   time-saving
   plans are complete
   plans contain cues for important data to document
   standardized language is easier to communicate and evaluate
   Disadvantages include
   plans are standard and not individualized
   language can be restrictive
   may not be enough room to write explanatory narrative.
   More than one standardized plan may be needed and plans would therefore be stapled together; the two plans may contain repetitive interventions and would need to be crossed out.
2. Education material: talking books, video cassettes, audio cassettes, computer programs, pamphlets, books.
   Teaching methods: discussion, role play, demonstration.
   The type of teaching method should be documented on the teaching plan, and the education material used for patient instruction should be documented, but the teaching plan or summary stays essentially the same. There is no significant difference in the plan when a nurse uses different methods or different resources.
3. Learning needs were not ranked in priority of importance; learning needs were not ranked in priority of sequence of basic to more complex; learning strengths and weaknesses were not assessed; the patient and family were not included in setting goals.
   To avoid these pitfalls nurses can use a standardized teaching form that includes on the form categories of strengths and weakness (or barriers to learning or special needs for learning) and patient and family inclusion in development of care plan. Ranking needs in priority of importance can be accomplished by using the sequence of physical, psychological, emotional, social, and spiritual needs categories. Role playing with another student will reinforce how to structure basic learning, then more complex learning; a sequence that facilitates ranking basis to complex is what, why, components of what to teach, precautions, how to respond in certain situations. In teaching skills, be sure to teach principles

and rationale, then demonstrate and have patient return demonstrate the skill, with guidance, and finally without coaching. Give patient education materials for reinforcement. Finally, complete documentation of patient teaching, outcomes, and response.
4. Medical orders for dressing change; status of wound including description with objective measurements. Information that would answer the following questions: Has Mrs. J. had any instruction in dressing change? What type of antibiotic has been prescribed and has Mrs. J. been taught about medication, administration, and side effects? What has the patient's and husband's response been to the body image change? Does Mrs. J. need and have family support or other caregiver for homemaker support during recuperation?
5. What activities of daily living can Mr. W. perform independently, or with assistance, and what are those for which he is completely dependent on caregivers? What speech problems does Mr. W. have, and does it include expressive or receptive aphasia? What means of communication is being used (such as a communication board) if Mr. J. cannot speak? What size Foley catheter? Has bladder training been started?

Learning to Document

1. *Cognitive learning outcome(s)*: Pt able to explain action and need for insulin; able to describe insulin injection procedure; able to list side effects of insulin; able to list rotation sites for insulin administration.
   Psychomotor learning outcome: Pt able to demonstrate appropriate insulin administration without coaching.
   Affective learning outcome: Pt able to inject insulin without apprehension or disabling anxiety.
2. See display, Discharge Planning Form, on page 250.
3. Among other information, key phrases documented on the discharge summary would include: identified needs of patient have been met (specify). Pt and family notified in writing of last day of service on (date). Pt's primary physician ordered (when required such as Medicare) or notified (in private care) of discontinuing of service. Appropriate referrals or recommendations made for future care (specify). Telephone numbers given for immediate access to health care or health care advice (specify).

CHAPTER 9

Fill in the Blank

1. Narrative nursing notes
2. Data base
3. Problem list
4. Chronologic
5. Process
6. Discharge summaries
7. The nursing process
8. Separate nursing care plan
9. Focus
10. Diagnostic related groups (medical diagnoses)

Matching Format and Rule

1. a
2. b
3. b
4. b

Matching Characteristic and Format

1. c
2. a
3. e
4. b
5. d

Multiple Choice

1. d
2. d
3. d
4. c
5. a

Challenge for Critical Thinking

1. Professionally, nurses are responsible and accountable for the care they provide; that care is communicated by documentation. Determining documentation methods defines how the professional nurse documents care and organizes nursing information for quality assurance, reimbursement, legal protection, research, and certifying and accrediting audits. As professionals, nurses should determine control over how they provide care and control over the method by which they communicate that care.
2. Different areas in the hospital have different levels of care, types of patients, and length of stay. Therefore, different areas have different and specific documentation needs. For example, the emergency department sees a variety of patients for a short period of time, so brief narrative notes may be the best method of documentation. Intensive care has numerous objective, technologic measurements that must be frequently documented, so flow sheets are a necessity for comparison of data; and the PIE system eliminates constantly needing to revise a care plan as the patient's condition rapidly changes. (There are many other examples.)
3. (Refer to text and Table 9–1.)
4. (Support preferences with advantages listed in the text. Original rationale for preference may also be acceptable, such as easy format to learn or easy to remember or fast to document.)
5. New government regulations, new reimbursement methods, new unit manager or top administration change, legal problem involving documentation, quality assurance deficiencies, and preparing for accreditation.

Learning to Document

1. See following displays on pages 250 to 252: Narrative Nursing Note, Problem-Oriented (SOAPE) Notes, and Focus Patient Care Notes.
2. See display, Critical Path Sample Answer, on page 253.

CHAPTER 10

Fill in the Blanks

1. Continuity of care and problem-solving
2. Can be based on the nursing process, legal and ethical principles apply, standards of care apply, principles of communication apply
3. Interest, attentiveness, respect, professional demeanor, sensitivity, acute perception
4. Preparation, or planning or organizing the report
5. Concentrate on what is being heard, eliminate distraction
6. Charge nurse reporter, group shared report, person-to-person report
7. Quality of the machine, the acoustics of the room
8. Physician–nurse, nurse–nurse, multidisciplinary team
9. Patient needs related to the specialty consultant
10. Veracity and confidentiality

Matching

1. e
2. d
3. c
4. b
5. a

Challenge for Critical Thinking

1. a. Background data and reason for care
   b. Primary medical and nursing diagnoses
   c. Explanation and status of current priority problems
   d. Changes in condition or in treatments
   e. Effective interventions or treatments of priority problems
   f. Patient outcomes and response to priority problems
   g. Progress toward expected outcomes in discharge planning
   h. Priority interventions of a timely nature
   For continuity of care a nurse needs to know (c) nursing interventions that have been implemented and are effective so that she can continue those interventions; and (h) interventions that are due so that progress can continue on a time-based plan.
2. The nurse would be liable due to negligence.
3. Walking rounds are most effective in observing and receiving information from the patient when the following conditions exist: the patient is not receiving a treatment; the patient is not experiencing discomfort, the patient is not eating a meal, the patient is not mentally preparing for the doctor's visit, the patient feels presentable in terms of appearance; and the patient is not anxious to get to the morning grooming routine.
4. Nursing camaraderie and stress reduction are always positive, but eating or a party atmosphere during report is distracting. Have a brief report, then bring out the food. Those nurses who have finished the shift may stay a short while, and nurses coming on the shift can enjoy the treats briefly and then during breaks.

5. (Refer to the section titled Change of Shift Report under the heading of Types of Reporting.)

6. Law and ethics are two forces that help people ensure rights, minimize potential harm, and guide human behavior. The force of the law and the persuasion of ethics are intertwined in legal issues of reporting. The laws are clear on certain issues relating to reporting. Legal transgressions are punishable by fine or imprisonment. Ethical considerations in reporting are not as clear, but they provide guidelines to determine what is right or best in a difficult situation. Ethical transgressions are subject to a person's conscience or occasionally to decisions rendered by a professional ethics committee.

7. Labeling patients by diagnoses and room number speeds up a report but depersonalizes a patient. The disadvantage of depersonalization far outweighs the benefit of speed. Also, nurses may feel that the reporter doesn't have a caring concern for patients, and they may also subconsciously withdraw from individualized and close nurse–patient relationships.

8. (Refer to the section titled Veracity under the heading Legal and Ethical Considerations in Reporting.)

9. Discern the nurse's professional responsibility in a situation, anticipate situations of concern, and limit liability by preventative action.

10. In both reporting and recording:
    - ▲ Information should be accurate, concise, organized, pertinent, current, and complete.
    - ▲ Language should be direct, simple, and geared to the level of the receiver.
    - ▲ Focus should be on the interchange and understanding of the information exchanged.
    - ▲ Attitudes or judgmental language should not enter into professional communication.
    - ▲ Nonprofessional, obscure, or inflammatory terms should be avoided.
    - ▲ Information should be presented in accordance to relationship of data; chronologic occurrence; or for summaries, in order of nursing process or critical decision-making.

Learning Skills in Reporting

1. Yes to the first and third question, refer to Similarity of Reporting Process and the Nursing Process. There should be a logical progression of data in the report that parallels the nursing process, and therefore reflects and supports the critical thinking and clinical decision-making that has occurred in the process.

2. This should be reported to the charge nurse (or head nurse) and to the physician. The truth should be told as the situation occurred. Depending on the organization's policy, an incident report may be required. Nursing notes should state that water was given and the patient vomited ('against medical orders' need not be written); the condition of the patient including vital signs should be documented q1h until the patient is stable, to show no patient injury occurred.

3. Usual schedule including naps, meals, snacks, and drinks; time and content of the next meal; preferred eating habits (finger food, sippie cup); usual ritual and favorite toys to settle her for a nap; how often diaper usually needs to be changed; her usual behavior; any behavioral indications of a problem; best way to console her if she cries (most babies like to be rocked or held and walked; some still use a pacifier at that age). A nurse would need the same information, but much of it would be documented in the initial assessment. The report should emphasize favorite juices and drinks to force fluids; how to keep the patient playing quietly to maintain bed rest; how the patient's behavior has been and any behavior that indicates pain or other symptoms. Visitors and what they are doing to help can also be important for the oncoming nurse to plan care.

4. Dr. Smith, this is Mary Miller, St. Thomas University student nurse. Your patient Sarah Sommers with the concussion and right fractured ulna is complaining her right hand feels tingly and the cast feels tight at her wrist. Her fingers are pale and cold and have 2+ edema. Capillary refill is over 3 sec. What would you like us to do? (Then Mary would repeat the order to have the cast reapplied. She will thank the doctor, give him an opportunity to ask any other questions or give any further orders and let him hang up first.)

5. 4/2/93 10:05 am t.c. to Dr. Smith to report pt c/o of R hand tingle and cast feeling tight at wrist. Reported fingers pale, cold, 2+ edema, capillary refill >3 sec. Doctor ordered reapply cast STAT. Cast room contacted and pt transported at 10:10 am.

6–10. Refer to chapter text to develop and critique reports and to compare advantages of different types of reports.

SAMPLE KARDEX

Vital signs Temp O R AX B/P Pulse & resp	9. am	Respiratory care	N/A
Resuscitation Status—CPR?	yes	Diet	1600 ADA
Living Will?	no	Fluids	64 oz / day
Notify physician if...	FBS ↑ 200	Weight	145 lbs
Sensory deficit	-0-	Treatments	-0-
Communication method and barriers	-0-	I & O	yes
Safety measures	Walk with assist to prevent falls	Consult/Regarding Date	soc. serv anxiety 3/25
Activity	OOB as tol.	Referrals Date	XYZ Home Health 3/25
Hygiene care Time preference	Shower c̄ stool after bkfst	Isolation	Date order: NA Date stop:
Bowel continence	yes	Bladder continence	Yes
Assistance needed in ADL	weak — help bathe & dress	Skin care	Dry — apply lotion prn

DIAGNOSTIC TESTS

Date Ordered	Test	Schedule Date	Preparation
3/25/93	qd FBS	3/26 thru 3/28	npo after 1200

Allergies ___ NKA ___

Diagnoses ___ Diabetes Mellitus ___

Physician ___ John Morris, MD ___ Phone ___ 100-1111 ___

Name ___ Cora Andrews ___ Room ___ 234 ___ Bed ___ 2 ___

SAMPLE VITAL SIGNS GRAPH

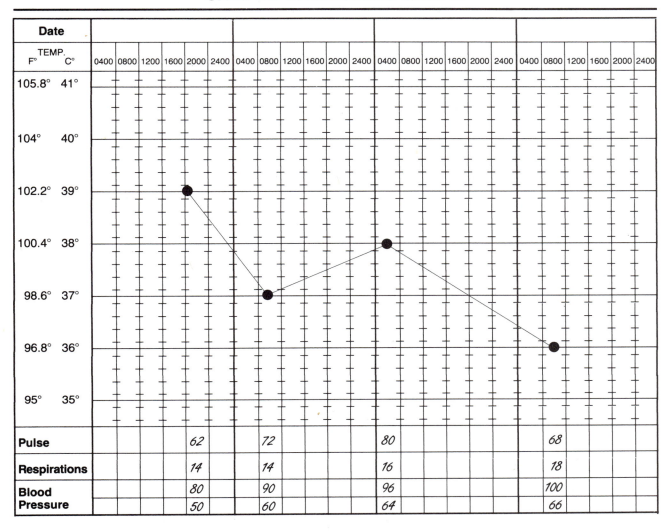

Date																									
TEMP. F° C°		0400	0800	1200	1600	2000	2400	0400	0800	1200	1600	2000	2400	0400	0800	1200	1600	2000	2400	0400	0800	1200	1600	2000	2400
Pulse					62				72						80						68				
Respirations					14				14						16						18				
Blood Pressure					80				90						96						100				
					50				60						64						66				

SKIN RISK ASSESSMENT FORM

Identify any patient at risk to develop skin conditions assessing the eight clinical condition parameters and assigning a score. Patient with a score of 8 or above should be considered at risk to develop skin conditions. Initiate prevention protocol.

Directions: Choose the number for each parameter that applies to the patient's status. Total the eight numbers to determine the patient's risk potential.

Clinical Condition Parameters	Dates & Year			
	9/30			
	Scores			
General Physical Condition (health problem)				
Good (minor) ... 0				
Fair (major but stable) ... 1	2			
Poor (chronic/serious not stable) ... 2				
Level of Consciousness (to commands)				
Alert (responds readily) ... 0				
Lethargic (slow to respond) ... 1				
Confused ... 2	0			
Semicomatose (responds only to verbal or painful stimuli) ... 3				
Comatose (no response to stimuli) ... 4				
Activity				
Ambulate without assistance ... 0				
Ambulate with assistance ... 1	3			
Chairfast ... 2				
Bedfast ... 3				
Mobility (extremities)				
Full active range ... 0				
Limited movement with assistance ... 1	3			
Moves only with assistance ... 2				
Immobile ... 3				
Incontinence (bowel and/or bladder)				
None ... 0				
Occasional (<2 per 24 h) ... 1	0			
Usually Incontinent (urine & stool, incl. catheter) ... 2				
Double Incontinence (urine & stool) ... 3				
Nutrition (for age and size)				
Good (eats/drinks adequately 3/4 of meal) ... 0				
Fair (eats/drinks less than 3/4 of meal) N/G, G, TUBE OR TPN ... 1	1			
Poor (unable/refuses to eat/drink—less than 1/2) ... 2				
Skin/Tissue Status				
Good (well nourished/skin intact) ... 0				
Fair (poorly nourished/skin intact) ... 1	1			
Poor (skin not intact) ... 2				
Predisposing Disease (diabetes, COPD, anemia, etc.)				
Absent ... 0				
1 disease present ... 1	1			
2 diseases present ... 2				
3 or more diseases present ... 3				
Total	11			
Signature & Title	Mod			

Suggested Preventive Protocol

8–10 Mild	Monitor skin closely. Turn & reposition q2h
11–15 Mod.	Special mattress; Pressure-relieving devices; elbow heel protectors, if indicated. Dietary intervention
16–22 Severe	Monitor skin daily. Lab work if indicated. Treatments as ordered.

Resident Name _____ Mynka, Myra _____ Room # ___ 101 ___   I.D. Number ___ 111-22-3333

NEUROLOGIC FLOW SHEET

PUPILS: SIZE 1m 2m 3m 4m 5m 6m

	Time	12:00 p	1:00	2:00	3:00	4:00											
Level of Consciousness	Alert																
	Oriented X3					X											
	Confused	X	X	X	X												
	Arouse to light pain																
	Arouse to deep pain																
	Comatose																
Pattern of Speech	Coherent					X											
	Incoherent																
	Slurred speech	X	X	X	X												
	Aphasic																
Motor Response	Facial symmetry																
	Obeys commands					X											
	Localizes pain																
	Withdraw from pain																
	Flaccid	X	X	X	X												
Motor Strength 0 to +4 Absent Strong	Right arm	0	0	0	0	0											
	Right leg	0	0	0	0	0											
	Left arm	0	0	0	0	+2											
	Left leg	0	0	0	0	+2											
	Equal grasp	0	0	0	0	0											
Pupils (see chart)	PERRLA	X	X	X	X	X											
	Right (size)	3	3	3	3	3											
	Left (size)	5	5	5	5	3											

COMPARING CLINICAL PROGRESS NOTES

Note Components	SOAPIE	PIE	DAR
Data	SO		D
Problem	A	P	
Intervention	PI	I	A
Evaluation	E	E	E

DAILY OBSERVATION FORM

ROBINSON MEMORIAL HOSPITAL
Patient Progress Notes

DAILY OBSERVATION RECORD

Date: *April 2, 1993*

								LEGEND	PULSE GRADING
B E H A V I O R / **L. O. C.**	Time:	*8:00 am*						P-Person	O-Absent
	Alert:							PL-Place	1+-Easily occuled
	Oriented	(P)(PL) T C	P PL T C	P PL T C	P PL T C	P PL T C		T-Time	2+-Occluded with
	Disoriented							C-Circumstance	mild pressure
	Lethargic	✓						+-Present	3+-Normal
	Unresponsive							––Absent	4+-Bounding
	Cooperative							R-Right	D-Doppler
	Uncooperative							L-Left	
	Anxious								**Patient Teaching**
	Eye Contact	Yes (No)	Yes No	Yes No	Yes No	Yes No			
S K I N	Temp: Warm								
	Hot								
	Cool	✓							
	Cold								
	Moisture: Dry								
	Moist	✓							
	Diaphoretic	✓							
	Turgor: Elastic								
	Non-Elastic								
	Color:	*Pale*							
	Integrity: Intact								
	Impaired								
C A R D I O V A S C U L A R	Heart Sounds: Regular	*70*							
	Irregular								
	Apical Radial Deficit	+ –	+ –	+ –	+ –	+ –		**Team Leader**	
	JVD @ 45	+ –	+ –	+ –	+ –	+ –		**Responsible**	
	Pulses	R L	R L	R L	R L	R L		7-3	
	Temporal								
	Carotid								
	Brachial							3-11	
	Radial	*65*							
	Femoral								
	Post. tibial							11-7	
	Dorsalis pedis								
	Calf tenderness:								
	on palpatation							OR	
	on dorsiflexion								
	Edema:	R L	R L	R L	R L	R L		7ᴬ-7ᴾ	
	Facial								
	ABD								
	Sacral							7ᴾ-7ᴬ	
	Arms								
	Hands	+2 +2							
	Legs	+2 +2							
	Ankles	+3 +3						Other	
	Pedal								

Signatures	EE	Ellen Eggland RN, MN		

Courtesy of Robinson Memorial Hospital, Ravenna, Ohio

TREATMENT FLOW SHEET

DATE _April 2, 1993_   TREATMENT FLOW SHEET

	7ᴬ	8ᴬ	9ᴬ	10ᴬ	11ᴬ	12ᴾ	1ᴾ	2ᴾ	3ᴾ	4ᴾ	5ᴾ	6ᴾ	7ᴾ	8ᴾ	9ᴾ	10ᴾ	11ᴾ	12ᴬ	1ᴬ	2ᴬ	3ᴬ	4ᴬ	5ᴬ	6ᴬ
Nursing Rounds																								
Activity: BR (1), BSC (2), Chair (3), Ambulate c Assist (4), Self Ambulate (5)		4																						
Bath: Self (1), Assist (2), Complete (3), Shower (4)		A																						
Back Care		✓																						
Oral Care																								
Pericare/Foley Care		✓																						
Turn and Reposition R-Right, S-Side, L-Left, B-Back		N/A																						
Bed in Prevention Mode		—																						
Restraints: Soft (1), Vest (2), Wrists (3), Ankles (4), Leathers (5), Remove q8O-check skin condition-then reapply (6), (R) Right, (L) Left		N/A																						
Side Rails: (▲▲), (▲▼), (▼▼)		1																						
Call Light in Reach		✓																						
Antiembolism Hose: Knee High (1), Thigh High (2), ICS (3)		1																						
Urine Color: Straw (1), Amber (2), Pink (3), Red (4), Orange (5), Tea (6), Clear (7), Cloudy (8), Sediment (9), Foley (10), Suprapubic (11), External Cath (12), Incontinent (13)		2 8 10																						
Oxygen		2ℓ																						
Cough/Deep Breathe (1), Incentive Spirometry (2)		1																						
Suctioning																								
	7ᴬ	8ᴬ	9ᴬ	10ᴬ	11ᴬ	12ᴾ	1ᴾ	2ᴾ	3ᴾ	4ᴾ	5ᴾ	6ᴾ	7ᴾ	8ᴾ	9ᴾ	10ᴾ	11ᴾ	12ᴬ	1ᴬ	2ᴬ	3ᴬ	4ᴬ	5ᴬ	6ᴬ

Initials	Signature	Initials	Signature	Initials	Signature
PA	Patty Adams, RN				

HEALTHCARE PERSONNEL

PATIENT INCIDENT REPORT

To Be Completed By Employee:

Patient name _Mrs. Mona Jilko_   Social Security Number _123-45-6789_

Address _111 Bellbottom Lane_

Diagnoses _CVA c̄ (R)sided lienuparesis_

Incident date _May 1, 1993_   Day _Sat._   Hour _12:00_ am/(pm)

Witnesses _Virginia Fleck, LPN_   Address _____ Phone _____

Necessary to notify family? Yes _____ No _X_ If yes, whom _Pt requested no call to dtr_

Other notified and when _Healthcare Personnel 12:10 pm. RN to visit today_

Exact location of incident _pt's bedroom at home_

Patient condition prior to accident/injury _Has been ambulating c̄ cane & no other assistance for past mo._ _Today c/o "dizziness & upset stomach."_

How injury/accident occurred _Told pt to stay in BR chair at noon for lunch — she said OK. When brought_ _in lunch 10 min later, pt found on floor inside BR door._

Type of injury (include nature of injury and body parts affected) _No c/o pain except R_ _wrist "a little stiff & sore." No reddened areas; skin intact; no bruises. (Ate lunch c̄ (L) hand due to soreness, but able to_ _knit s̄ c/o pain or stiffness at 2 pm)._

Treatment received including where, doctor's name, date and time (attach treatment report).
None

If patient has insurance:

Carrier _____ Policy No. _____

Employee's Signature _Virginia Fleck, LPN_   Today's Date _5-1-93_

DISCHARGE PLANNING FORM

Assessment	Plan	Interventions	Evaluation
Summary of Discharge Planning Sessions: Date: 3/29/93 *Bed to chair transfer* *TPN care* *taught by RN and* *Carole Gable, dietitian* 3/31/93 *PCA procedure* *Disc of home care* *referrals: XYZ and* *TQI-IV* *Review of TPN* 4/2/93 *Review of PCA, Questions* *& answers re: care* *Written instructions given* *re TPN, PCA, meds,* *nutrition & dssg change*	Consult: ☒ Social Service *3/31* ☒ Home Health Care *3/31* ☒ Nutrition Services *3/29* ☐ Physical Therapy ☐ Occupational Therapy ☒ Pastoral Care *3/29* ☒ IV Therapy Co *3/31* ☐ ☐ Patient Education Re: ☒ *TPN* ☒ *PCA* ☒ *dssg Δ's* ☒ *Meds (see list attached)* Family/Significant Other Education: ☒ *husband* ☐ ☐	Consult/Services Scheduled: *Soc Serv 3/31* ✓ *XYZ Home Health Care 4/1* ✓ *TQI IV Therapy Co 4/1* ✓ *Rev Robt Hunt 3/29* ✓ *Nutrition Dept 3/29* ✓ ☒ Home-Going Equipment: *1 wk supply of syringes* *Telfa & Kling bandages* *Hosp bed, w/c, BSC* *ordered for home* ☒ See Patient Education Record/Progress Notes	☒ Patient Ready for Discharge To *Home* On *Apr 2, 1993* *with home care assist* ☒ Patient/Family able to manage care. Understand care instructions and follow-up plan. ☒ *Mutually set goals:* *1) independence in care mgmt c̄ supervision of home care RN.* *2) Continued relief from pain (maintain below +4)* *3) assistance c̄ ADL and homemaking* *Nancy Jones* _____ RN Signature

NARRATIVE NURSING NOTE

Date/Time	Nursing Notes
1/5/93 8³⁰ am	*Pt c/o ½ hr postprandial "heartburn," a burning sensation in epigastric area c̄ constant, dull +6*
	pain that feels worse when she lies down. No c/o N/V. —
	Mylanta 30 cc po administered per prn order and head of bed elevated to 45°.
9⁰⁰ am	*Pt states relief from heartburn to +2 pain. —————— J. Reff, RN*

PROBLEM-ORIENTED (SOAPE) NOTES

Date	Time	No.	Problem	Patient Progress Notes
1/5/93	830 am	1	Pain	S: Pt c/o "heartburn," a constant, dull, burning sensation in
				upper abdomen (+6 pain)
				O: Pt. grimacing, leaning forward and holding hand against
				epigastric area.
				A: Pain R/T reflux gastric secretions
				P: Admin Mylanta 30 cc po prn as ordered.
				Head of bed elevated 45°. J. Reff, RN
1/5/93	900 am	1	Pain	E: Pt states pain — relieved to +2 level
				————————————————J. Reff, RN

PIE NURSING NARRATIVE NOTE	
Date/Time	**Nursing Notes**
1/5/93 830 am	P: Pain +2 "heartburn" in epigastric area ————————————
	I: Medicated c̄ 30 cc Mylanta and elevated head of bed to 45° ————J. Reff, RN
1/5/93 900 am	E: Pt states relief from pain to +2. ————————————J. Reff, RN

SAMPLE FOCUS PATIENT CARE NOTES

Date/Time	Focus	Patient Care Notes
1/5/93　830 am	Pain	D: Pt c/o "heartburn" +6 pain and burning sensation in epigastric area. No c/o
		N/V. Pt. grimacing in pain, leaning forward and holding stomach
		A: Administered Mylanta 30 cc po prn as ordered.
		Elevated head of bed 45°. —————————————J. Reff, RN
1/5/93　900 am	Pain	R: Pt states relief from pain to +2 level —————————J. Reff, RN

CRITICAL PATH SAMPLE ANSWER

Primary Diagnosis _____ Joint Replacement (Knee) _____

DRG Code _____ 471 _____

LOS _____ 12.3 days _____

1993	Post-Op Day 1–Date: 3/16	Post-Op Day 2–Date: 3/17	Post-Op Day 3–Date: 3/18
Consults			XYZ Home Health RN to visit pt.
Tests		X-ray R knee	
Patient activities	OOB in chair in pm	No wt bear R leg Crutch walk c̄ assist as tol	No wt bear R leg walk c̄ crutch and assist 15 ft.
Teaching	Reinforce C & DB " " transfer technique	Reinforce crutch walk technique. Meds admin & s.e.	S/S of infection symptoms to report to MD
Treatments	C & DB q 2 h	C & DB q 4 h DSD change am	
Medication	Percodan 5 mg T̈T tab q 6 h	Percodan 5 mg T̈T tab q 6 h prn	Percodan 5 mg T̄ tab q 6 h prn
Diet	NPO	Clear liq	liquids
Discharge planning		Refer to Soc Serv for home care	

McKenzie, C., RN, Torkelson, N. G., MS, RN, Holt, M. A., BSN, RN. *Case & cost: Nursing case management improves both.* Nursing Management 20(10) October, 1989:30–34.

VARIATION	CAUSE	ACTION TAKEN
3/17 Perceived constipation	Habitual abuse of enemas	Incr po liquids to 1000 cc ad lib Call to Dr. Jones who ordered regular diet on Day 3 as tol. and Colace 240 mg po qd

Index

Page numbers followed by f indicate illustrations; t following a page number indicates tabular material.